Kenneth B. Gordon

Eric M. Ruderman

Editors

Psoriasis and Psoriatic Arthritis

An Integrated Approach

Kenneth B. Gordon
Eric M. Ruderman
Editors

Psoriasis and Psoriatic Arthritis

An Integrated Approach

With 47 Figures and 36 Tables

Springer

Kenneth B. Gordon, MD
Division of Dermatology
Loyola University
Stritch School of Medicine
2160 S. First Ave., Building 112, Room 342
Maywood, IL 60153
USA

Eric M. Ruderman, MD
Division of Rheumatology
Northwestern University
Feinberg School of Medicine
675 N. St. Clair St.
Chicago, IL 60611
USA

Library of Congress Control Number: 2004113294

ISBN 3-540-21280-9 Springer Berlin Heidelberg New York

Springer is a part of Springer Science+Business Media
springeronline.com

Printed in Germany

Editor: Marion Philipp
Desk Editor: Irmela Bohn
Production: ProEdit GmbH, 69126 Heidelberg, Germany
Cover: Frido Steinen-Broo, EStudio Calamar, Spain
Typesetting: K. Detzner, 67346 Speyer, Germany

Printed on acid-free paper SPIN 113908012 21/3111 ML 5 4 3 2 1

Preface

Dermatologists and rheumatologists alike are confronted with patients suffering from both psoriasis and psoriatic arthritis, and are often asked to address the disease with which they are least familiar. In our experience, proper care of either ailment requires a working knowledge of both. Working together to manage these patients, we have found that the most effective treatments must account for all manifestations of disease, whether skin or joint, and that this approach is the best way to ensure satisfied patients with the most unrestricted quality of life.

Our goal with this book is to bring current information about psoriasis and psoriatic arthritis together in a form that is useful for a satisfactory understanding of the pathophysiology, clinical aspects, and therapy of both diseases. Ideally, the integrated approach of this text will give specialists the necessary tools to work together effectively in the same office or in consultation. While this type of coordinated care strikes us as the best approach, we recognize that all dermatologists and rheumatologists will not have this luxury, and we hope this book will also serve as a useful review of those disease elements both within and outside the reader's own area of expertise.

This book is dedicated to our families: Dafna, Danny, and Jake Gordon, and Stacey Empson and Lucy Ruderman. We thank them for their patience in helping us through this endeavor.

Kenneth B. Gordon, MD
Eric M. Ruderman, MD

December 2004

Contents

List of Contributors

Mahreen Ameen
St. Johns Institute of Dermatology
St. Thomas' Hospital
London
UK

Milan J. Anadkat, MD
Division of Dermatology
Washington University School of Medicine
St. Louis, MO
USA

Jonathan N.W.N. Barker, MD
St. Johns Institute of Dermatology
St. Thomas' Hospital
London
UK

Jennifer Barton, MD
University of Rochester Medical Center
Rochester, NY
USA

Clifton O. Bingham, MD
Johns Hopkins University
Baltimore, MD
USA

Brian K. Bonish, MD
Loyola University of Chicago
Medical Center
Skin Disease Research Laboratory
Cardinal Bernardin Cancer Center
Maywood, IL
USA

Jennifer C. Cather, MD
University of Texas Southwestern Medical
School Dallas
Dallas, TX
USA

Daniel O. Clegg, MD
Division of Rheumatology
University of Utah Medical Center
Salt Lake City, UT
USA

Jennifer Dempsey, MD
Vanderbilt University Medical School
Dermatology Consultants
Nashville, TN
USA

Christa L. Doherty, BSc (Hons)
QEII Health Sciences Centre
Halifax, Nova Scotia
Canada

Steven R. Feldman, MD, PhD
Wake Forest University School of Medicine
Medical Center Boulevard
Winston-Salem, NC
USA

Dafna D. Gladman, MD FRCPC
Center for Prognosis Studies
Toronto Hospital Western Division
Toronto, ON
Canada

Kenneth B. Gordon, MD
Division of Dermatology
Loyola University
Stritch School of Medicine
Maywood, IL
USA

Joan Guitart, MD
Northwestern University
Department of Dermatology
Chicago, IL
USA

Michael P. Heffernan, MD
Division of Dermatology
Washington University School of Medicine
St. Louis, MO
USA

Philip Helliwell, MD
Academic Unit of Musculoskeletal Disease
University of Leeds
Leeds
UK

Christopher Jackson, MD
Division of Rheumatology
University of Utah Medical Center
Salt Lake City, UT
USA

Christine C. Jacobson, AB
Department of Dermatology
Stanford University School of Medicine
Stanford, CA
USA

Ja Huen Jung, MD
UCSD
Rheumatology Division
Department of Medicine
La Jolla, CA
USA

Arthur F. Kavanaugh, MD
UCSD
Rheumatology Division
Department of Medicine
La Jolla, CA
USA

Alexa Kimball, MD, MPH
Dermatology Clinical Studies Unit
Massachusetts General and Brigham
and Women's Hospitals
Boston, MA
USA

Richard G.B. Langley, MD, FRCPC
QEII Health Sciences Centre
Halifax, Nova Scotia
Canada

Mark Lebwohl, MD, FACP
Department of Dermatology
The Mt. Sinai Medical Center
New York, NY
USA

Philip J. Mease, MD
Seattle Rheumatology Associates
University of Washington
Seattle, WA
USA

M. Alan Menter
Division of Dermatology
Baylor University Medical Center
University of Texas Southwestern Medical
School Dallas
Dallas, TX
USA

Scott J. Murray, MD, FRCPC
QEII Health Sciences Centre
Halifax, Nova Scotia
Canada

Brian J. Nickoloff, MD, PhD
Loyola University Medical Center
Maywood, IL
USA

Bettina M. Prinz Vavricka, MD
Department of Dermatology
University Hospital Zurich
Zurich
Switzerland

Rachel Quinby, MD
Charlottesville, VA
USA

Proton Rahman, MD
Rheumatology
St. Claires Mercy Hospital
St. Johns, NF
Canada

Stephen R. Rapp, PhD
Department of Psychiatry
and Behavioral Medicine
Wake Forest University School of Medicine
Winston-Salem, NC
USA

Soumya M. Reddy, MD
Rheumatology & Medicine
Hospital for Joint Diseases
New York, NY
USA

Christopher T. Ritchlin, MD
Allergy Immunology Rheumatology
University of Rochester Medical Center
Rochester, NY
USA

Eric M. Ruderman, MD
Division of Rheumatology
Department of Medicine
Northwestern University
Feinberg School of Medicine
Chicago, IL
USA

Jennifer Soung
Department of Dermatology
The Mt. Sinai Medical Center
New York, NY
USA

Bruce E. Strober, MD, PhD
Associate Director
Dermatopharmacology Unit
New York University
School of Medicine
New York, NY
USA

Zuhre Tutuncu, MD
UCSD
Rheumatology Division
Department of Medicine
La Jolla, CA
USA

Michael D. Zanolli, MD
Vanderbilt University Medical School
Dermatology Consultants
Nashville, TN
USA

Introduction

I

Kenneth B. Gordon, Eric M. Ruderman

Psoriasis and psoriatic arthritis are among the more common inflammatory diseases of the skin and joints respectively. Unfortunately, despite the fact that these diseases so frequently coexist, they have commonly been considered separate entities. Dermatologists managing a patient's psoriasis often would fail to inquire about joint pain or stiffness, let alone make a diagnosis of psoriatic arthritis. Likewise, rheumatologists, concentrating on minimizing the discomfort and disability associated with inflammatory arthritis, would be relatively indifferent to the emotional and physical morbidity associated with the skin disease. This disconnect in the care of patients with both psoriasis and psoriatic arthritis almost certainly led to less than optimal therapy.

How did the diagnostic and therapeutic disconnect between psoriasis and psoriatic arthritis develop? On the surface, one might assume that since dermatologists focus primarily on the skin and rheumatologists treat the joints, the tunnel vision associated with the primary organ system precluded a deeper understanding of the diseases and their impact. However, dermatologists and rheumatologists have long cooperated in the treatment of connective tissue diseases such as systemic lupus erythematosis and dermatomyositis. Cooperative clinics were developed in university settings to treat the various manifestations of these diseases as a whole. Patients in such clinics and, indeed, those treated in other settings as well, would generally receive therapy that considered all of the organ systems involved in their illness. The driving force behind this cooperation was the recognition that connective tissue diseases had significant physical and emotional implications for the patient, and that a team approach was necessary for optimal benefit.

Psoriasis and psoriatic arthritis have historically been considered to be different from other systemic connective tissue diseases, with less significant long-term consequences. Until the past 10–15 years, psoriasis was felt to be a strictly cutaneous disease, best treated in most circumstances with topical medications. Only the most severe cases of psoriasis were felt to merit more aggressive, systemic treatment. In the same manner, psoriatic arthritis, even after being recognized as a separate entity, was viewed as a more benign cousin of rheumatoid arthritis, with fewer long-term sequelae and unlikely progression to permanent joint damage. As practitioners have learned that the presence of skin or joint disease is of no great significance, it is perhaps not surprising that many simply chose to ignore it except in the most obvious cases. After all, if the patient were bothered by these particular manifestations of their disease, wouldn't he or she pursue care with the appropriate specialist anyway?

Much has changed in the past two decades to make this thought process obsolete. Psoriasis is now recognized as a systemic, immune-mediated condition that can have a tremendous impact on the patient, both physically and emotionally. Acceptance of aggressive treatments for psoriasis has risen in both patients and physicians. Likewise, the potentially devastating permanent joint destruction that can be associated with psoriatic arthritis has become commonly recognized. With greater understanding of the far-reaching consequences of both these conditions has come a greater imperative that their independent elements be recognized early, and not ignored by practitioners focusing solely on the organ system of greatest importance to their primary specialty.

Perhaps the greatest reason for dermatologists and rheumatologists to understand both psoriasis and psoriatic arthritis and cooperate in their management lies in the area of therapy. With increasing recognition of the common elements in the inflammatory pathophysiology of psoriasis and psoriatic arthritis has come the realization that many treatments could have a significant impact on both conditions. Clinical experience, however, has shown that some treatments for psoriasis, such as systemic retinoids, may have limited impact on joint disease. Likewise, some drugs that have been shown to be effective agents in psoriatic arthritis, such as sulfasalazine, have limited benefit for the skin. Finally, some medications, such as methotrexate or tumor necrosis factor antagonists, may produce benefit in both skin and joints. Disconnected care for the patient with both skin and joint disease may lead to polypharmacy, whereas an approach that recognizes the importance of both diseases may be both more efficient and more effective.

Much of the impetus for this book developed from our recognition of this disconnect in our own practices. For a number of years, we would refer patients with significant skin and/or joint disease to each other after treating the condition with which each of us was most familiar. Only after recognizing that our therapy could frequently be more effective with better communication did we begin to see patients together. We found that the information that we shared as clinicians primarily interested in the skin or the joints was not only beneficial for the patients we managed in our joint clinic, but for those we saw in our general practice as well.

The experience of teaching and learning together was the driving force in the development of this text. We actively sought to make this book comprehensive when dealing with the individual diseases. Thus, the chapters taken individually would make a complete textbook of either psoriasis or psoriatic arthritis. However, we believe the whole should be considered as greater than the sum of the parts. The chapters are purposely juxtaposed so the clinician can readily compare the issues that govern the understanding of psoriatic disease of both the skin and the joints. This format closely resembles the discussions we had as we worked together in our clinic. We found that much of the information will be similar with regard to these diseases, but the differences are central to optimal care for our patients. Our hope is that primary care physicians, dermatologists, and rheumatologists, along with trainees in all specialties that may encounter patients with psoriasis or psoriatic arthritis, will be able to use this text to develop a greater appreciation of the elements involved in treating these two diseases, just as we learned from each other.

Genetics II

A Psoriasis

Mahreen Ameen,
Jonathan N.W.N. Barker

Contents

1 Introduction

A genetic basis for psoriasis vulgaris has long been recognised by clinicians based on observations that psoriasis clusters in some families although the mode of inheritance does not follow Mendelian patterns. In segregation analyses of large multigenerational families no clear inheritance pattern is seen and therefore psoriasis belongs to a group termed genetically complex or multifactorial diseases. In multifactorial diseases, susceptible individuals may have several disease genes which act in a concerted fashion but require environmental trigger factors to bring about disease pathogenesis.

2 Epidemiological Studies

More robust support for a genetic basis of psoriasis came from large-scale epidemiological studies such as Lomholt's classic study of psoriasis on the Faroe Islands [32] followed by Hellgren's study in Sweden [22]. These revealed a high incidence of psoriasis in relatives of psoriatics compared with the general population or with matched control subjects; Lomholt reported a 91% family occurrence in patients with psoriasis: Hellgren's data showed the prevalence of psoriasis to be 7.8% in first-degree relatives compared with a 3.14% prevalence in matched controls, and 1.97% in the population overall. Later American and Danish twin studies showed high concordance of psoriasis in monozygotic (MZ) twins compared with dizygotic (DZ) twins, strongly implicating genetic factors [9, 18]. The Danish Twin Registry showed a 63% concordance for psoriasis in MZ twins compared with 15% for DZ twins corresponding to an estimated heritability of 91% [9]. Similar figures were obtained by Farber et al. [18], who also noted that in MZ twins the clinical presentation is similar in age of onset, severity and course, features not observed in DZ twins, suggesting that genetic factors may play a role in these clinical variables. Given that concordance rates do not reach 100% (even when older twins are examined) suggests that environmental factors must be necessary for disease expression. The heritability of psoriasis, or the proportion of phenotypic variability attributable to genetic factors, has been estimated to range from 60–90% [15].

3 Association with the Human Leucocyte Antigens (HLA)

Given the autoimmune nature of psoriasis early genetic studies from the 1970s focussed on association with the Major Histocompatability Complex (MHC) located on the short arm of chromosome 6 in the region of 6p21.3. The MHC is the most gene dense region of the human genome and contains genes encoding for class I and II human leucocyte antigens (HLA). Association with HLA-B13 was first identified and later with other class I antigens, HLA-B17, -B37, -B57, -Cw6 and -Cw7, and class II antigens HLA-DR4 and –DR7 [7, 46]. Of these the largest and most consistently reported relative risk has been with HLA-Cw6, and association has been shown in many ethnically and geographically diverse groups including Indian, Chinese and Japanese populations [3, 7, 46, 51]. Furthermore a significantly higher frequency of HLA-Cw6 has been found associated with early onset (-type I) psoriasis which has a strong genetic component, as compared with late onset (type II) psoriasis (85% versus 14% [13]) providing further support that HLA-Cw6 is implicated in the genetic basis of psoriasis. HLA-B57 represents the next most strongly associated HLA antigen with psoriasis.

4 Psoriasis Associated MHC Haplotypes

The MHC genes characteristically display strong linkage disequilibrium (LD) because of low recombination (the crossing over of alleles during meiosis) frequencies between them. Hence in the presence of LD genes are more likely to be inherited together as haplotypes. Recombination between the HLA-B and -C alleles is very rare resulting in the formation of conserved or ancestral haplotypes [14]. A number of psoriasis-associated MHC haplotypes have been identified which demonstrate stronger disease association than their component alleles. Schmitt-Egenholf et al. [42] first reported association of early onset psoriasis with an extended haplotype (EH) 57.1: Cw6-B57-DRB1*0701-DQA1*0201-DQB1*0303 (DQB1*0303 is an allele encoding the DQ9 molecule) which contains the two major risk alleles for psoriasis susceptibility, HLA-Cw6 and –B57. Other HLA risk haplotypes for psoriasis have also been identified: EH13.1, Cw6-B13-DRB1*0701 and EH37.1, Cw6-B37-DRB1*1001 [25, 26]. These haplotypes have been shown to confer different risk for psoriasis within and between populations [25] suggesting that genetic factors residing within these haplotypes may be responsible for disease risk. Furthermore the identification of a haplotype linked with psoriasis that does not contain the HLA-Cw6 allele, AH8.1 (HLA-Cw7-B8-DRB1*0301-DQB1*02) [26], and HLA-Cw7 disease association in some populations, notably the Japanese [3], suggest that HLA-C may not be the true disease locus for psoriasis but a marker in LD with a major non-HLA susceptibility gene residing on the high-risk haplotypes. A multilocus model (the involvement of more than one gene) for inheritance of psoriasis was therefore proposed [15].

5 Multilocus Model

This model was derived by applying the method of Risch [40] to calculate λ_R –1 for both Lomholt's and Hellgren's data, where λ_R is the risk ratio and is defined as the risk of disease in a relative of degree R in relation to the population prevalence. Risch demonstrated that for a single gene disease or disease caused by the additive effect of several genes, λ_R –1 decreases by a factor of two with each degree of relationship. However if several genes interact epistatically then their individual contributions become multiplicative and λ_R –1 decreases by more than a factor of two with each degree of relationship. Calculations show that λ_R –1 decreases by a factor of 7 in patients from the Faroe islands and by a factor of 6 in patients from Sweden, consistent with a multilocus model of disease inheritance [15]. Furthermore Risch reported that if the risk ratio for first degree relatives is at least four, and there is at least one major loci, then it is possible to search for the genes by genetic linkage studies, paving the way for genome-wide scans of psoriasis.

6 Genome-Wide Scans

Since the late 1990s several genome-wide scans have been performed using both parametric (i.e. model-based) and non-parametric approaches in order to detect linkage with any psoriasis susceptibility loci. Polymorphic markers distributed evenly across the genome were utilised to study the cosegregation of a trait and genetic marker. Studies have utilised either extended kindreds or affected sib pair (ASP) families to investigate distortion of frequency of allele sharing from expected values if random segregation exists. A criterion LOD score (logarithm of the odds ratio, a measure of genetic linkage) of 3.6 was required for a definitive declaration of linkage [29]. A number of candidate loci for psoriasis have now been identified (*PSORS1–9*, psoriasis susceptibility 1–9), although not all have been independently confirmed by other groups (Table 1). However, in complex disease genetics it is not uncommon for a linkage result found by one group not be confirmed by other groups, even if the linkage is real. Conversely, confirmation of linkage by independent groups does not give definitive proof of the existence of a gene. Possible explanations for this include locus heterogeneity (different loci contributing to the disease phenotype in different populations), epistasis (where genes interact with each other in a multiplicative fashion) between loci and allelic heterogeneity (each disease locus may have a number of causal alleles). Despite these, a consensus was reached that linkage findings in complex diseases require confirmation in independent data sets [35].

To date robust evidence for linkage has been replicated for chromosome 6p21 (*PSORS1*) [10, 11, 16, 25, 36, 48], 17q25 (*PSORS2*) [16, 23, 36, 41, 47] and 1q (*PSORS4*) [7, 11].

7 PSORS1

The strongest evidence of linkage has been established for *PSORS1* locus (OMIM 177900) on chromosome 6p21.3, which contains the MHC.

Table A1. Psoriasis susceptibility loci identified by genetic linkage studies

Locus name	Chromosomal location	Linkage studies
PSORS1 (OMIM 177900)	6p21.3	[10, 11, 16, 25, 30, 36, 41, 48, 49, 51]
PSORS2 (OMIM 602723)	17q24–25	[16, 23, 36, 41, 47]
PSORS3 (OMIM 601454)	4q34	[33, 41]
PSORS4 (OMIM 603935)	1q21	[7, 11]
PSORS5 (OMIM 604316)	3q21	[17, 41]
PSORS6 (OMIM 605364)	19p13-q13	[31, 49]
PSORS7 (OMIM 605606)	1p35-p34	[49]
PSORS8	16q12–13	[24, 36]
PSORS9 (OMIM 607857)	4q	[7, 41, 51]
	2p14	[7, 49]
	2q	[48]
	7	[49]
	8q	[48]
	14q	[7, 49]
	15	[41]
	20p	[36, 48]

Database OMIM (Online Mendelian Inheritance in Man)

Trembath et al. [48] first identified significant linkage to this MHC region following a two-stage genome scan on 106 affected sib-pairs from 68 Caucasian families from the UK using a non-parametric statistical approach (LOD=6.5, $p=5.8\times10^{-7}$). Nair et al. [36] also identified significant linkage in a genome-wide scan of 86 nuclear and 29 extended families with 182 independent sib-pairs from USA and Germany (LOD=3.52, $p=2.9\times10^{-5}$). Burden et al. [10] obtained a maximum LOD score of 4.63 under a dominant inheritance model with 70% penetrance and 5% phenocopies from family material collected from Scotland. Veal et al. [49] performed a genome-wide screen of 284 Caucasian affected sib-pairs of UK origin using non-parametric statistics, identifying significant linkage (LOD=4.7, $p=2\times10^{-6}$). Hence significant linkage to *PSORS1* has been reported in several studies of different populations (Table 1) thereby fulfilling the criteria for confirmed linkage for this locus [35].

To date no functional role has been assigned to HLA-C. Furthermore given that HLA-Cw6 is not present in all psoriatic individuals and not all HLA-Cw6-bearing haplotypes confer equal risk for psoriasis, the strong HLA-Cw6 association found in many populations may be secondary to strong LD with a nearby gene on the same chromosome. Linkage analyses however of family cohorts used in genome-wide scans is a relatively blunt tool which is only able to localise broad chromosomal regions of interest as linkage can extend over several megabases of DNA on each side of the gene. LD mapping has therefore been used to narrow the size of a disease candidate region assigned by linkage analysis and studies have now been performed in Caucasian and Japanese populations [6, 37, 38]. By alignment of the different minimal intervals, the overlap between these studies points to a LD region in the proximal segment of the MHC class I region of approximately 300 kb around HLA-C.

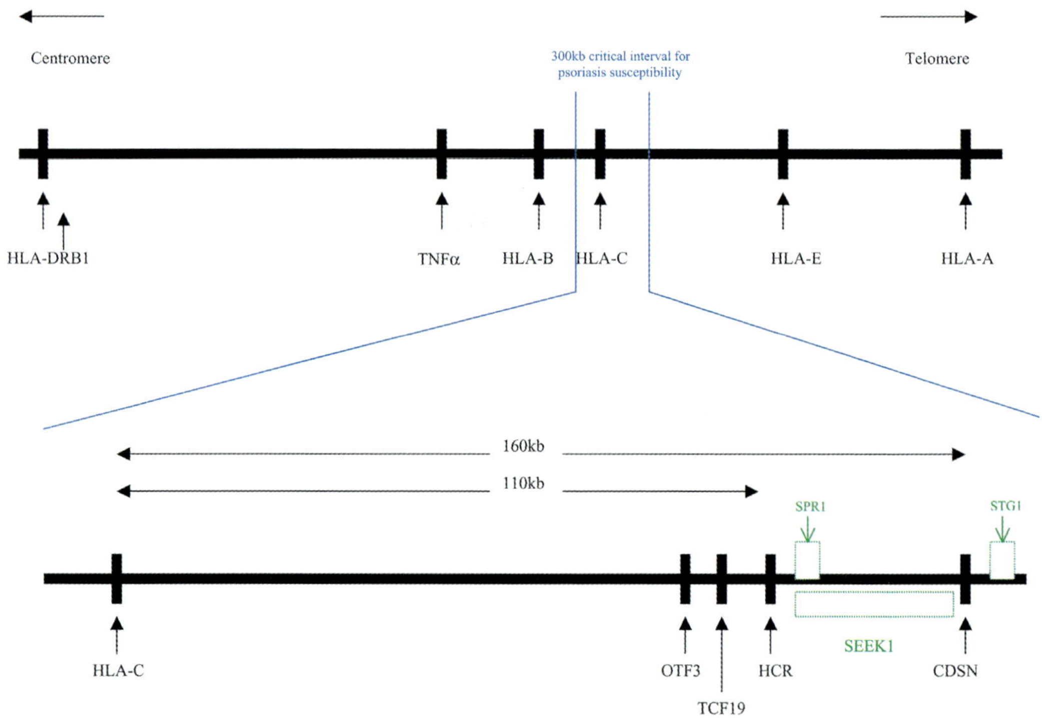

Fig. A1. PSORS1 on chromosome 6p21.3 depicting five known candidate genes and three predicted genes

8 PSORS1 Genes

The refined *PSORS1* interval has been completely sequenced and other than HLA-C (OMIM 142840) four other genes have been characterised:

- Octamer-binding transcription factor-3, OTF3 (POU5F1; OMIM 164177)
- TCF19 (SC1; OMIM 600912)
- HCR (PG8; OMIM 605310)
- CDSN ('S' gene; OMIM 602593)

In addition the presence of three more genes (SEEK1, SPR1 and STG1) has been predicted [5, 38] (Fig. 1) and the region also contains four pseudogenes (NOB4, NOB5, HCGIX-3 and HCGII-2).

Candidate gene analysis using both case-control as well as robust family-based association studies such as the transmission disequilibrium test (TDT) has demonstrated disease association for the genes encoding HCR, CDSN and OTF3 (Table 2). Although a single OTF3 allele has shown association in a Spanish cohort [19] it is an unlikely candidate for psoriasis susceptibility as the gene encodes for a transcriptional factor involved in embryonic stem cells lineage commitment. There is strong genetic and functional evidence implicating HCR and CDSN in psoriasis pathogenesis. They have been sequenced for single nucleotide polymorphisms (SNPs) which are inherited biallelic single base pair differences and the most common polymorphic variant.

9 Corneodesmosin (CDSN; OMIM 602593)

The CDSN gene lies 160 kb telomeric of HLA-C in the class I region and encodes for a late differentiation epidermal desmosomal glycoprotein which is expressed exclusively in cornified epithelia and shares structural homology with other cutaneous proteins such as keratin [52]. CDSN is important in corneocyte cohesion and its proteolysis is believed to play a major role in desquamation [44]. Abnormally high CDSN expression has been observed in psoriasis as well as other hyperproliferative skin disorders [21] and restricted control of its synthesis is diminished in psoriatic skin [2]. The CDSN gene is highly polymorphic, a feature shared with other MHC-located genes and as with other genes the CDSN SNPs are approximately equally divided between synonymous and non-synonymous changes. Non-synonymous SNPs inducing amino acid changes may modify sites for epidermal proteases giving rise to the characteristic epidermal features of psoriasis. Alternatively changes in amino acid charges may alter CDSN structure thereby interfering with function [20].

Linkage and association with psoriasis vulgaris has been demonstrated for an allele of the

Table A2. Candidate gene analysis of *PSORS1* on chromosome 6p

Gene	Allele/SNP	Population	Study analysis	Odds ratio (OR)	*P* value	Reference
CSDN	+1243	Britain	Case-control	2.66	2×10^{-9}	[45]
CDSN	+619: +1243	Britain	Family-based TDT	–	2.8×10^{-6}	[1]
CDSN	+619: +1243	Germany and USA	Family-based TDT	–	0.0085	[26]
CDSN	+619: +1236: +1243	Germany	Family-based TDT	–	0.0031	[43]
HCR CDSN	+307: +325: +1723: +2327 +619: +1243	Britain, Finland, Sweden, Italy, Spain, Gujarati Indian	Case-control and family-based TDT	2.5 (1.9–3.3) 2.0 (1.6–2.5)	1×10^{-10} 4×10^{-9}	[5]
OTF3	β-Allele (*Hin*dIII)	Spain	Case-control	3.76	<0.0003	[19]

CDSN gene defined by SNPs +619 (Ser→Phe) and +1243 (Ser→Leu) which give amino acid substitutions [1, 27, 45]. Given the high CDSN polymorphism content, SNP haplotypes rather than single alleles are likely to influence protein structure. A high-risk haplotype of CDSN which includes SNPs +619: +1236: +1243 has shown significant association for psoriasis vulgaris [43]. Therefore based on its genomic position in close proximity to HLA-C and putative biological function CDSN is an attractive candidate gene for psoriasis susceptibility.

10 CR (PG8; OMIM 605310)

The HCR gene is located only 110 kb telomeric of HLA-C within the critical region for psoriasis susceptibility. It encodes for a plectin-like protein with α-helical coiled-coil rod domains. It is ubiquitously expressed in all human tissues but is upregulated in psoriatic epidermis [4]. Sequencing analysis demonstrates that it is also highly polymorphic and genetic studies have shown strong association in several populations with a four-SNP haplotype (+307: +325: +1723: +2327) redefined as allele HCR WWCC [5]. Three of the amino acid substitutions specifying this high-risk haplotype (Arg→Trp at HCR-307, Arg→Trp at HCR-325 and Gly→Cys at HCR 1723) are predicted to induce secondary structural alterations of the HCR protein. In addition functional studies suggest that HCR is a regulator of keratinocyte differentiation and proliferation providing further support for HCR candidacy in psoriasis pathogenesis [5].

The MHC is subject to strong LD effects, which make it difficult to define the individual contributions of candidate genes. Veal et al. [50] however performed a family-based analysis using a dense SNP-based map and showed that HLA-C and CDSN SNPs do not show LD when non-disease bearing chromosomes are analysed. They identified a rare susceptibility haplotype (cluster D), originating from a double recombination event that replaced HCR risk alleles while preserving HLA-C and CDSN disease associated SNPs, which suggests that CDSN SNPs in conjunction with HLA-C risk alleles confer disease susceptibility. This has also been demonstrated in an Indian Gujarati cohort [12].

11 Non-MHC Loci

The contribution of the *PSORS1* locus to the relative risk of developing psoriasis is calculated to be approximately 35–50% [48] suggesting that non-MHC loci must exist harbouring disease alleles necessary for disease expression. Several of the other loci have also been replicated but not achieved genome-wide significance. This may be because these loci have only minor effects and therefore their detection is likely to require even larger cohorts and more dense genetic marker panels. Some of these non-MHC candidate loci for psoriasis susceptibility however are biologically interesting with putative functional roles in psoriasis pathogenesis.

The candidate interval on 19p (*PSORS6*, OMIM 605364) contains the gene that codes for ICAM-1, a ligand for lymphocyte function-associated (LFA) antigens that acts as a major cell adhesion molecule mediating leucocyte migration in psoriasis. *PSORS4* on chromosome 1q21 contains the Epidermal Differentiation Complex, a cluster of genes expressed during epithelial differentiation [34]. It also contains a number of other skin expressed genes including loricrin, involucrin and filaggrin, as well as psoriasin which is overexpressed in psoriatic lesions and acts as a potent and selective chemotactic inflammatory protein for CD4+ T cells. Several immune related genes have been mapped to 1p (*PSORS7*) including the gene encoding EPS15, a highly specific intracellular substrate for the epidermal growth factor receptor which is overexpressed in psoriatic epidermis [39]. Recently two genes have been identified within *PSORS2* (17q24-q25), SLC9A3R1 and NAT9, a new member of the *N*-acetyltransferase family [23]. Of the two, SLC9A3R1 is a more plausible candidate for involvement in psoriasis pathogenesis as it is a phosphoprotein implicated in diverse aspects of epithelial membrane biology.

Epistasis has also been demonstrated between candidate loci. Epistasis with HLA has been described for 1q21 [11] and Veal et al. [49] suggested possible epistatic interactions between *PSORS1* and chromosomal regions 2p and 14q. Some psoriasis susceptibility loci coincide with loci identified in genome-wide scans of other autoimmune and inflammatory diseases such as chromosomes 1q for atopic dermatitis, 3q21 and 17q24.3 for rheumatoid arthritis and 16p for inflammatory bowel disease [8]. This suggests that clinically distinct autoimmune diseases may be controlled by a common set of susceptibility genes. Indeed a common susceptibility locus on chromosome 16 could explain the strong clinical concomitance of psoriasis and Crohn's disease. Of particular interest a recent genome scan for psoriatic arthritis has identified linkage with chromosome 16q (*PSORAS1*, OMIM 607507)) [28], a locus that it shares with psoriasis vulgaris [24, 36]. It has also been suggested that inflammatory diseases may arise from an overlapping set of susceptibility loci as with the case of psoriasis vulgaris and atopic eczema [8].

12 Conclusion

Numerous studies support a major role for *PSORS1* in psoriasis vulgaris and research continues in an effort to identify the primary candidate gene for psoriasis susceptibility within this locus. However this region containing the MHC is subject to strong LD effects making it extremely difficult to dissect out the role of individual candidate genes. Further resolution of this region is proving to be extremely difficult and therefore other approaches will have to be explored in order to define susceptibility genes. Studies indicating a functional role of some of these disease-associated SNPs would provide further and robust evidence for their involvement. In addition demonstration of candidate gene association in diverse ethnic populations (a trans-racial gene mapping approach that has been successfully used for other complex diseases such as diabetes) as well as other clinical subtypes of psoriasis would also lend further credence.

Non-MHC genes may also be implicated in disease pathogenesis and the overall genetic basis of psoriasis is likely to be complicated with different combinations of genes in different individuals and populations required for the varied clinical manifestations of psoriasis. Despite the complexities of genetic research in psoriasis the efforts are considered extremely worthwhile as the elucidation of its genetic basis will shed further light on its underlying pathogenesis and holds the promise of future pharmacogenetic and pharmacogenomic applications.

References

1. Allen MH, Veal C, Faassen A, Powis SH, Vaughan RW, Trembath RC, Barker JN (1999) A non-HLA gene within the MHC in psoriasis. Lancet 353:1589–1590
2. Allen M, Ishida-Yamamoto A, McGrath J, Davison S, Lizuka H, Simon M, et al. (2001) Corneodesmosin expression in psoriasis vulgaris differs from normal skin and other inflammatory skin disorders. Lab Invest 81:969–976
3. Asahina A, Akazaki S, Nakagawa H, Kuwata S, Tokunaga K, Ishibashi Y, Juji T (1991) Specific nucleotide sequence of HLA-C is strongly associated with psoriasis vulgaris. J Invest Dermatol 97:254–258
4. Asumalahti K, Laitinen T, Itkonen-Vatjus R, Lokki ML, Suomela S, Snellman E, et al. (2000) A candidate gene for psoriasis near HLA-C, HCR (Pg8), is highly polymorphic with a disease-associated susceptibility allele. Hum Mol Genet 9:1533–1542
5. Asumalahti K, Veal C, Laitinen T, Suomela S, Allen M, Elomaa O, et al. (2002) Coding haplotype analysis supports HCR as the putative susceptibility gene for psoriasis at the MHC PSORS1 locus. Hum Mol Genet 11:589–597
6. Balendran N, Clough RL, Arguello JR, Barber R, Veal C, Jones AB, et al. (1999) Characterisation of the major susceptibility region for psoriasis at chromosome 6p21.3. J Invest Dermatol 113:322–328
7. Bhalerao J, Bowcock AM (1998) The genetics of psoriasis: a complex disorder of the skin and immune system. Hum Mol Genet 7:1537–1545
8. Bowcock AM, Shannon W, Du F, Duncan J, Cao K, Aftergut K, et al. (2001) Insights into psoriasis and other inflammatory diseases from large-scale gene expression studies. Hum Mol Genet 10:1793–1805
9. Brandrup F, Holm N, Grunnet N, Henningsen K, Hansen HE (1982) Psoriasis in monozygotic twins: variations in expression in individuals with identical genetic constitution. Acta Derm Venereol 62:229–236

10. Burden AD, Javed S, Bailey M, Hodgins M, Conor M, Tillman D (1998) Genetics of psoriasis: paternal inheritance and a locus on chromosome 6p. J Invest Dermatol 110:958–960
11. Capon F, Novelli G, Semprini S, Clementi M, Nudo M, Vultaggio P, et al. (1999) Searching for psoriasis susceptibility genes in Italy: genome scan and evidence for a new locus on chromosome 1. J Invest Dermatol 112:32–35
12. Capon F, Toal IK, Evans JC, Allen MH, Patel S, Tillman D, et al. (2003) Haplotype analysis of distantly related populations implicates corneodesmosin in psoriasis susceptibility. J Med Genet 40:447–452
13. Christophers E, Henseler T (1990) Psoriasis type I and type II are subtypes of nonpustular psoriasis. In: Roenigk HH, Maibach HI (eds) Psoriasis, 2nd edn. Marcel Dekker, New York, pp 15–21
14. Degli-Esposti MA, Leaver AL, Christiansen FT, Witt CS, Abraham LJ, Dawkins RL (1992) Ancestral haplotypes: conserved population MHC haplotypes. Hum Immunol 34:242–252
15. Elder JT, Nair RP, Guo SW, Henseler T, Christophers E, Voorhees JJ (1994) The genetics of psoriasis. Arch Dermatol 130:216–224
16. Enlund F, Samuelsson L, Enerback C, Inerot A, Wahlstrom J, Yhr M, et al. (1999a) Analysis of three suggested psoriasis susceptibility loci in a large Swedish set of families: confirmation of linkage to chromosome 6p (HLA region), and to 17q, but not to 4q. Hum Hered 49:2–8
17. Enlund F, Samuelsson L, Enerback C, Inerot A, Wahlstrom J, Yhr M, et al. (1999b) Psoriasis susceptibility locus in chromosome region 3q21 identified in patients from southwest Sweden. Eur J Hum Genet 7:783–790
18. Farber EM, Nall L, Watson W (1974) Natural history of psoriasis in 61 twin pairs. Arch Dermatol 109: 207–211
19. Gonzalez S, Martinez-Borra J, Sanchez del Rio J, Santos-Juanes J, Lopez-Vazquez A, Blanco-Gelaz M, Lopez-Larrea C (2000) The OTF3 gene polymorphism confers susceptibility to psoriasis independent of the association of HLA-Cw*0602. J Invest Dermatol 115:824–828
20. Guerrin M, Vincent C, Simon M, Tazi Ahnini R, Fort M, Serre G (2001) Identification of six novel polymorphisms in the human corneodesmosin gene. Tissue Antigens 57:32–38
21. Haftek M, Simon M, Kanitakis J, Marechal S, Claudy A, Serre G, Schmitt D (1997) Expression of corneodesmosin in the granular layer and stratum corneum of normal and diseased epidermis. Br J Dermatol 137:863–864
22. Hellgren L (1967) Psoriasis: The prevalence in sex, age and occupational groups in total populations in Sweden. Morphology, inheritance and association with other skin and rheumatic diseases. Almquist and Wiksell, Stockholm
23. Helms C, Cao L, Krueger JG, Wijsman EM, Chamian F, Gordon D, et al. (2003) A putative RUNX1 binding site variant between SLC9A3R1 and NAT9 is associated with susceptibility to psoriasis. Nat Genet 35: 349–356
24. International Psoriasis Genetics Consortium (2003) The International Psoriasis Genetics Study: Assessing linkage to 14 candidate susceptibility loci in a cohort of 942 affected sib pairs. Am J Hum Genet 73 :430–437
25. Jenisch S, Henseler T, Nair RP, Guo S, Westphal E, Stuart P, et al. (1998) Linkage analysis of human leukocyte antigen (HLA) markers in familial psoriasis: strong disequilibrium effects provide evidence for a major determinant in the HLA-B/-C region. Am J Hum Genet 63:191–199
26. Jenisch S, Westphal E, Nair RP, Stuart P, Voorhees JJ, Christophers E, et al. (1999a) Linkage disequilibrium analysis of familial psoriasis: identification of multiple disease-associated MHC haplotypes. Tissue Antigens 53:135–146
27. Jenisch S, Koch S, Henseler T, Nair RP, Elder JT, Watts CE, et al. (1999b) Corneodesmosin gene polymorphism demonstrates strong linkage disequilibrium with HLA and association with psoriasis vulgaris. Tissue Antigens 54:439–449
28. Karason A, Gudjonsson JE, Upmanyu R, Antonsdottir AA, Hauksson VB, Runasdottir EH, et al. (2003) A susceptibility gene for psoriatic arthritis maps to chromosome 16q: evidence for imprinting. Am J Hum Genet 72:125–131
29. Lander E, Kruglyak L (1995) Genetic dissection of complex traits: guidelines for interpreting and reporting linkage results. Nat Genet 11:241–247
30. Leder RO, Farber EM, Mansbridge J, Hallmayer J (1994) Genetic mapping of the psoriasis susceptibility locus – retrospective analysis of 84 kindreds shows linkage to polymorphic class-I HLA Loci. J Invest Dermatol 102:530
31. Lee YA, Ruschendorf F, Windemuth C, Schmitt-Egenolf M, Stadelmann A, Nurnberg G, et al. (2000) Genome-wide scan in German families reveals evidence for a novel psoriasis-susceptibility locus on chromosome 19p13. Am J Hum Genet 67:1020–1024
32. Lomholt G (1963) Psoriasis: Prevalence, spontaneous course and genetics: a census study on the prevalence of skin diseases on the Faroe Islands, GEC Gad, Copenhagen
33. Mathews D, Fry L, Powles A, Weber J, McCarthy M, Fisher E, et al. (1996) Evidence that a locus for familial psoriasis maps to chromosome 4q. Nature Genet 14:231–233
34. Mischke D, Korge BP, Marenholz I, Volz A, Ziegler A (1996) Genes encoding structural proteins of epidermal cornification and S-100 calcium binding proteins form a gene complex ("epidermal differentiation complex") on human chromosome 1q21. J Invest Dermatol 106:989–992
35. Morton NE (1998) Significance levels in complex inheritance. Am J Hum Genet 62:690–697
36. Nair RP, Henseler T, Jenisch S, Stuart P, Bichakjian CK, Lenk W, et al. (1997) Evidence for two psoriasis

susceptibility loci (HLA and 17q) and two novel candidate regions (16q and 20p) by genome-wide scan. Hum Mol Genet 6:1349–1356

37. Nair RP, Stuart P, Henseler T, Jenisch S, Chia NV, Westphal E, et al. (2000) Localization of psoriasis susceptibility locus PSORS1 to a 60-kb interval telomeric to HLA-C. Am J Hum Genet 66:1833–1844
38. Oka A, Tamiya G, Tomizawa M, Ota M, Katsuyama Y, Makino S, et al. (1999) Association analysis using refined microsatellite markers localizes a susceptibility locus for psoriasis vulgaris within a 111 kb segment telomeric to the HLA-C gene. Hum Mol Genet 8:2165–2170
39. Oyama N, Sekimata M, Nihei Y, Iwatsuki K, Homma Y, Kaneko F (1998) Different growth properties in response to epidermal growth factor and interleukin-6 of primary keratinocytes derived from normal and psoriatic lesional skin. J Dermatol Sci 16:120–128
40. Risch N (1990) Linkage strategies for genetically complex traits, I: multilocus models. Am J Hum Genet 46:222–228
41. Samuelsson L, Enlund F, Torinsson A, Yhr M, Inerot A, Enerback C, et al. (1999) A genome-wide search for genes predisposing to familial psoriasis by using a stratification approach. Hum Genet 105:523–529
42. Schmitt-Egenolf M, Eiermann TH, Boehncke WH, Stander M, Sterry W (1996) Familial juvenile onset psoriasis is associated with the human leucocyte antigen (HLA) class 1 side of the extended haplotype Cw6-B57-DRB1*0701-DQA1*0201-DQB1*0303: a population- and family-based study. J Invest Dermatol 106:711–714
43. Schmitt-Egenolf M, Windemuth C, Hennies HC, Albis-Camps M, von Engelhardt B, Wienker T, et al. (2001) Comparative association analysis reveals that corneodesmosin is more closely associated with psoriasis than HLA-Cw*0602-B*5701 in German families. Tissue Antigens 57:440–446
44. Simon M, Jonca N, Guerrin M, Haftek M, Bernard D, Caubet C, et al. (2001) Refined characterisation of corneodesmosin proteolysis during terminal differentiation of human epidermis and its relationship to desquamation. J Biol Chem 276:20292–20299
45. Tazi Ahnini R, Camp NJ, Cork MJ, Mee JB, Keohane SG, Duff GW, Giovine FS (1999) Novel genetic association between the corneodesmosin (MHC S) gene and susceptibility to psoriasis. Hum Mol Genet 8:1135–1140
46. Tiilikainen A, Lassus A, Karvonen J, Vartiainen P, Julin M (1980) Psoriasis and HLA-Cw6. Br J Dermatol 102:179–184
47. Tomfohrde J, Silverman A, Barnes R, Fernandez-Vina MA, Young M, Lory D, et al. (1994) Gene for familial psoriasis susceptibility mapped to the distal end of human chromosome 17q. Science 264:1141–1145
48. Trembath RC, Clough RL, Rosbotham JL, Jones AB, Camp RD, Frodsham A, et al. (1997) Identification of a major susceptibility locus on chromosome 6p and evidence for further disease loci revealed by a two stage genome-wide search in psoriasis. Hum Mol Genet 6:813–820
49. Veal CD, Clough RL, Barber RC, Mason S, Tillman D, Ferry B, et al. (2001) Identification of a novel psoriasis susceptibility locus at 1p and evidence of epistasis between PSORS1 and candidate loci. J Med Genet 38:7–13
50. Veal CD, Capon F, Allen MH, Heath EK, Evans JC, Jones A, et al. (2002) Family-based analysis using a dense single nucleotide polymorphism-based map defines genetic variation at PSORS1, the major psoriasis-susceptibility locus. Am J Hum Genet 71:554–564
51. Zhang XJ, He PP, Wang ZX, Zhang J, Li YB, Wang HY, et al. (2002) Evidence for a major psoriasis susceptibility locus at 6p21 (PSORS1) and a novel candidate region at 4q31 by genome-wide scan in Chinese Hans. J Invest Dermatol 119:1361–1366
52. Zhou Y, Chaplin DD (1993) Identification in the HLA class I region of a gene expressed late in keratinocyte differentiation. Proc Natl Acad U S A 90:9470–9473

II

B Psoriatic Arthritis

Proton Rahman, Dafna D. Gladman

Contents

1 Introduction

Psoriatic arthritis (PsA) is a complex genetic disorder that results from an interplay between multiple genetic and environmental factors. Although the exact pathogenesis of PsA is unclear, there is a substantial contribution of genetic factors to the etiology of PsA [1]. Cumulative evidence not only implicates genetic determinants for disease susceptibility, but they are also important for disease expression [2, 3]. Evidence for the genetic basis of PsA is based on data gathered from family based investigations, population based studies, association studies with HLA antigens, genome wide linkage scans, and positional candidate gene studies within and outside the major histocompatibility (MHC) region.

The marked increase in the prevalence of psoriasis in first degree relatives of probands with PsA [4], along with the immunological overlaps between these two diseases [5], is highly suggestive of shared genetic factors between psoriasis and PsA. Thus, supporting evidence for the genetic burden of PsA also comes from studies in the genetics of psoriasis, especially since the latter disease has been studied more extensively [5]. The greater emphasis on the genetics of psoriasis is in part due to a higher prevalence of psoriasis, which facilitates the recruitment of affected sibling pairs for genome wide linkage analysis. As PsA occurs in approximately one in three to five subjects with psoriasis, the occurrence of affected sibling pairs in PsA is approximately 25-fold less prevalent.

2 Genetic Epidemiology of Psoriatic Arthritis

The present flurry of genetic studies in PsA has partially surfaced as a result of the convincing epidemiological studies that have noted a striking familiality to PsA.

Population Based Studies: Estimating the Genetic Burden

The prevalence of PsA is higher in individuals who have a first degree relative with PsA than in individuals who do not have an affected first degree relative. The landmark study indicating the strong familial clustering of PsA was performed by Moll and Wright in 1973 [4]. In this study, first- and second-degree relatives of 88 patients with PsA ascertained from a hospital population were systematically assessed. Sampling of the PsA probands was consecutive and non-selective. Of the probands with PsA, 12.5% had at least one relative with confirmed PsA. Of the 181 first-degree relatives assessed, 10 relatives had PsA, including 5 siblings. Thus the overall prevalence of PsA among first-degree relatives was 5.5%. As the authors estimated the prevalence of PsA in the UK population to be 0.1%, the magnitude of genetic contribution for affected first-degree relatives (λ_1) was 55, as defined by Risch's method [6]. This estimate is substantially higher than the relative risk for psoriasis, which is 4 to 10 (reviewed in [7]). The most conservative estimate for the relative risk of siblings (λ_s) would be 27, if we assume that all first-degree relatives assessed were siblings. This magnitude of recurrence risk for an affected sibling suggests a strong familial predisposition for PsA. Other published studies assessing the familial tendency are small and often have inadequate controls. However, as reviewed by Moll and Wright, these studies also noted familial clustering of PsA [4].

Another common measure used to gauge the magnitude of genetic burden is heritability, which is defined as the proportion of variability in a trait attributed to a genetic factor. At present there are no published reports quantifying the heritability of PsA.

The extent to which familial aggregation of PsA is due to genetic or environmental factors can be assessed by comparing the concordance rate of monozygotic versus dizygotic twins. Unlike psoriasis, there are no twin studies in PsA. However, Moll and Wright reported on a triplet born with an identical twin and a non identical third triplet [4]. Both identical twins developed psoriasis, with one having spondylitis and the other polyarthritis. The non identical twin had no psoriasis or arthritis. With respect to psoriasis, there is a three fold increased risk of psoriasis in monozygotic twins as compared to fraternal twins (reviewed in [6]). However, as the concordance for psoriasis is never 100% among monozygotic twins, and can be as low as 35%, the data suggests that environmental factors also play an important role (reviewed in [6]). The same scenario is likely to be the case in PsA.

Family Studies: Determining Mode of Inheritance

Although there are no formal segregation analyses in PsA, it is universally acknowledged that PsA is a complex disease with a multifactorial pattern of inheritance. Some investigators have described large multiplex families that appear to segregate in an autosomal dominant fashion, with multiple individuals affected in multiple generations. Even for these selected families, a multifactorial inheritance model cannot be ruled out.

A non-Mendelian mode of transmission, referred to as genomic imprinting, has also been proposed for psoriasis and PsA [8, 9]. Genomic imprinting refers to an epigenetic effect that causes differential expression of a gene depending on the sex of the transmitting parent. The imprinting process dictates the expression of a gene from only one affected parent of certain sex rather than both genes of a homologous pair. The classic disorder recognized to be a consequence of genomic imprinting is the Prader-Willi Syndrome (reviewed in [10]). More recently, some autoimmune diseases have also been suspected of harbouring imprinted genes (reviewed in [10]).

Parent of origin effect has been demonstrated clinically in PsA [9]. In a clinic-based study, we systematically identified 95 probands with an affected parent. Sixty-two of these probands (0.65) had an affected father and 33 (35%) had an affected mother [9]. As the proportion of paternal transmission 0.65 was significantly greater than 0.5 (p=0.001), an excess paternal transmission was implicated in PsA. Similar trends were noted in the probands' offspring and second-degree relatives. Furthermore, a recent linkage study in PsA noted significant linkage only when assessing the transmission of alleles of paternal origin [11]. In a related study, but from a different cohort, we reported that if there was already 1 affected child in the family, the corresponding risk for another sibling affected was 0.10, 0.22 and 0.31 if no parents were affected, the mother was affected, or the father was affected, respectively [12]. Thus, the presence of this epigenetic phenomenon should be considered for incorporation in the genetic model for linkage studies, as its inclusion may influence the evidence for a linkage.

Stratifying PsA in an Attempt to Decrease Genetic Heterogeneity

The elucidation of genetic factors for most complex diseases is complicated by genetic heterogeneity. This is especially true for PsA, given the marked clinical heterogeneity of the disorder. Stratification of complex disease by clinical subset, may not only decrease clinical heterogeneity but also reduce the genetic heterogeneity. Indeed, this has been the experience in psoriasis. Henseler and Christophers in 1985 noted that type I psoriasis, defined by the onset of psoriasis prior to age 40, was much more genetic, as a greater proportion of patients had a family history of psoriasis, stronger HLA associations (HLA-Cw6, HLA-DR7, HLA-B13 and HLA-Bw57), and more severe psoriasis [13].

In a complimentary study in PsA, we noted a similar trend, although our findings have yet to be replicated due to a paucity of studies [14]. We stratified 508 PsA patients, of which 397 had their onset of psoriasis prior to the age of 40 and 111 later. PsA patients with early onset psoriasis were more likely to have a family history of psoriasis (47% vs 25%) and PsA (12.9% vs 5.4%). Significant differences in other clinical features such as skin lesions preceding joint lesions (81.3% vs 48.6%), and lower number of actively inflamed joints at presentation (9.2 vs 12.0) was noted in the early onset group. A differential expression of HLA antigens (HLA-B17, HLA-Cw6) was also observed. In light of these findings, inclusion of the age of onset of psoriasis as a potential stratification variable may also reduce the effect of heterogeneity in studies of PsA.

3 MHC – Candidate Region in PsA

For over two decades it has been recognized that selected alleles at the HLA loci render individuals at an increased risk for PsA. Multiple case control studies have demonstrated an association between HLA antigens and PsA in many different populations [15–21]. A summary of the evidence pertaining to the MHC as a candidate region in PsA is presented below.

HLA Association Studies

As most HLA studies reported in PsA were done prior to 1990, HLA typing was primarily performed with serologic techniques. While HLA Class II alleles have been reported in PsA, the findings are not as convincing as those with Class I antigens, encoded by the HLA-A, -B, and -C loci of the MHC genomic region. HLA antigens B13, B16 and its splits B38 and B39, as well as B17 and Cw6 are associated with psoriasis, with or without arthritis, while HLA-B27, B7 and HLA-B38 and -B39 are associated with PsA [17, 22]. The association with HLA-B38 and –B39 has been replicated in multiple populations [17, 22, 23]. HLA-B27 was associated with back involvement while HLA-B38 and -B39 occurred more frequently among patients with peripheral polyarthritis [15, 17, 21]. HLA-Cw*0602 is increased among with PsA compared to controls and is associated with an earlier age of onset of psoriasis [24, 25].

Class II antigens, encoded by the HLA-D region of the MHC, have been reported to be increased in patients with PsA in some studies. Associations of HLA-DR4 with PsA [15, 17, 18] have been reported, but several investigators found no HLA-D associations with PsA [19, 20]. Furthermore, PsA probands with RA-like symmetric polyarthritis were noted to have a similar frequency of HLA-DR4 as patients with rheumatoid arthritis [22].

Gladman et al. investigated the distribution of HLA-DRB1*04 alleles in 90 HLA-DR4+ patients with PsA, 90 HLA-DR4+ patients with rheumatoid arthritis and 90 HLA-DR4+ healthy controls. HLA-DRB1*0401 was significantly higher in rheumatoid arthritis than in PsA or controls ($p<0.01$) whereas HLADRB1*0402 was higher among patients with PsA [26]. However, HLA-DRB1 "shared epitope" alleles were associated with radiological changes in patients with PsA [27]. Molecular techniques using

RFLP analysis of class II genes in PsA demonstrated an association with the DRB1*0701 (DR7a) gene but not with T-cell receptor genes [28].

HLA Antigens as Prognostic Markers

To identify HLA markers for disease progression in PsA, Gladman et al. systematically assessed PsA probands over a 14-year period who had serological HLA typing for Class I and II antigens [2]. Progression of damage was defined as transition into higher damage states, defined by the number of damaged joints. The best multivariate model identified the HLA antigens B27 when DR7 was present, and DQw3 when DR7 was not present, as predicting disease progression across all transitions. HLA-B39 was associated with progression only in early disease. In a follow up study by Gladman et al. they studied 292 PsA probands to determine whether the addition of all serologically defined HLA antigens to a baseline model further influences the predisposition to disease progression in PsA [3]. The above model identified HLA-B22 as "protective" for disease progression. The authors concluded that selected HLA antigens are risk factors for disease progression.

Mapping Studies in the MHC Region

Excess HLA haplotype sharing has been demonstrated in affected sibling pairs with PsA [29]. Specifically, genomic DNA from 46 sibling pairs of probands affected with PsA were amplified in PCR using locus specific primers homologous to nucleotide sequences for each of the HLA-A, -B, -C, -DR and DQ loci. PCR amplicons were identified by reverse line blot assay using Sequence Specific Oligonucleotide (SSO) probes. Evidence for excessive haplotype sharing was examined through Green and Woodrow's test. Of the 46 sibling pairs affected with PsA, the sharing of 2, 1, or 0 haplotypes for the PsA affected sibling pairs was 14, 27, and 5 respectively (p=0.04). Thus, sibling pair analysis also implicates the HLA region on chromosome 6p as a candidate region in PsA.

Martinez-Borra et al. set out to map the locus for susceptibility to psoriasis in PsA by comparing the associations found in PsA patients with those detected in matched patients with psoriasis alone [30]. They analyzed several polymorphic markers and genes spanning from the microsatellite C1×2×5 located 19 kb centromeric to HLA-C, to the corneodesmosing gene (CDSN), located 147 kb telomeric to HLA-C. By comparing the susceptibility regions associated with the two diseases, an overlapping interval of 100 kb between HLA-C and OTF3 was identified, and this region was felt to be a critical candidate region in PsA.

4 Candidate Genes in the MHC Region

There is evidence that other genes in the HLA region on chromosome 6p may be important. To date association studies have been reported for the following candidate genes in PsA: MICA, TNF-α, TAP, and SEEK1.

MICA

A family of polymorphic genes, referred to as the MHC class I-related chain-related genes (MICA) maps to the HLA region. MICA resides 47 kb centromeric to the HLA-B locus. The high degree of linkage disequilibrium between MICA alleles and those closely linked to HLA-B genes, as well as the pattern of MICA tissue expression, implicate MICA as a potential candidate gene in PsA (as reviewed in [31]). Gonzalez et al. noted a higher frequency of the tri-nucleotide repeat polymorphism MICA-A9 in 65 Spanish PsA patients as compared to 177 healthy controls [31]. The authors noted that the increase in MICA-A9 detected in PsA patients was not in linkage disequilibrium (LD) with HLA-Cw*0602. As MICA-A9 was not associated with uncomplicated psoriasis vulgaris (psoriasis without arthritis), this suggests that MICA-A9 is associated just with PsA. Gonzalez et al. confirmed their finding in an independent Jewish population [32]. Among 52 PsA patients and

73 control patients they noted that the MICA-A9 polymorphism was found in 56% of the PsA patients and 27% of the controls (RR=3.3, $pc<0.0009$). In this cohort the MICA-A9 polymorphism was found to be in linkage disequilibrium with HLA-B alleles. The reports by Gonzalez et al. suggest that MICA, or genes in linkage disequilibrium may be involved in the pathogenesis of PsA.

TNFα

The tumor necrosis factor alpha (TNF-α) gene is located 250 kb centromeric from HLA-B. TNF-α levels, as well as levels of interleukin-1 (IL-1), IL-15, and IL-10, are increased in synovial fluid and synovial membranes of PsA patients compared with osteoarthritis patients. In view of the location and proposed biologic effect of TNF-α it has been speculated that polymorphisms within this locus may contribute to the susceptibility to PsA [33, 34]. Polymorphisms in the promoter region involving the substitution of G/A at positions 308 and 238 have figured prominently in various studies.

Hohler et al. assessed TNF-α promoter polymorphisms by sequence-specific oligonucleotide hybridization in Caucasian patients with juvenile onset psoriasis, PsA, and in healthy controls. A mutation at position 238 of the TNF-α promoter was present in 23 of 60 patients (38%; $p<0.0001$; $p[\text{corr}]<0.008$) with juvenile onset psoriasis and in 20 of 62 patients (32%; $p<0.0003$; $p[\text{corr}]<0.03$) with PsA, compared with seven of 99 (7%) Caucasian controls [35]. Meanwhile the mutation at position 308 was found in similar proportions of PsA patients and controls. Hohler et al. confirmed their finding in an independent population and also noted a marked decrease in the TNF-α 308 allele in PsA patients as compared to healthy controls [36].

The TNF associations in PsA reported by Hohler et al. have not been universally replicated across various populations. Gonzalez et al. reported no association with TNF-α 238 and 308 in 52 PsA subjects and 73 controls from a Jewish population [32]. In a more recent Irish study, Balding et al. reported no association with TNF-α 308 in 147 Irish PsA subjects and 389 controls. However, the presence of early onset of psoriasis, joint erosions and more rapidly progressive disease were associated with the 308 genotype [37]. Finally, Al-Heresh et al. noted no association between TNF-α 238 and 308 for their entire PsA cohort of 124 probands. However, in this study, the 238 allele was absent in the spondyloarthropathy group, and increased in patients with peripheral polyarthritis. The authors noted that the latter finding can be accounted for by linkage disequilibrium, as all patients with 238 allele were positive for HLA-Cw*0602 [38].

TAP

The ATP-binding cassette transporter TAP translocates peptides from the cytosol to awaiting MHC class I molecules in the endoplasmic reticulum. TAP is made up of the TAP1 and TAP2 polypeptides. As TAP genes are essential in class I antigen presentation they were considered as possible candidates for susceptibility genes (as reviewed in [39]). Hohler et al. examined 60 patients with juvenile onset psoriasis, 63 psoriatic arthritis patients, and 101 controls for polymorphisms in TAP1 and TAP2 [39]. Although a weak association was noted with the TAP1*0101 allele in psoriasis patients, statistical significance was lost after correction for multiple testing. No differences were noted for any of TAP gene polymorphisms in PsA.

SEEK1

Recently, a Swedish study noted a strong association between mutations in SEEK1 and PsA. SEEK1, the function of which is unknown, is located just telomeric to the HCR gene and is expressed in psoriatic skin [40]. The SNP +39604 in exon 2 of SEEK1 demonstrated the most striking association with the psoriasis population as compared to controls (66% vs 22%, $p<0.0001$). This finding was independent of HLA-Cw*0602.

We examined the possible association between SNP +39604 in exon 2 of SEEK1 and

PsA, in two distinct populations, a founder population from Newfoundland and an admixed population from Toronto [41]. Seventy-two PsA patients and 73 ethnically matched controls from Newfoundland and 79 PsA patients and 68 controls from Toronto were enrolled. The genotype frequency for the mutant (*T*) allele was 51% among Newfoundlanders with PsA and 34% in the controls (p=0.04). In the Toronto cohort, the genotype frequency for the T allele was 35% for PsA patients and 40% in controls (p=ns). Thus there is a modest association between SEEK1 mutation and PsA in the Newfoundland cohort, which was not replicated in the Toronto PsA cohort. The disparity between the Newfoundland and Toronto cohorts may be due to an enhanced signal to noise ratio in the Newfoundland founder population; alternatively, this allele may be in linkage disequilibrium with HLA-Cw*0602 in the Newfoundland population.

5 Candidate Regions Outside the MHC

Linkage Studies

A common strategy employed to elucidate genetic determinants of a complex disease is positional cloning. In this strategy investigators attempt to isolate the disease gene by its chromosomal location without any prior knowledge of the position or function of the gene. Positional cloning requires a collection of families with multiple affected individuals so that linkage analysis can be performed. This can be done by constructing a model that explains the inheritance of disease in the pedigrees, and then estimating the recombination fraction for a given pedigree. This is referred to as the traditional, or recombinant based, method. An alternative approach for linkage analysis is to identify affected family members (typically affected sibling pairs), and assess the allele sharing. This is referred to as the allele sharing, or non-parametric, method. The latter method is based on the premise that, in the presence of linkage between a marker and disease, sets of relatives who share the same disease status will be more alike at the marker locus than one would expect if the two loci were segregating independently.

To date, only one genome wide scan has been completed in PsA. This study localized a candidate region for PsA on chromosome 16q [11]. In this Icelandic study, 178 patients were identified with PsA. Using their Icelandic genealogy database the authors were able to connect 100 of these patients into 39 families for linkage analysis. This genome scan was performed using 1,000 microsatellite markers. Following the initial linkage scan and addition of extra markers the strongest evidence for linkage was observed on chromosome 16, with an LOD score of 2.17 at the marker D16S3038. The investigators then stratified the linkage analysis using only paternal transmissions to affected individuals, and obtained an LOD score of 4.19 at marker D16S267. Using maternal transmissions only, the maximum LOD score was 1.03 at marker D16S3089. The authors concluded that there is a susceptibility gene for PsA within the 16q locus that may be involved in paternal transmission of PsA.

Other potential candidate regions that warrant consideration in PsA include those that have demonstrated significant linkage in psoriasis. To date, the psoriasis susceptibility loci that have been mapped using linkage strategies include : PSORS1 on 6p21.3, PSORS2 on 17q, PSORS3 on 4q, PSORS4 on 1cen-q21, PSORS5 on 3q21, PSORS6 on 19p, PSORS7 on 1p, and PSORS9 on 4q31 [42–49]. Additional putative psoriasis candidate loci have been reported on 16q and 20p [50]. The loci on 6p and 17q have been replicated with independent linkage studies [48, 50]. See Chap. II.A for a more detailed discussion of the susceptibility loci in psoriasis.

Positional Candidate Genes

CARD15–16q12

CARD15 is a member of the CED4/APAF1 family of apoptosis regulators, and has been mapped to 16q12. CARD15 is expressed predominantly in monocytes. CARD15 functions as an intracellular toll-like receptor (TLR), which binds bacterial components and activates NF-κB. CARD15 mutations have been implicated in altering recognition of bacterial lipopolysaccharide (LPS) [51]. This hypothesis has been supported by functional experiments as 1007-fs mutations decreased NF-kB activation by LPS [52]. CARD15 has now definitively been shown to be associated with Crohn's disease [53, 54]. The possibility of a common susceptibility gene between psoriasis/PsA and Crohn's disease is supported by epidemiological studies that note a four- to eightfold increased incidence of psoriasis and psoriatic arthritis in subjects with CD [50, 55] and a linkage study in PsA that reported significant linkage at a region overlapping the loci for CARD15 [11]. In addition, a recent study from the International Psoriasis Genetics Consortium reported that the strongest evidence of allele sharing outside the MHC region was found on chromosome 16q [56].

We recently screened 187 PsA patients and 136 controls from the Newfoundland population for the three common independent sequence variants of CARD15 (R702W, leu1007-fsinsC and G908R) [57]. These variants were detected by polymerase chain reaction using allele-specific primers and visualized through gel electrophoresis. CARD15 variants were significantly more frequent in the PsA patients (OR 2.97, 1.61–5.47; p=0.0005) and this was independent of HLA-Cw*0602. However, we have not been able to replicate this finding in the more admixed Toronto cohort It is possible that the CARD15 variant noted to be associated with PsA in the Newfoundland population may be in linkage disequilibrium with another gene in the 16q12 region.

IL-1 2q12–2q13

As noted previously, IL-1 is seen in significantly higher concentrations in the serum, synovial fluid, and synovial membrane of PsA patients, as compared to osteoarthritis patients and healthy volunteers. IL-1 is a potent pro-inflammatory cytokine that occurs as IL-1α and IL-1β. The biological activity of IL-1α and IL-1β is initiated by its binding with type 1 IL-1 receptor (as reviewed in [58]). The action of IL-1 is inhibited by IL-1 receptor antagonist (IL-ra). The loci for these genes are found in a cluster on chromosome 2q12 to 2q13 [59]. Ravinddran et al. genotyped polymorphisms in IL-1α -889 genotype, IL-1β +3953, and IL-1 receptor R1 +970 genes in 140 patients with PsA and 100 controls. The frequency of IL-1α –889C allele and CC homozygotes was significantly increased in PsA. There was no association with the other IL-1 polymorphisms. The authors concluded that the IL-1 gene complex may play a role in the development of PsA, or that it may be in linkage disequilibrium with another gene on chromosome 2q12 to 2q13. However, an independent study of 147 Irish PsA patients and 389 controls noted no association with IL-1β +3953 and IL-1 receptor antagonist gene polymorphisms [37]. In this cohort, IL-1 polymorphisms did not predispose to development of PsA.

KIR 19q13.4

Natural Killer (NK) cells are bone marrow derived lymphocytes involved in the surveillance and killing of foreign or infected cells through a mechanism involving recognition of HLA molecules by an extremely diverse set of receptors on the cell surface [60]. NK receptors include Killer cell Ig-like receptors (*KIRs*), which are coded for on chromosome 19q13.4. A recent observation in an animal model for psoriasis led to a hypothesis that that the direct activation of T cells bearing NK receptors for MHC class I triggers psoriasis [61]. A similar mechanism may be operating in PsA. NK cell activity in the peripheral blood was shown to be lower than in the synovium in patients with PsA [62]. Martin et al. recently demonstrated that individuals with genes encoding activating *KIR*s, but lacking HLA-C alleles that encode the corresponding ligands for those receptors, are relatively susceptible to developing PsA [63], suggesting that disease expression may depend on the *KIR* phenotype.

6 Conclusion

In summary, there is a clear genetic contribution to PsA. Although there are distinct immunological and genetic differences between psoriasis and PsA, many genetic determinants are likely to be shared between these two diseases. The MHC region has consistently been identified as a high priority candidate region in PsA. Strong association has been noted with HLA antigens and other candidate genes that reside within this region. HLA antigens are important not only for disease susceptibility but also for disease expression. There also has been a recent expansion of the number of critical regions and candidate genes suspected in PsA susceptibility from outside the MHC region. The strong genetic contribution to PsA, coupled with rapidly advancing sequencing and bio-informatic platforms, means that elucidation of the major genetic determinants for PsA within and outside the MHC region should soon be feasible.

References

1. Gladman DD, Rahman P (2001) Psoriatic arthritis. In: Ruddy S, Harris ED, Sledge CB, Budd RC, Sergent JS (eds) Kelly's textbook of rheumatology, 6th edn. WB Saunders, Philadelphia, pp 1071–1079
2. Gladman DD, Farewell VT (1995) The role of HLA antigens as indicators of progression in psoriatic arthritis (PsA): multivariate relative risk model. Arthritis Rheum 38:845–850
3. Gladman DD, Farewell VT, Kopciuk K, Cook RJ (1998) HLA antigens and progression in psoriatic arthritis. J Rheumatol 25;730–733
4. Moll JM, Wright V (1973) Familial occurrence of PsA. Ann Rheum Dis 32:181–201
5. Bhalerao J, Bowcock AM (1998) The genetics of psoriasis: a complex disorder of the skin and immune system. Hum Mol Genet 7:10:1537–1545
6. Risch N (1990) Linkage strategies for genetically complex traits. 1. Multilocus model. Am J Hum Genet 46:222–228
7. Elder JT, Nair RP, Guo SW, Hensler T, Christophers E, Voorhees JJ (1994) The genetics of psoriasis. Arch Dermatol 130:216–224
8. Traupe H, van Gurp PJ, Happle R, Boezeman J, van de Kerkhof PC (1992) Psoriasis vulgaris, fetal growth, and genomic imprinting. Am J Med Genet 42:649–654
9. Rahman P, Gladman DD, Schentag C, Petronis A (1999) Excessive paternal transmission in psoriatic arthritis (PsA). Arthritis Rheum 42:1228–1231
10. Morison IM, Reeve AE (1998) A catalogue of imprinted genes and parent of origin effects in humans and animals. Hum Mol Genet 7:10:1599–1609
11. Karason A, Gudjonsson JE, Upmanyu R, Antonsdottir AA, Hauksson VB, Runasdottir EH, Jonsson HH, Gudbjartsson DF, Frigge ML, Kong A, Stefansson K, Valdimarsson H, Gulcher JR (2003) A susceptibility gene for psoriatic arthritis maps to chromosome 16p: evidence for imprinting. Am J Hum Genet 72:125–131
12. Rahman P, Gladman D, Khraishi M, Hamilton S, Tobin Y, Hefferton D, Alderdice CA (2003) Influence of parental history on the recurrence risk of siblings with psoriatic arthritis. J Rheumatol 30:1885
13. Henseler T, Christophers E (1985) Psoriasis of early and late onset: characterization of two types of psoriasis vulgaris. J Am Acad Dermatol 13:450–456
14. Rahman P, Gladman DD, Schentag CT (1999) Immunogenetic profile of patients with psoriatic arthritis varies according to the age of onset of psoriasis. Arthritis Rheum 42:822–833
15. Eastmond CJ (1994) Genetics and HLA antigens. In: Baillière's clinical rheumatology. Psoriatic arthritis. In: Wright V, Helliwell P (eds) Baillière Tindall, London, pp 263–276
16. Gerber LH, Murray CL, Perlman SG, Barth WF, Decker JL, Nigra TA, Mann DL (1982) Human lymphocyte antigens characterizing psoriatic arthritis and its alleles. J Rheumatol 9:703–707
17. Espinoza LR, Vasey FB, Gaylord SW, et al. (1982) Histocompatibility typing in the seronegative spondyloarthropathies; a survey. Semin Arthritis Rheum 11:375–381
18. Kantor SM, Hsu SH, Bias WB, Arnett FC (1984) Clinical and immunologic subsets of psoriatic arthritis. Clin Exp Rheumatol 2:105–109
19. Beaulieu AD, Roy R, Mathon G, Morissette J, Latulippe L, Lang JY, Mathieu JP, Brunet D, Hebert J, Archambault H, et al. (1983) Psoriatic arthritis: risk for patients with psoriasis – a study based on histocompatibility antigen frequencies. J Rheumatol 10:633–636
20. McKendry RJR, Sengar DPS, Des Groseilliers JP, Dunne JV (1984) Frequency of HLA antigens in patients with psoriasis or psoriatic arthritis. Can Med Assoc J 130:411–415
21. Salvarani C, Macchioni PL, Zizzi F, Mantovani W, Rossi F, Baricchi R, Ghirelli L, Frizziero L, Portioli I (1989) Clinical subgroups in Italian patients with psoriatic arthritis. Clin Exp Rheumatol 7:391–396
22. Gladman DD, Anhorn KA, Schachter RK, Mervart H (1982) HLA antigens in psoriatic arthritis. J Rheumatol 13:586–592

23. Trabace S, Cappellacci S, Ciccarone P, Liaskos S, Polito R, Zorzin L (1994) Psoriatic arthritis: a clinical, radiological and genetic study of 58 Italian patients. Acta Derm Venereol Suppl (Stockh). 186:69–70
24. Gladman DD, Cheung C, Michener G, Wade JA (1999) HLA C-locus alleles in psoriatic arthritis. Hum Immunol 60:259–261
25. Al-Haresh AM, Proctor J, Jones SM, Dixey J, Cox B, Welsh K, McHugh N (2002) Tumour necrosis factor-α polymorphisms and the HLA-Cw*602 allele in psoriatic arthritis. Rheumatology 41:525–530
26. Gladman DD, Farewell VT, Rahman P, Schentag CT, Pellet F, Ng CM, Wade JA (2001) HLA-DRB1*04 alleles in psoriatic arthritis (PsA): comparison with rheumatoid arthritis and healthy controls. Hum Immunol 62:1239–1244
27. Korendowych E, Dixey J, Cox B, Jones S, McHugh N (2003) The influence of the HLA-DRB1 rheumatoid arthritis shared epitope on the clinical characteristics and radiological outcome of psoriatic arthritis. J Rheumatol 30:96–101
28. Sakkas LI, Loqueman N, Bird H, Vaughan RW, Welsh KI, Panayi GS (1990) HLA class II and T cell receptor gene polymorphism in psoriatic arthritis and psoriasis. J Rheumatol 17:487–490
29. Gladman DD, Farewell VT, Pellett F, Schentag C, Rahman P (2003) HLA is a candidate region for psoriatic arthritis. evidence for excessive HLA sharing in sibling pairs. Hum Immunol 64:887–889
30. Martinez-Borra J, Gonzalez S, Santos-Juanes J, Sanchez del Rio J, Torre-Alonso JC, Lopez-Vazquez A, Blanco-Gelaz MA, Lopez-Larrea C (2003) Psoriasis vulgaris and psoriatic arthritis share a 100 kb susceptibility region telomeric to HLA-C. Rheumatology 42:1089–1092
31. Gonzalez S, Martinez-Borra J, Torre-Alonso JC, Gonzalez-Roces S, Sanchez del Rio J, Rodriguez Perez A, Brautbar C, Lopez-Larrea C (1999) The MICA-A9 triplet repeat polymorphism in the transmembrane region confers additional susceptibility to the development of psoriatic arthritis and is independent of the association of Cw*0602 in psoriasis. Arthritis Rheum 42:1010–1016
32. Gonzalez S, Brautbar C, Martinez-Borra J, Lopez-Vazquez A, Segal R, Blanco-Gelaz MA, Enk CD, Safriman C, Lopez-Larrea C (2001) Polymorphism in MICA rather than HLA-B/C genes is associated with psoriatic arthritis in the Jewish population. Hum Immunol 62:632–638
33. Danning CL, Illei GG, Hitchon C, Greer MR, Boumpas DT, McInnes IB (2000) Macrophage-derived cytokine and nuclear factor kappaB p65 expression in synovial membrane and skin of patients with psoriatic arthritis. Arthritis Rheum 43:1244–1256
34. Partsch G, Steiner G, Leeb BF, Dunky A, Broll H, Smolen JS (1997) Highly increased levels of tumor necrosis factor-alpha and other proinflammatory cytokines in psoriatic arthritis synovial fluid. J Rheumatol 24:518–523
35. Hohler T, Kruger A, Schneider PM, Schopf RE, Knop J, Rittner C, Meyer zum Buschenfelde KH, Marker-Hermann E (1997) A TNF-alpha promoter polymorphism is associated with juvenile onset psoriasis and psoriatic arthritis. J Invest Dermatol 109:562–565
36. Hohler T, Grossmann S, Stradmann-Bellinghausen B, Kaluza W, Reuss E, de Vlam K, Veys E, Marker-Hermann E (2002) Differential association of polymorphisms in the TNFalpha region with psoriatic arthritis but not psoriasis. Ann Rheum Dis 61:213–218
37. Balding J, Kane D, Livingstone W, Mynett-Johnson L, Bresnihan B, Smith O, FitzGerald O (2003) Cytokine gene polymorphisms: association with psoriatic arthritis susceptibility and severity. Arthritis Rheum 48:1408–1413
38. Al-Heresh AM, Proctor J, Jones SM, Dixey J, Cox B, Welsh K, McHugh N (2002) Tumour necrosis factor-alpha polymorphism and the HLA-Cw*0602 allele in psoriatic arthritis. Rheumatology 41:525–530
39. Hohler T, Weinmann A, Schneider PM, Rittner C, Schopf RE, Knop J, Hasenclever P, Meyer zum Buschenfelde KH, Marker-Hermann E (1996) TAP-polymorphisms in juvenile onset psoriasis and psoriatic arthritis. Hum Immunol 51:49–54
40. Holm SJ, Carlen LM, Mallbris L, Stahle-Backdahl M, O'Brien KP (2003) Polymorphisms in the SEEK1 and SPR1 genes on 6p21.3 associated with psoriasis in the Swedish population. Exp Dermatol 12:435–444
41. Rahman P, Tobin Y, Peddle L, Snelgrove T, Pellet F, Hamilton S, Alderdice C, Khraishi M, Schentag C, Gladman D (2004) Association of SEEK1 and psoriatic arthritis in two distinct Caucasian populations. J Rheumatol (abstract)
42. Trembath RC, Clough RL, Rosbotham J L, Jones AB, Camp RDR, Frodsham A, Browne J, Barber R, Terwilliger J, Lathrop GM, Barker JNWN (1997) Identification of a major susceptibility locus on chromosome 6p and evidence for further disease loci revealed by a two stage genome-wide search in psoriasis. Hum Mol Genet 6:813–820
43. Tomfohrde J, Silverman A, Barnes R, Fernandez-Vina MA, Young M, Lory D, Morris L, Wuepper KD, Stastny P, Menter A, Bowcock A (1994) Gene for familial psoriasis susceptibility mapped to the distal end of human chromosome 17q. Science 264:1141–1145
44. Matthews D, Fry L, Powles A, Weber J, McCarthy M, Fisher E, Davies K, Williamson R (1996) Evidence that a locus for familial psoriasis maps to chromosome 4q. Nature Genet 14:231–233
45. Capon F, Novelli G, Semprini S, Clementi M, Nudo M, Vultaggio P, Mazzanti C, Gobello T, Botta A, Fabrizi G, Dallapiccola B (1999) Searching for psoriasis susceptibility genes in Italy: genome scan and evidence for a new locus on chromosome 1. J Invest Derm 112:32–35

46. Enlund F, Samuelsson L, Enerback C, Inerot A, Wahlstrom J, Yhr M, et al. (1999) Psoriasis susceptibility locus in chromosome region 3q21 identified in patients from southwest Sweden. Eur J Hum Genet 7:783–790
47. Lee Y-A, Ruschendorf F, Windemuth C, Schmitt-Egenolf M, Stadelmann A, Nurnberg G, et al. (2000) Genomewide scan in German families reveals evidence for a novel psoriasis-susceptibility locus on chromosome 19p13. Am J Hum Genet 67:1020–1024
48. Veal CD, Clough RL, Barber RC, Mason S, Tillman D, Ferry B, et al. (2001) Identification of a novel psoriasis susceptibility locus at 1p and evidence of epistasis between PSORS1 and candidate loci. J Med Genet 38:7–13
49. Zhang X-J, He P-P, Wang Z-X, Zhang J, Li Y-B, Wang H-Y, et al. (2002) Evidence for a major psoriasis susceptibility locus at 6p21 (PSORS1) and a novel candidate region at 4q31 by genome-wide scan in Chinese Hans. J Invest Derm 119:1361–1366
50. Nair RP, Henseler T, Jenisch S, Stuart P, Bichakjian CK, Lenk W, et al. (1997) Evidence for two psoriasis susceptibility loci (HLA and 17q) and two novel candidate regions (16q and 20p) by genome-wide scan. Hum Mol Genet 6:1349–1356
51. Ogura Y, Bonen DK, Inohara N, Nicolae DL, Chen FF, Ramos R, Britton H, Moran T, Karaliuskas R, Duerr RH, Achkar JP, Brant SR, Bayless TM, Kirschner BS, Hanauer SB, Nunez G, Cho JH (2001) A frameshift mutation in NOD2 associated with susceptibility to Crohn's disease. Nature 411:603–606
52. Hugot J-P, Cho JH (2002) Update on genetics of inflammatory bowel disease. Curr Opin Gastroenterol 18:410–415
53. Lesage S, Zouali H, Cezard JP, Colombel JF, Belaiche J, Almer S, Tysk C, O'Morian C, Gassull M, Binder V, Finkel Y, Modigliani R, Gower-Rousseau C, Marcy J, Merlin F, Chamaillard M, Jannot AS, Thomas G, Hugot JP (2002) CARD15/NOD2 mutational analysis and genotype-phenotype correlation in 612 patients with inflammatory bowel disease. Am J Hum Genet 70:845–857
54. Vermeire S, Wild G, Kocher K, Cousineau J, Dufresne L, Bitton A, Langelier D, Pare P, Lapointe G, Cohen A, Daly MJ, Rioux JD (2002) CARD15 genetic variation in a Quebec population: prevalence, genotype-phenotype relationship, and haplotype structure. Am J Hum Genet 71:74–83
55. Lee FI, Bellary SV, Francis C (1990) Increased occurrence of psoriasis in patients with Crohn's disease and their relatives. Am J Gastroenterol 85:962–963
56. International Psoriasis Genetics Consortium (2003) The International Psoriasis Genetics Study: assessing linkage to 14 candidate susceptibility loci in a cohort of 942 affected sib pairs. Am J Hum Genet 73:430–437
57. Rahman P, Bartlett S, Siannis F, Pellett FJ, Farewell VT, Peddle L, Schentag CT, Alderdice CA, Hamilton S, Khraishi M, Tobin Y, Hefferton D, Gladman DD (2003) CARD15: a pleiotropic autoimmune gene that confers susceptibility to psoriatic arthritis. Am J Hum Genet 73:677–681
58. Ravindran JS, Owen P, Lagan A, Lewis J, Korendowych E, Welsh K, McHugh N (2004) Interleukin 1{alpha}, interleukin 1{beta} and interleukin 1 receptor gene polymorphisms in psoriatic arthritis. Rheumatology 43:22–26
59. Nicklin MJ, Barton JL, Nguyen M, FitzGerald MG, Duff GW, Kornman K (2002) A sequence-based map of the nine genes of the human interleukin-1 cluster. Genomics 79:718–725
60. Trowsdale J (2001) Genetic and functional relationships between MHC and NK receptor genes. Immunity 16:363–374
61. Nickoloof BJ, Wrone-Smith T, Bonich B, Procelli SA (1999) Response of murine and normal human skin to injection of allogenetic blood-derived psoriatic immunocytes: detection of T cells expressing receptors typically present on natural killer cells including CD94, CD158 and CD161. Arch Dermatol 135: 546–552
62. McQueen FM, Skinner MA, Krissansen GW, Robinson E, Tan PL (1994) Natural killer cell function and expression of beta 7 integrin in psoriatic arthritis. J Rheumatol 21:2266–2273
63. Martin MP, Nelson G, Lee J-H, Pellett F, Gao X, Klitz W, Wade J, Wilson M, Trowsdale J, Gladman D, Carrington M (2002) Susceptibility to psoriatic arthritis: influence of activating killer immunoglobulin-like receptor genes in the absence of their corresponding HLA ligands. J Immunol 169:2818–2822

Immunopathogenesis III

A Psoriasis

Brian K. Bonish, Brian J. Nickoloff

Contents

1 Introduction

For over 100 years, psoriatic plaques were known to possess key cellular components including epidermal hyperplasia accompanied by an inflammatory cell-rich infiltrate. Initially, the striking clinical presentation of thick, silvery plaques and scale led investigators to focus on the keratinocyte component and dysregulated cell proliferation within the epidermis as the cause of psoriasis. Since typical plaques have thickened skin and parakeratotic scale, a loss of the granular cell layer, increased epidermal cell layers and increased mitotic figures in the basal keratinocytes, it was not unreasonable for clinicians to initially treat psoriasis using agents to stop or reduce keratinocyte proliferation. Also, since psoriasis is largely confined to the skin, most skin biologists would assume that keratinocytes must be primarily involved in the disease process. However, it still remains to be determined if psoriasis represents a skin disorder because of a fundamental abnormality in the epidermal keratinocyte, or primarily in a specific skin-seeking subset of immunocytes.

The T-cell infiltrates in psoriasis have a nonrandom patterns of migration including CD8+ T cells present in the epidermis, and CD4+ T cells in the dermis. Besides T cells, other immunocyte subsets include increased numbers of neutrophils, dermal dendritic cells, macrophages, and mast cells. Focus began to shift towards this immune infiltrate as the primary pathogenic process in 1979, with the serendipitous observation that cyclosporine improved psoriasis in a patient with rheumatoid arthritis [23]. With the advent of monoclonal antibodies in the 1980s, combined with immunohistochemistry, it became possible to characterize the pathologic immunology in psoriasis with greater refinement and with a more comprehensive set of findings. Based on additional observations as described later, it is now widely accepted that psoriasis is a T-cell-mediated disease, and that these pathogenic T cells drive the epidermal hyperplasia. Whether the pathogenic T cells are reactive against self-antigens, or non-self antigens, remains to be determined. It is of central importance that, before psoriasis can be classified as an autoimmune disease, it will be necessary to determine the nature of the antigen responsible for mediating the T-cell activation event that triggers the onset of lesion formation.

Continued use of the tools of molecular biology has allowed us to continually refine our knowledge of the immunopathological basis of psoriasis. This molecular approach has provided much needed information about the pathways and gene expression profiles in psoriasis. Unfortunately, although we have learned many details, the specific cause of this disease remains unknown. Despite improvements in treatment options, including the recent advent of specific immunologic therapy, there is still no cure. However, new therapeutic targets are emerging with our new understanding and a transition from serendipitous drug development to more selective targeting of key molecular mediators has occurred in this rapidly changing field of active basic and clinical investigation.

2 Immunopathology of Psoriasis

Over time various models to explain psoriasis have covered a broad range of cell types. The inclusion of various cell types should not be surprising given the vast confederacy of cells present within the plaque ranging from resident epidermal keratinocytes derived from the ectoderm to bone marrow derived cells such as dendritic cells and T lymphocytes. Some of the earliest theories of the immunopathogenesis of psoriasis featured the response of skin to environmentally derived stimuli such as trauma and infection. These theories focused primarily on the epidermal keratinocyte [64]. A later model highlighted the potential role of fibroblasts because some clinicians viewed psoriasis as a perpetual wound healing response [51, 78]. By this theory, fibroblasts activated in the dermis were viewed as the genesis of psoriatic plaques as by driving keratinocyte proliferation [102]. Defects in neutrophils have been proposed [117]. Mast cells have been noted to have increased interferon-gamma (IFN-γ) in psoriatic patients [2]. As psoriatic plaques are often symmetrical, it has been suggested that nerve conduction pathways play a role through the factors they release [96]. Support for this hypothesis is derived from clinical observation that plaques fail to develop in denervated skin [40]. There is also increased vascularity in psoriatic plaques and defects in endothelial cells have been observed [71]. It is not currently known if psoriatic plaques are dependent on the increased vascularity, which is highly characteristic of skin lesions.

Despite the myriad cell types contributing to psoriasis, it is widely accepted that T-lymphocytes play a central role in the immunopathology of psoriasis [10, 24, 29, 116]. Therapies that target T cells specifically, such as anti-CD4 antibodies and interleukin-2 toxin (IL-2) conjugates have been shown to improve psoriasis [11, 46, 47]. Many studies have demonstrated the importance of specific T-cell subsets and dendritic antigen presenting cells (APCs) in psoriatic plaques [12, 45, 46, 58, 63, 76, 80, 81, 105, 111, 115].

In an attempt to assimilate this immunological-based information into one theory, the cytokine network model has been proposed [81]. In this model, external stimuli such as trauma, or internal stimuli such as infections including HIV-1, neuropeptides, or ingested medications (beta-blockers, lithium), trigger activation of immunocytes, which in turn set up a cascade of cytokines with tumor necrosis factor-alpha (TNF-α) from APCs and keratinocytes and IFN-γ from activated Th-1 type lymphocytes. Since the original depiction of the cytokine network focused on IFN-γ and TNF-α, many dozens of cytokines, chemokines, and growth factors that may play a significant role have been added.

Psoriasis has a strong genetic component, and in many families, several affected patients can be traced through multiple generations. The genetics of this disease are described in detail in later chapters. Briefly, 40% of patients with psoriasis have family members who are also affected, and monozygotic twins have a 70% concordance [10, 102]. The strongest genetic association in psoriasis is with the MHC class I allele Cw6*0602, occurring most commonly in early onset (Type 1) psoriasis. Even in the case of Cw6*0602, however, it estimated that only 10% of Caucasians with Cw6*0602 develop psoriasis. Extensive mapping by several laboratories and the International Psoriasis Genetic Consortium have mapped at least nine susceptibility regions, designated PSORS1-PSORS9 [30]. Extensive genetic studies have narrowed the region (PSOSR1) on 6p21 down to a region between HLA-Cw6 and corneodesmosin. It is quite possible that there is linkage disequilibrium with another gene or gene cluster within this region. Genetic disequilibrium with the Ig-like killer cell-inhibitory receptors (KIR) have recently been reported [73]. These receptors are expressed on natural killer (NK) cells and NK-T cells and are important for regulation of activation of these cells through recognition of MHC-1 surface proteins. Another major region associated in some studies with psoriasis could also have an immunologic importance. PSORS2 located on17q24-q25 and contains the genes SLC9A3R1 and NAT9 [50]. Despite the possible role for many different proteins, the current consensus is that the most likely primary genetic determinant responsible for psoriasis involves expression of the HLA-Cw6 0602 allele. From an immunological perspective, any model for psoriasis has to be able to explain why this MHC class I allele is so important to the pathogenesis of psoriasis.

3 T Cells and Inflammatory Pathways in Psoriasis

T-Cell Signalling

One central requirement of an immunocyte/cytokine based model of psoriasis is that the critical T-cell populations must be active in the skin. There are a large number of proteins involved in signaling between T cells and APCs (professional and others, including keratinocytes) that mediate this activity. One of the fundamental principles of T-cell activation is that at least two different signals must be present for optimal T-cell proliferation and cytokine release. The first signal, termed signal 1, is the appropriate antigen, and is presented to T cells by APCs in the context of either MHC class I or class II molecules (or in the case of glycolipids in the context of non-classical MHC molecules such as CD1d). In addition, to signal 1, the T cell must also receive so-called costimulatory signals for optimal proliferation and cytokine release. Several such molecules include CD80 and CD86 expressed by APCs which bind CD28 on T cells. In addition, interactions between adhesion molecules like LFA-1 and ICAM-1 are also important for costimulation. For psoriasis studies, it has not been possible to unequivocally establish the identity of the antigen in signal 1, but it is still possible to intervene therapeutically by interfering with the costimulatory signals. An illustration of the receptors discussed here is shown in Fig. A1. The interface between the T cell and an APC has been described as an immunological synapse [28]. These discrete clusters of surface proteins and signaling machinery mediate the function of immune cells [8, 65]. Real-time focal imaging has demonstrated the existence of these structures [35]. Components of the immunological synapse include a ring of adhesion molecules (LFA-1), binding to ICAM-1 on an adjacent cell [36, 88]. The relevance of this to psoriasis is demonstrated by the fact that efalizumab (anti-LFA-1) which blocks the interaction of LFA-1 with ICAM-1 has improved psoriatic lesions in a multi-center randomized placebo controlled trial [67]. Beyond the adhesion molecule component of the synapse, there is a requirement for engagement of costimulatory molecules which include CD2:LFA-3 [77, 90] and CD28:CD80/CD86 (B7.1/B7.2) [6]. Blockade of the CD2:LFA-3 interaction has been effectively demonstrated to improve lesions of psoriasis through the use of an LFA-3 Ig fusion (alefacept) [37]. CTLA4-Ig which blocks CD28/CD80/CD86 has also been used to therapeutic effect [1]. Directly targeting T cells with immunotherapy using anti-CD3 [121], and anti-CD4 is also effective [47]. An IL-2 receptor directed diphtheria-toxin (denileukin diftitox) is also capable of improving the symptoms of psoriasis [11, 46]. Taken together, the basic and clinical research studies indicate that specifically targeting the protein interactions involved in signal 2 can have a profound impact on the activity of psoriasis.

Beyond the external signaling components of the synapse there are a number of internal signal transduction pathways with potential relevance to the immunopathology of psoriasis. Alterations in the intracellular signal transduction system have been proposed to alter central tolerance. Breakdown of negative thymic selection leads to auto-reactive T cells in the periphery which could play a role in psoriasis

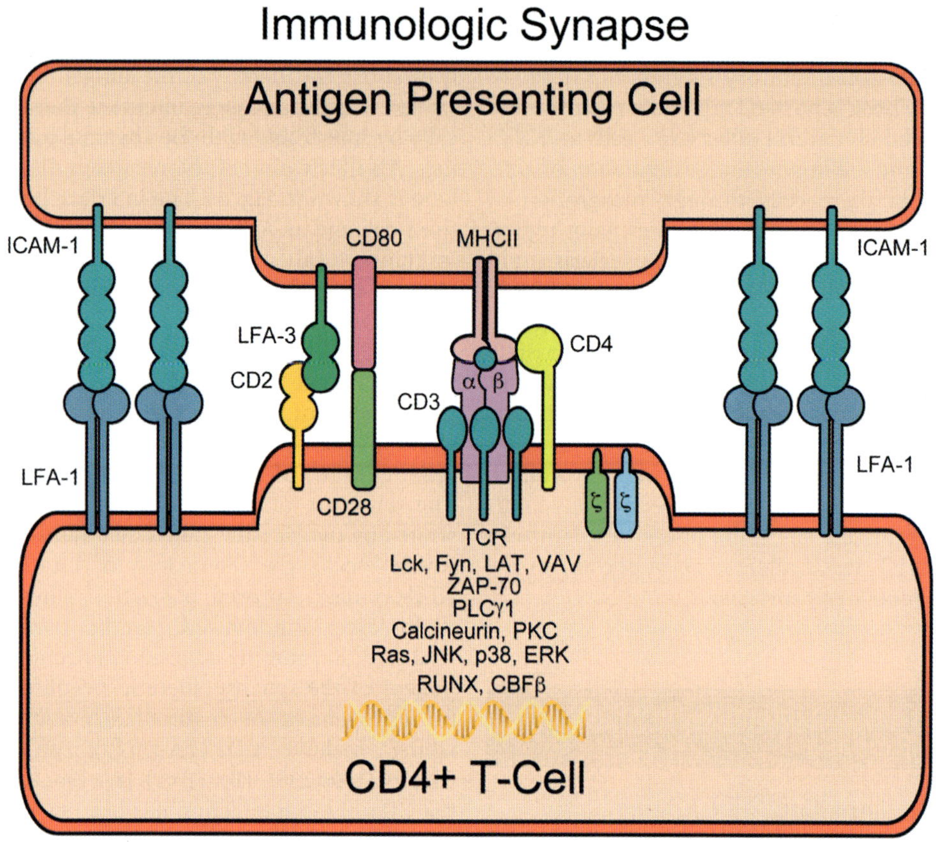

Fig. A1. Surface molecules present at the surface of dendritic APCs and T cells that contribute to T-cell activation

[123]. ZAP-70 is a protein tyrosine kinase involved in cell activation and found in both T cells and NK cells. Mice with mutations in ZAP-70 have been shown to develop rheumatoid arthritis like disease [103]. The clinical manifestations of these mice were altered by MHC locus mutations analogous to PSOR1 and PSOR2. Immune-receptor tyrosine based activation motif (ITAM) mutations have been identified in the TCR-ζ chain of 2.5% of rheumatoid arthritis patients in an SH2 region that interacts with ZAP-70.

Inflammatory Pathways in Psoriasis

Models of the cytokine pathways in psoriasis have been modified as new information has become available [16, 81, 82]. Originally, models were focused on the prostaglandin and arachidonic acid pathways leading to attempts at fish oil therapy [62, 120]. More recent models have focused on cytokines, as it became clear that cytokines were more likely to mediate acute and chronic inflammation in skin compared to arachidonic acid-derived molecules. As mentioned above, the pathogenesis of psoriasis can be broken down into a number of cellular and cytokine signaling events. In Fig. A2 we present a current working model for the immunopathogenesis of psoriasis. An initial danger signal probably arises from the keratinocytes themselves as portrayed in the current model [82]. The well-known Koebner phenomenon arising from abrasion to the skin has been shown to change the epidermal maturation pathway [72]. The exact mechanism that stimulates the keratinocyte to produce a danger signal is unclear

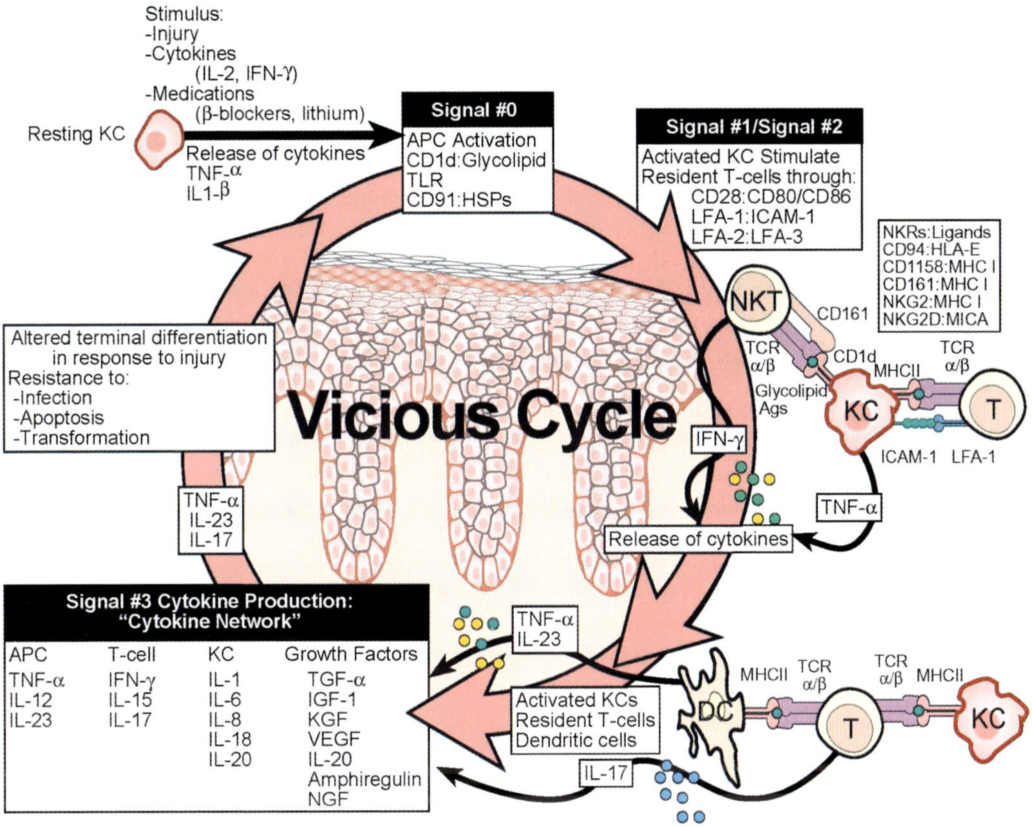

Fig. A2. Working model for immunopathogenesis of psoriasis

[74], but several following events probably lead to the activation of resting APCs [110]. These cells in turn provide signal 1 to resident T cells [14]. This signal must be accompanied by sufficient co-stimulatory signals and trigger release of preformed cytokines or rapid cytokine production of IL-1 and tumor necrosis factor-alpha (TNF-α) [84]. In addition dendritic cells constitutively expressing MHC II (HLA-DR) and can provide stimulation [29]. Even bacterial products from skin flora, normally separated from the immune system by an intact barrier function could serve as a stimuli [13]. A number of superantigens have been shown to be capable of stimulating T cells [70, 86, 112]. Also the release of heat shock proteins (HSPs) from epidermal keratinocytes that could bind to CD91 expressed by dendritic APCs and send a danger signal [17, 33].

Another potential signaling pathway for keratinocytes and dendritic APCs is through exposure to glycolipids that can bind CD1d and stimulate NK T cells [22, 41]. Immune cells can also engage toll-like receptors expressed by dendritic APCs [32]. The production of TNF-α can stimulate a number of cell types, providing targets for therapy [3].

Recently gene array technology has provided profiles of gene expression in psoriatic plaques [26, 93]. Many of the genes up regulated in plaques are inflammatory cytokines providing additional amplification of the inflammatory signals. Among these is high mobility group B1 (HMGB1) that binds to receptor RAGE [93]. HMGB1 can influence TNF-α regulation [127] and has been demonstrated to be important in the regulation of other inflammatory diseases [79]. APCs are likely responsible for the production of cytokines TNF-α [89], IL-12 [56], and IL-23 [4]. IL-23 may be playing a more dominant role in immunocyte recruitment in psoriasis than IL-12. IL-23 and IL-12 share a common subunit, p40, but there is now data that the unique IL-23 subunit p19 is expressed longer and more strongly than that of IL-12 [68]. T cells present in plaques likely produce the increase in expression of IFN-γ [15], IL-15 [101, 118], and IL-17 among other T-cell-derived cytokines [5]. Keratinocytes are the source of IL-1, IL-6, IL-8 [16, 56], IL-18 [94], and IL-20 [18] to name a few.

Chemokines are small molecular weight proteins that play a key role in immunocyte recruitment into the skin. Gene arrays also demonstrate changes in a number of chemokine and chemokine receptors of relevance to psoriasis by combining data obtained from immunostaining and molecular profiling it is possible to document. There are change in levels of expression of a large number of chemokines including: TARC (CCL17), MIG (CXCL9), IP10 (CXCL10), MDC (CCL22), RANTES (CCL5) as recently reviewed in Krueger [63]. Besides these chemokines that are accepted as playing a pathogenic role in psoriasis, additional reports have suggested the importance of other chemokines including: CXCR2 [66], CXCR3, CCR4 [100], CCL27-CCR10 [55], MIP3alpha (CCL20), MIP3beta (CCL19) and CCR6 [54].

Besides cytokines and chemotactic polypeptides, there are a larger number of mitogenic factors present within psoriatic plaques. Elevated growth factors found within psoriatic plaques include transforming growth factor alpha (TGF-α), insulin like growth factor 1 (IGF-1), keratinocyte growth factor (KGF), vascular endothelial growth factor (VEGF), nerve growth factor (NGF), amphiregulin, and IL-20 [63]. As further genomic and pharmacogenomic profiling or psoriatic lesions occurs, it is highly likely that even more cytokines, chemokines and growth factors will be added to these lists.

4 Animal Models of Psoriasis

Psoriasis has a complex inheritance pattern and its development and severity is likely the result of the interaction of several genes and environmental factors. Some support for this comes from the fact that several animal models with single gene mutations have been described, but all fail to have all the relevant features of the human disease [85]. It appears that many transgenic mice contain red and scaly skin or tails, but further microscopic and immunologic analysis demonstrate that these transgenic mice do not contain bona fide psoriatic characteristics. There are several recent reviews of various mouse mutation models that have been proposed for psoriasis [106, 125].

As mentioned earlier, psoriasis was once thought to be a disease of epidermal keratinocytes [38, 64]. Bone marrow transplant literature early on suggested immunocytes might be culpable after some psoriatic patient's disease resolved after autologous transplant [31, 59, 60]. Formal proof for the role of bone marrow-derived immunocytes was provided in the form of a severe combined immunodeficiency (SCID) mouse:human skin chimera model. In this animal model, symptomless (PN) human skin from psoriatic patients is grafted onto SCID mice. After engraftment, the injection of immunocytes taken from psoriatic patients were capable of transforming PN skin into a stable plaque (PP) [19, 43, 87, 97, 124, 126]. The SCID model's demonstration of PN to PP conversion was with CD4 and not CD8+ T cells [87]. This result was supported by other investigators using a different mouse inflammatory model [61]. That CD4+ T cells could cause plaques was an unexpected result as HLA-Cw6 is associated with psoriasis, suggesting a MHC class I pathology [30, 46, 113]. This led to a search for receptors on CD4+ cells that can recognize MHC class I molecules. Such receptors exist on NK cells and a subset of T cells (NK-T cells) and there is evidence to suggest they may play a role in psoriasis [44, 92].

The SCID mouse:human skin chimera model also provides a useful clinical screening tool for therapeutic agents [34] (Tables A1, A2). Nu-

Table A1. Pre-clinical testing using SCID-Hu model

Validation	Agents	Target	Therapeutic response
1. Dam et al. [34]	Vit D3	Immunocytes	+
	CsA	NFAT	+
	IL-10	Th-1 cytokines	–
Therapeutic assessment			
1. Hicke et al. [53]	LD201 1t1 (aptamers)	L-selectin	+ (only SCID)
2. Zeigler et al. [128]	Anti-CD11a Ab	LFA-1/ICAM-1	+
3. Schon et al. [107]	Efomycine M	E and P-selectins	+
4. Zollner et al. [129]	PS-159 (lactacystin)	Proteasome inhibitor	+
5. Boehncke et al. [21]	SEA (F47A/D227A)	Bacterial superantigens	+
6. Villadsen et al. [118]	Anti-IL-15 mAb	IL-15	

Table A2. Use of SCID-Hu for pre-clinical testing of therapeutic agents in psoriasis

Locus	Chromosome	Associated disease
PSOR1	6p21	Asthma
PSOR2	17q25	Eczema
PSOR3	4q	
PSOR4	1q21	Eczema
PSOR5	3q21	Rheumatoid arthritis
PSOR6	19p13	
PSOR7	1p	
PSOR8	Withdrawn	
PSOR9	4q31–34	

merous reports of engrafted psoriatic plaques responding to have been published [20, 21, 53, 107, 118, 128, 129]. This model provides a more complex and realistic environment in which to test these agents than can be generated by tissue culture or transgenic animals alone. Table A1 provides a summary of published studies documenting the utility of this animal model for psoriasis.

Another animal model of psoriasis has been described using AGR129 mice. These mice are deficient in type I and type II interferon receptors and recombinant activating gene 2 (RAG2) [119]. PN skin grafted to these mice develop plaques without exogenous CD4+ T cells. There is local proliferation of T cells with expression of TNF-α. The resident dermal T cells and APCs are sufficient for induction of psoriatic plaques. One theory as to why these plaques develop is that AGR129 mice lack NK cells and possibly can not reject the resident CD4+ T cells or APCs in the grafted skin [48].

The lack of interferon receptors may also allow a specific milieu of cytokines (including IL-7) to flourish that would otherwise be shut down, leading to activation of the resident T cells in the graft. This model also supports the role for TNF-α proposed in the cytokine network model [81]. The AGR129 mouse model also confirms SCID mouse model results where sustained plaques are possible to exist due to ongoing local immune reactions [91]. This model is also the first spontaneous mouse model of an autoimmune disease process, and as such lends itself to testing agents that may prevent rather than treat plaque formation.

Our understanding of the immunopathology of psoriasis is confirmed by the effectiveness of different specific immunotherapeutics. At least three different broad categories of intervention have been successful [25]. First is the prevention of cytokine release. Calcineurin inhibitors such as cyclosporine A, tacrolimus (1996; [99]), sirolimus (rapamycin) [98] and pimecrolimus (ASM981) [95] are effective in reducing the severity of psoriatic disease. A second approach is blocking the effectiveness of cytokines after release. TNF-α inhibitors have been very effective agents. Studies have demonstrated that anti-TNF-α antibodies such as MAb backbone changed infliximab [8] and the humanized adalimunab [104] work well as do solubilized TNF-α receptors such as etanercept [69,75,109]. A third approach has been less successful. Recombinant Th-2 cytokines have been employed to attempt to nullify the Th-1 phenotype of psoriasis. Studies examining IL-10 [9], IL-11 [93,114] and IL-4 [42] were able to demonstrate a moderate effect.

III

5 Conclusion

It is now accepted that psoriasis is an immune-mediated disease. Genetic studies show a strong association with the MHC class I Cw6*0602 allele, although inheritance is complex and likely multifactorial. CD4+ T cells have been shown to be capable of inducing disease in animal models, and newer animal models with AGR129 mice demonstrate that all of the needed cell types for plaque development are present in symptomless psoriatic skin [27]. Finally, many of the cytokines believed to be important in psoriasis have been confirmed in patients by the use of specific immunologic agents. Future studies are required to identify the antigen that incites local immune reactions, the gene(s) that mediate its transmission from one generation to the next, and a better understanding of the interaction between heredity and environment in the immunopathogenesis of psoriasis. As new molecular details are identified, it will be possible to design newer and better therapeutic agents for psoriasis.

■ **Acknowledgements.** The authors would like to thank Ms. Stephanie Hiffman for manuscript preparation. The authors would also like to thank the NIH for partial support of the psoriasis research conducted in Dr. Nickoloff's laboratory (AR 40065).

References

1. Abrams JR, Kelley SL, Hayes E, Kikuchi T, Brown MJ, Kang S, Lebwohl MG, Guzzo CA, Jegasothy BV, Linsley PS, Krueger JG (2000) Blockade of T lymphocyte costimulation with cytotoxic T lymphocyte-associated antigen 4-immunoglobulin (CTLA4Ig) reverses the cellular pathology of psoriatic plaques, including the activation of keratinocytes, dendritic cells, and endothelial cells. J Exp Med 192:681–694
2. Ackermann L, Harvima IT, Pelkonen J, Ritamaki-Salo V, Naukkarinen A, Harvima RJ, Horsmanheimo M (1999) Mast cells in psoriatic skin are strongly positive for interferon-gamma. Br J Dermatol 140:624–633
3. Aggarwal BB (2003) Signalling pathways of the TNF superfamily: a double-edged sword. Nat Rev Immunol 3:745–756
4. Aggarwal S, Ghilardi N, Xie MH, de Sauvage FJ, Gurney AL (2003) Interleukin-23 promotes a distinct CD4T cell activation state characterized by the production of interleukin-17. J Biol Chem 278: 1910–1914
5. Albanesi C, Scarponi C, Cavani A, Federici M, Nasorri F, Girolomoni G (2000) Interleukin-17 is produced by both Th1 and Th2 lymphocytes, and modulates interferon-gamma- and interleukin-4-induced activation of human keratinocytes. J Invest Dermatol 115:81–87
6. Alegre ML, Frauwirth KA, Thompson CB (2001) T-cell regulation by CD28 and CTLA-4. Nat Rev Immunol 1:220–228
7. Anton v.d. M, Davis SJ, Shaw AS, Dustin ML (2000) Cytoskeletal polarization and redistribution of cell-surface molecules during T cell antigen recognition. Semin Immunol 12:5–21
8. Antoni C, Manger B (2002) Infliximab for psoriasis and psoriatic arthritis. Clin Exp Rheumatol 20: S122–S125
9. Asadullah K, Sterry W, Stephanek K, Jasulaitis D, Leupold M, Audring H, Volk HD, Docke WD (1998) IL-10 is a key cytokine in psoriasis. Proof of principle by IL-10 therapy: a new therapeutic approach. J Clin Invest 101:783–794
10. Austin LM, Ozawa M, Kikuchi T, Walters IB, Krueger JG (1999) The majority of epidermal T cells in psoriasis vulgaris lesions can produce type 1 cytokines, interferon-gamma, interleukin-2, and tumor necrosis factor-alpha, defining TC1 (cytotoxic T lymphocyte) and TH1 effector populations: a type 1 differentiation bias is also measured in circulating blood T cells in psoriatic patients. J Invest Dermatol 113:752–759
11. Bagel J, Garland WT, Breneman D, Holick M, Littlejohn TW, Crosby D, Faust H, Fivenson D, Nichols J (1998) Administration of DAB389IL-2 to patients with recalcitrant psoriasis: a double-blind, phase II multicenter trial. J Am Acad Dermatol 38: 938–944

12. Baker BS, Griffiths CE, Lambert S, Powles AV, Leonard JN, Valdimarsson H, Fry L (1987) The effects of cyclosporin A on T lymphocyte and dendritic cell sub-populations in psoriasis. Br J Dermatol 116:503–510
13. Baker BS, Brown DW, Fischetti VA, Ovigne JM, Porter W, Powles A, Fry L (2001) Skin T cell proliferative response to M protein and other cell wall and membrane proteins of group A streptococci in chronic plaque psoriasis. Clin Exp Immunol 124: 516–521
14. Banchereau J, Steinman RM (1998) Dendritic cells and the control of immunity. Nature 392:245–252
15. Barker JN, Karabin GD, Stoof TJ, Sarma VJ, Dixit VM, Nickoloff BJ (1991a) Detection of interferon-gamma mRNA in psoriatic epidermis by polymerase chain reaction. J Dermatol Sci 2:106–111
16. Barker JN, Mitra RS, Griffiths CE, Dixit VM, Nickoloff BJ (1991b) Keratinocytes as initiators of inflammation. Lancet 337:211–214
17. Basu S, Binder RJ, Ramalingam T, Srivastava PK (2001) CD91 is a common receptor for heat shock proteins gp96, hsp90, hsp70, and calreticulin. Immunity 14:303–313
18. Blumberg H, Conklin D, Xu WF, Grossmann A, Brender T, Carollo S, Eagan M, Foster D, Haldeman BA, Hammond A, Haugen H, Jelinek L, Kelly JD, Madden K, Maurer MF, Parrish-Novak J, Prunkard D, Sexson S, Sprecher C, Waggie K, West J, Whitmore TE, Yao L, Kuechle MK, Dale BA, Chandrasekher YA (2001) Interleukin 20: discovery, receptor identification, and role in epidermal function. Cell 104:9–19
19. Boehncke WH, Dressel D, Zollner TM, Kaufmann R (1996) Pulling the trigger on psoriasis. Nature 379:777
20. Boehncke WH, Kock M, Hardt-Weinelt K, Wolter M, Kaufmann R (1999) The SCID-hu xenogeneic transplantation model allows screening of anti-psoriatic drugs. Arch Dermatol Res 291:104–106
21. Boehncke WH, Hardt-Weinelt K, Nilsson H, Wolter M, Dohlsten M, Ochsendorf FR, Kaufmann R, Antonsson P (2001) Antagonistic effects of the staphylococcal enterotoxin a mutant, SEA(F47A/D227A), on psoriasis in the SCID-hu xenogeneic transplantation model. J Invest Dermatol 116: 596–601
22. Bonish B, Jullien D, Dutronc Y, Huang BB, Modlin R, Spada FM, Porcelli SA, Nickoloff BJ (2000) Overexpression of CD1d by keratinocytes in psoriasis and CD1d-dependent IFN-gamma production by NK-T cells. J Immunol 165:4076–4085
23. Borel JF, Gunn HC (1986) Cyclosporine as a new approach to therapy of autoimmune diseases. Ann N Y Acad Sci 475:307–319
24. Bos JD (1988) The pathomechanisms of psoriasis; the skin immune system and cyclosporin. Br J Dermatol 118:141–155
25. Bos WH, Farber EM (1997) Joseph Stalin's psoriasis: its treatment and the consequences. Cutis 59: 197–199
26. Bowcock AM, Shannon W, Du F, Duncan J, Cao K, Aftergut K, Catier J, Fernandez-Vina MA, Menter A (2001) Insights into psoriasis and other inflammatory diseases from large-scale gene expression studies. Hum Mol Genet 10:1793–1805
27. Boyman O, Hefti HP, Conrad C, Nickoloff BJ, Suter M, Nestle FO (2004) Spontaneous development of psoriasis in a new animal model shows an essential role for resident T cells and tumor necrosis factor-{alpha}. J Exp Med 199:731–736
28. Bromley SK, Burack WR, Johnson KG, Somersalo K, Sims TN, Sumen C, Davis MM, Shaw AS, Allen PM, Dustin ML (2001) The immunological synapse. Annu Rev Immunol 19:375–396
29. Brown DW, Baker BS, Ovigne JM, Hardman C, Powles AV, Fry L (2000) Skin CD4+ T cells produce interferon-gamma in vitro in response to streptococcal antigens in chronic plaque psoriasis. J Invest Dermatol 114:576–580
30. Capon F, Munro M, Barker J, Trembath R (2002) Searching for the major histocompatibility complex psoriasis susceptibility gene. J Invest Dermatol 118:745–751
31. Cooley HM, Snowden JA, Grigg AP, Wicks IP (1997) Outcome of rheumatoid arthritis and psoriasis following autologous stem cell transplantation for hematologic malignancy. Arthritis Rheum 40:1712–1715
32. Curry JL, Qin JZ, Bonish B, Carrick R, Bacon P, Panella J, Robinson J, Nickoloff BJ (2003a) Innate immune-related receptors in normal and psoriatic skin. Arch Pathol Lab Med 127:178–186
33. Curry JL, Qin JZ, Robinson J, Nickoloff BJ (2003b) Reactivity of resident immunocytes in normal and prepsoriatic skin using an ex vivo skin-explant model system. Arch Pathol Lab Med 127: 289–296
34. Dam TN, Kang S, Nickoloff BJ, Voorhees JJ (1999) 1alpha,25-dihydroxycholecalciferol and cyclosporine suppress induction and promote resolution of psoriasis in human skin grafts transplanted on to SCID mice. J Invest Dermatol 113:1082–1089
35. Dustin ML, Colman DR (2002) Neural and immunological synaptic relations. Science 298:785–789
36. Dustin ML, Springer TA (1988) Lymphocyte function-associated antigen-1 (LFA-1) interaction with intercellular adhesion molecule-1 (ICAM-1) is one of at least three mechanisms for lymphocyte adhesion to cultured endothelial cells. J Cell Biol 107: 321–331
37. Ellis CN, Krueger GG (2001) Treatment of chronic plaque psoriasis by selective targeting of memory effector T lymphocytes. N Engl J Med 345:248–255
38. Ellis CN, Fradin MS, Messana JM, Brown MD, Siegel MT, Hartley AH, Rocher LL, Wheeler S, Hamilton TA, Parish TG (1991) Cyclosporine for plaque-type psoriasis. Results of a multidose, double-blind trial. N Engl J Med 324:277–284
39. European FK 506 Multicentre Psoriasis Study Group (1996) Systemic tacrolimus (FK 506) is effective for the treatment of psoriasis in a double-

blind, placebo-controlled study. Arch Dermatol 132:419–423
40. Farber EM, Nickoloff BJ, Recht B, Fraki JE (1986) Stress, symmetry, and psoriasis: possible role of neuropeptides. J Am Acad Dermatol 14:305–311
41. Gerlini G, Hefti HP, Kleinhans M, Nickoloff BJ, Burg G, Nestle FO (2001) Cd1d is expressed on dermal dendritic cells and monocyte-derived dendritic cells. J Invest Dermatol 117:576–582
42. Ghoreschi K, Mrowietz U, Rocken M (2003) A molecule solves psoriasis? Systemic therapies for psoriasis inducing interleukin 4 and Th2 responses. J Mol Med 81:471–480
43. Gilhar A, David M, Ullmann Y, Berkutski T, Kalish RS (1997) T-lymphocyte dependence of psoriatic pathology in human psoriatic skin grafted to SCID mice. J Invest Dermatol 109:283–288
44. Gilhar A, Ullmann Y, Kerner H, Assy B, Shalaginov R, Serafimovich S, Kalish RS (2002) Psoriasis is mediated by a cutaneous defect triggered by activated immunocytes: induction of psoriasis by cells with natural killer receptors. J Invest Dermatol 119:384–391
45. Gottlieb AB (1988) Immunologic mechanisms in psoriasis. J Am Acad Dermatol 18:1376–1380
46. Gottlieb SL, Gilleaudeau P, Johnson R, Estes L, Woodworth TG, Gottlieb AB, Krueger JG (1995) Response of psoriasis to a lymphocyte-selective toxin (DAB389IL-2) suggests a primary immune, but not keratinocyte, pathogenic basis. Nat Med 1: 442–447
47. Gottlieb AB, Lebwohl M, Shirin S, Sherr A, Gilleaudeau P, Singer G, Solodkina G, Grossman R, Gisoldi E, Phillips S, Neisler HM, Krueger JG (2000) Anti-CD4 monoclonal antibody treatment of moderate to severe psoriasis vulgaris: results of a pilot, multicenter, multiple-dose, placebo-controlled study. J Am Acad Dermatol 43:595–604
48. Grandjean I, Duban L, Bonney EA, Corcuff E, Di Santo JP, Matzinger P, Lantz O (2003) Are major histocompatibility complex molecules involved in the survival of naive CD4+ T cells? J Exp Med 198: 1089–1102
49. Guilhou JJ, Meynadier J, Clot J (1978) New concepts in the pathogenesis of psoriasis. Br J Dermatol 98:585–592
50. Helms C, Cao L, Krueger JG, Wijsman EM, Chamian F, Gordon D, Heffernan M, Daw JA, Robarge J, Ott J, Kwok PY, Menter A, Bowcock AM (2003) A putative RUNX1 binding site variant between SLC9A3R1 and NAT9 is associated with susceptibility to psoriasis. Nat Genet 35:349–356
51. Heng MC, Kloss SG, Kuehn CS, Chase DG (1985) The sequence of events in psoriatic plaque formation after tape-stripping. Br J Dermatol 112: 517–532
52. Henseler T, Christophers E (1995) Disease concomitance in psoriasis. J Am Acad Dermatol 32: 982–986
53. Hicke BJ, Watson SR, Koenig A, Lynott CK, Bargatze RF, Chang YF, Ringquist S, Moon-McDermott L, Jennings S, Fitzwater T, Han HL, Varki N, Albinana I, Willis MC, Varki A, Parma D (1996) DNA aptamers block L-selectin function in vivo. Inhibition of human lymphocyte trafficking in SCID mice. J Clin Invest 98:2688–2692
54. Homey B, Dieu-Nosjean MC, Wiesenborn A, Massacrier C, Pin JJ, Oldham E, Catron D, Buchanan ME, Muller A, deWaal MR, Deng G, Orozco R, Ruzicka T, Lehmann P, Lebecque S, Caux C, Zlotnik A (2000) Up-regulation of macrophage inflammatory protein-3 alpha/CCL20 and CC chemokine receptor 6 in psoriasis. J Immunol 164:6621–6632
55. Homey B, Alenius H, Muller A, Soto H, Bowman EP, Yuan W, McEvoy L, Lauerma AI, Assmann T, Bunemann E, Lehto M, Wolff H, Yen D, Marxhausen H, To W, Sedgwick J, Ruzicka T, Lehmann P, Zlotnik A (2002) CCL27-CCR10 interactions regulate T cell-mediated skin inflammation. Nat Med 8:157–165
56. Hong K, Chu A, Ludviksson BR, Berg EL, Ehrhardt RO (1999) IL-12, independently of IFN-gamma, plays a crucial role in the pathogenesis of a murine psoriasis-like skin disorder. J Immunol 162: 7480–7491
57. International Psoriasis Genetics Study (2003) Assessing linkage to 14 candidate susceptibility loci in a cohort of 942 affected sib pairs. Am J Hum Genet 73:430–437
58. Jones JL, Berth-Jones J, Fletcher A, Hutchinson PE (1994) Assessment of epidermal dendritic cell markers and T-lymphocytes in psoriasis. J Pathol 174:77–82
59. Jowitt SN, Yin JA (1990) Psoriasis and bone marrow transplantation. BMJ 300:1398–1399
60. Kanamori H, Tanaka M, Kawaguchi H, Yamaji S, Fujimaki K, Tomita N, Fujisawa S, Ishigatsubo Y (2002) Resolution of psoriasis following allogeneic bone marrow transplantation for chronic myelogenous leukemia: case report and review of the literature. Am J Hematol 71:41–44
61. Kess D, Peters T, Zamek J, Wickenhauser C, Tawadros S, Loser K, Varga G, Grabbe S, Nischt R, Sunderkotter C, Muller W, Krieg T, Scharffetter-Kochanek K (2003) CD4+ T cell-associated pathophysiology critically depends on CD18 gene dose effects in a murine model of psoriasis. J Immunol 171:5697–5706
62. Kragballe K, Duell EA, Voorhees JJ (1986) Selective decrease of 15-hydroxyeicosatetraenoic acid (15-HETE) formation in uninvolved psoriatic dermis. Arch Dermatol 122:877–880
63. Krueger JG (2002) The immunologic basis for the treatment of psoriasis with new biologic agents. J Am Acad Dermatol 46:1–23
64. Krueger GG, Bergstresser PR, Lowe NJ, Voorhees JJ, Weinstein GD (1984) Psoriasis. J Am Acad Dermatol 11:937–947
65. Krummel MF, Davis MM (2002) Dynamics of the immunological synapse: finding, establishing and solidifying a connection. Curr Opin Immunol 14: 66–74

66. Kulke R, Bornscheuer E, Schluter C, Bartels J, Rowert J, Sticherling M, Christophers E (1998) The CXC receptor 2 is overexpressed in psoriatic epidermis. J Invest Dermatol 110:90–94
67. Lebwohl M, Tyring SK, Hamilton TK, Toth D, Glazer S, Tawfik NH, Walicke P, Dummer W, Wang X, Garovoy MR, Pariser D (2003) A novel targeted T-cell modulator, efalizumab, for plaque psoriasis. N Engl J Med 349:2004–2013
68. Lee E, Trepicchio WL, Oestreicher JL, Pittman D, Wang F, Chamian F, Dhodapkar M, Krueger JG (2004) Increased expression of interleukin 23 p19 and p40 in lesional skin of patients with psoriasis vulgaris. J Exp Med 199:125–130
69. Leonardi CL, Powers JL, Matheson RT, Goffe BS, Zitnik R, Wang A, Gottlieb AB (2003) Etanercept as monotherapy in patients with psoriasis. N Engl J Med 349:2014–2022
70. Leung DY, Walsh P, Giorno R, Norris DA (1993) A potential role for superantigens in the pathogenesis of psoriasis. J Invest Dermatol 100:225–228
71. Lowe PM, Lee ML, Jackson CJ, To SS, Cooper AJ, Schrieber L (1995) The endothelium in psoriasis. Br J Dermatol 132:497–505
72. Mansbridge JN, Knapp AM (1987) Changes in keratinocyte maturation during wound healing. J Invest Dermatol 89:253–263
73. Martin MP, Nelson G, Lee JH, Pellett F, Gao X, Wade J, Wilson MJ, Trowsdale J, Gladman D, Carrington M (2002) Cutting edge: susceptibility to psoriatic arthritis: influence of activating killer Ig-like receptor genes in the absence of specific HLA-C alleles. J Immunol 169:2818–2822
74. Matzinger P (2002) The danger model: a renewed sense of self. Science 296:301–305
75. Mease PJ, Goffe BS, Metz J, VanderStoep A, Finck B, Burge DJ (2000) Etanercept in the treatment of psoriatic arthritis and psoriasis: a randomised trial. Lancet 356:385–390
76. Mehlis SL, Gordon KB (2003) The immunology of psoriasis and biologic immunotherapy. J Am Acad Dermatol 49:S44–S50
77. Miller GT, Hochman PS, Meier W, Tizard R, Bixler SA, Rosa MD, Wallner BP (1993) Specific interaction of lymphocyte function-associated antigen 3 with CD2 can inhibit T cell responses. J Exp Med 178:211–222
78. Morhenn VB (1988) Keratinocyte proliferation in wound healing and skin diseases. Immunol Today 9:104–107
79. Nathan C (2002) Points of control in inflammation. Nature 420:846–852
80. Nestle FO, Turka LA, Nickoloff BJ (1994) Characterization of dermal dendritic cells in psoriasis. Autostimulation of T lymphocytes and induction of Th1 type cytokines. J Clin Invest 94:202–209
81. Nickoloff BJ (1991) The cytokine network in psoriasis. Arch Dermatol 127:871–884
82. Nickoloff BJ (1999) The immunologic and genetic basis of psoriasis. Arch Dermatol 135:1104–1110
83. Nickoloff BJ (2001) Creation of psoriatic plaques: the ultimate tumor suppressor pathway. A new model for an ancient T-cell-mediated skin disease. Viewpoint. J Cutan Pathol 28:57–64
84. Nickoloff BJ, Naidu Y (1994) Perturbation of epidermal barrier function correlates with initiation of cytokine cascade in human skin. J Am Acad Dermatol 30:535–546
85. Nickoloff BJ, Wrone-Smith T (1997) Animal models of psoriasis. Nat Med 3:475–476
86. Nickoloff BJ, Wrone-Smith T (1998) Superantigens, autoantigens, and pathogenic T cells in psoriasis. J Invest Dermatol 110:459–460
87. Nickoloff BJ, Wrone-Smith T (1999) Injection of pre-psoriatic skin with CD4+ T cells induces psoriasis. Am J Pathol 155:145–158
88. Nickoloff BJ, Lewinsohn DM, Butcher EC, Krensky AM, Clayberger C (1988) Recombinant gamma interferon increases the binding of peripheral blood mononuclear leukocytes and a Leu-3+ T lymphocyte clone to cultured keratinocytes and to a malignant cutaneous squamous carcinoma cell line that is blocked by antibody against the LFA-1 molecule. J Invest Dermatol 90:17–22
89. Nickoloff BJ, Karabin GD, Barker JN, Griffiths CE, Sarma V, Mitra RS, Elder JT, Kunkel SL, Dixit VM (1991) Cellular localization of interleukin-8 and its inducer, tumor necrosis factor-alpha in psoriasis. Am J Pathol 138:129–140
90. Nickoloff BJ, Mitra RS, Green J, Shimizu Y, Thompson C, Turka LA (1993) Activated keratinocytes present bacterial-derived superantigens to T lymphocytes: relevance to psoriasis. J Dermatol Sci 6:127–133
91. Nickoloff BJ, Kunkel SL, Burdick M, Strieter RM (1995) Severe combined immunodeficiency mouse and human psoriatic skin chimeras. Validation of a new animal model. Am J Pathol 146:580–588
92. Nickoloff BJ, Bonish B, Huang BB, Porcelli SA (2000) Characterization of a T cell line bearing natural killer receptors and capable of creating psoriasis in a SCID mouse model system. J Dermatol Sci 24:212–225
93. Oestreicher JL, Walters IB, Kikuchi T, Gilleaudeau P, Surette J, Schwertschlag U, Dorner AJ, Krueger JG, Trepicchio WL (2001) Molecular classification of psoriasis disease-associated genes through pharmacogenomic expression profiling. Pharmacogenomics J 1:272–287
94. Ohta Y, Hamada Y, Katsuoka K (2001) Expression of IL-18 in psoriasis. Arch Dermatol Res 293:334–342
95. Rappersberger K, Komar M, Ebelin ME, Scott G, Burtin P, Greig G, Kehren J, Chibout SD, Cordier A, Holter W, Richter L, Oberbauer R, Stuetz A, Wolff K (2002) Pimecrolimus identifies a common genomic anti-inflammatory profile, is clinically highly effective in psoriasis and is well tolerated. J Invest Dermatol 119:876–887

96. Raychaudhuri SP, Rein G, Farber EM (1995) Neuropathogenesis and neuropharmacology of psoriasis. Int J Dermatol 34:85–693
97. Raychaudhuri SP, Dutt S, Raychaudhuri SK, Sanyal M, Farber EM (2001) Severe combined immunodeficiency mouse-human skin chimeras: a unique animal model for the study of psoriasis and cutaneous inflammation. Br J Dermatol 144:931–939
98. Reitamo S, Spuls P, Sassolas B, Lahfa M, Claudy A, Griffiths CE (2001) Efficacy of sirolimus (rapamycin) administered concomitantly with a subtherapeutic dose of cyclosporin in the treatment of severe psoriasis: a randomized controlled trial. Br J Dermatol 145:438–445
99. Reynolds NJ, Al Daraji WI (2002) Calcineurin inhibitors and sirolimus: mechanisms of action and applications in dermatology. Clin Exp Dermatol 27:555–561
100. Rottman JB, Smith TL, Ganley KG, Kikuchi T, Krueger JG (2001) Potential role of the chemokine receptors CXCR3, CCR4, and the integrin alphaEbeta7 in the pathogenesis of psoriasis vulgaris. Lab Invest 81:335–347
101. Ruckert R, Asadullah K, Seifert M, Budagian VM, Arnold R, Trombotto C, Paus R, Bulfone-Paus S (2000) Inhibition of keratinocyte apoptosis by IL-15: a new parameter in the pathogenesis of psoriasis? J Immunol 165:2240–2250
102. Saiag P, Coulomb B, Lebreton C, Bell E, Dubertret L (1985) Psoriatic fibroblasts induce hyperproliferation of normal keratinocytes in a skin equivalent model in vitro. Science 230:669–672
103. Sakaguchi N, Takahashi T, Hata H, Nomura T, Tagami T, Yamazaki S, Sakihama T, Matsutani T, Negishi I, Nakatsuru S, Sakaguchi S (2003) Altered thymic T-cell selection due to a mutation of the ZAP-70 gene causes autoimmune arthritis in mice. Nature 426:454–460
104. Scheinfeld N (2003) Adalimumab (HUMIRA): a review. J Drugs Dermatol 2:375–377
105. Schlaak JF, Buslau M, Jochum W, Hermann E, Girndt M, Gallati H, Meyer zum Buschenfelde KH, Fleischer B (1994) T cells involved in psoriasis vulgaris belong to the Th1 subset. J Invest Dermatol 102:145–149
106. Schon MP (1999) Animal models of psoriasis – what can we learn from them? J Invest Dermatol 112:405–410
107. Schon MP, Krahn T, Schon M, Rodriguez ML, Antonicek H, Schultz JE, Ludwig RJ, Zollner TM, Bischoff E, Bremm KD, Schramm M, Henninger K, Kaufmann R, Gollnick HP, Parker CM, Boehncke WH (2002) Efomycine M, a new specific inhibitor of selectin, impairs leukocyte adhesion and alleviates cutaneous inflammation. Nat Med 8:366–372
108. Sigmundsdottir H, Sigurgeirsson B, Troye-Blomberg M, Good MF, Valdimarsson H, Jonsdottir I (1997) Circulating T cells of patients with active psoriasis respond to streptococcal M-peptides sharing sequences with human epidermal keratins. Scand J Immunol 45:688–697
109. Smith CA, Davis T, Wignall JM, Din WS, Farrah T, Upton C, McFadden G, Goodwin RG (1991) T2 open reading frame from the Shope fibroma virus encodes a soluble form of the TNF receptor. Biochem Biophys Res Commun 176:335–342
110. Soumelis V, Reche PA, Kanzler H, Yuan W, Edward G, Homey B, Gilliet M, Ho S, Antonenko S, Lauerma A, Smith K, Gorman D, Zurawski S, Abrams J, Menon S, McClanahan T, Waal-Malefyt RR, Bazan F, Kastelein RA, Liu YJ (2002) Human epithelial cells trigger dendritic cell mediated allergic inflammation by producing TSLP. Nat Immunol 3:673–680
111. Szabo SK, Hammerberg C, Yoshida Y, Bata-Csorgo Z, Cooper KD (1998) Identification and quantitation of interferon-gamma producing T cells in psoriatic lesions: localization to both CD4+ and CD8+ subsets. J Invest Dermatol 111:1072–1078
112. Travers JB, Hamid QA, Norris DA, Kuhn C, Giorno RC, Schlievert PM, Farmer ER, Leung DY (1999) Epidermal HLA-DR and the enhancement of cutaneous reactivity to superantigenic toxins in psoriasis. J Clin Invest 104:1181–1189
113. Trembath RC, Clough RL, Rosbotham JL, Jones AB, Camp RD, Frodsham A, Browne J, Barber R, Terwilliger J, Lathrop GM, Barker JN (1997) Identification of a major susceptibility locus on chromosome 6p and evidence for further disease loci revealed by a two stage genome-wide search in psoriasis. Hum Mol Genet 6:813–820
114. Trepicchio WL, Ozawa M, Walters IB, Kikuchi T, Gilleaudeau P, Bliss JL, Schwertschlag U, Dorner AJ, Krueger JG (1999) Interleukin-11 therapy selectively downregulates type I cytokine proinflammatory pathways in psoriasis lesions. J Clin Invest 104:1527–1537
115. Uyemura K, Yamamura M, Fivenson DF, Modlin RL, Nickoloff BJ (1993) The cytokine network in lesional and lesion-free psoriatic skin is characterized by a T-helper type 1 cell-mediated response. J Invest Dermatol 101:701–705
116. Valdimarsson H, Baker BS, Jonsdottir I, Powles A, Fry L (1995) Psoriasis: a T-cell-mediated autoimmune disease induced by streptococcal superantigens? Immunol Today 16:145–149
117. Van De Kerkhof PC (2000) Neutrophils in psoriasis: cause or effect? Clin Exp Dermatol 25:165
118. Villadsen LS, Schuurman J, Beurskens F, Dam TN, Dagnaes-Hansen F, Skov L, Rygaard J, Voorhorst-Ogink MM, Gerritsen AF, van Dijk MA, Parren PW, Baadsgaard O, van de Winkel JG (2003) Resolution of psoriasis upon blockade of IL-15 biological activity in a xenograft mouse model. J Clin Invest 112:1571–1580
119. Vollstedt S, Franchini M, Alber G, Ackermann M, Suter M (2001) Interleukin-12- and gamma interferon-dependent innate immunity are essential and sufficient for long-term survival of passively immunized mice infected with herpes simplex virus type 1. J Virol 75:9596–9600

120. Voorhees JJ (1977) Pathophysiology of psoriasis. Annu Rev Med 28:467–473
121. Weinshenker BG, Bass BH, Ebers GC, Rice GP (1989) Remission of psoriatic lesions with muromonab-CD3 (orthoclone OKT3) treatment. J Am Acad Dermatol 20:1132–1133
122. Weitz-Schmidt G, Welzenbach K, Brinkmann V, Kamata T, Kallen J, Bruns C, Cottens S, Takada Y, Hommel U (2001) Statins selectively inhibit leukocyte function antigen-1 by binding to a novel regulatory integrin site. Nat Med 7:687–692
123. Werlen G, Hausmann B, Naeher D, Palmer E (2003) Signaling life and death in the thymus: timing is everything. Science 299:1859–1863
124. Wrone-Smith T, Nickoloff BJ (1996) Dermal injection of immunocytes induces psoriasis. J Clin Invest 98:1878–1887
125. Xia YP, Li B, Hylton D, Detmar M, Yancopoulos GD, Rudge JS (2003) Transgenic delivery of VEGF to mouse skin leads to an inflammatory condition resembling human psoriasis. Blood 102:161–168
126. Yamamoto T, Matsuuchi M, Katayama I, Nishioka K (1998) Repeated subcutaneous injection of staphylococcal enterotoxin B-stimulated lymphocytes retains epidermal thickness of psoriatic skin-graft onto severe combined immunodeficient mice. J Dermatol Sci 17:8–14
127. Yang H, Wang H, Tracey KJ (2001) HMG-1 rediscovered as a cytokine. Shock 15:247–253
128. Zeigler M, Chi Y, Tumas DB, Bodary S, Tang H, Varani J (2001) Anti-CD11a ameliorates disease in the human psoriatic skin-SCID mouse transplant model: comparison of antibody to CD11a with cyclosporin A and clobetasol propionate. Lab Invest 81:1253–1261
129. Zollner TM, Podda M, Pien C, Elliott PJ, Kaufmann R, Boehncke WH (2002) Proteasome inhibition reduces superantigen-mediated T cell activation and the severity of psoriasis in a SCID-hu model. J Clin Invest 109:671–679

III

B Psoriatic Arthritis

Jennifer Barton,
Christopher T. Ritchlin

Contents

1 Introduction

Psoriatic arthritis is an inflammatory arthritis that can be distinguished from rheumatoid arthritis by unique clinical manifestations, characteristic radiographic findings and the absence of rheumatoid factor [1]. Patients often present with focal inflammation at multiple sites involving the skin, joints, and tendon insertion sites or entheses. Potentially revealing clues to the pathogenesis of PsA are provided by several observations, which include the strong family history of psoriasis in many psoriatic arthritis patients, the association of skin and joint disease with class I major histocompatability alleles, the equal frequency in men and women, and reports that skin and joint inflammation can be triggered or worsened by a variety of environmental factors. Taken together, these elements are compatible with a polygenetic disorder that is modulated by external stimuli. Unfortunately, until recently, the disease mechanisms underlying joint inflammation in the psoriatic joint were largely unknown. Recent advances in immunology, molecular biology and imaging techniques, however, have provided a new understanding of key events fostering inflammation in psoriatic skin and joints. Moreover, the arrival of targeted biological therapies has greatly improved treatment responses and provided novel opportunities for understanding the contribution of specific effector cell populations to ongoing inflammation and defining the role of both pro- and anti-inflammatory cytokines in vivo [2].

2 Immunopathology

Mounting evidence supports the concept that distinct disease mechanisms underlie susceptibility and progression of psoriatic as compared to rheumatoid arthritis. Yet several barriers are encountered when examining pathogenic events in psoriatic arthritis. These include the relative paucity of animal models, heterogeneous disease subsets, and the possibility that factors related to the underlying psoriasis may mask or confound those related to arthritis. Nevertheless, seminal pathophysiologic insights have resulted from careful study of four principle anatomic sites of disease involvement- the psoriatic plaque, the synovial membrane, the enthesis, and the cartilaginous and bony structures in the psoriatic joint.

Psoriatic Plaque

As discussed in Chap. IIIA, psoriasis was traditionally viewed as a hyperproliferative disorder, and research efforts focused on the keratinocyte, a cell considered paramount in the pathobiology of plaque formation [3]. The emphasis has gradually shifted, however, in part, based on compelling evidence from the SCID mouse:human skin chimera model demonstrating that T lymphocytes are critical effector cells necessary and sufficient for induction of psoriasis [4]. Additional evidence favoring the importance of the T lymphocyte in psoriasis arose from reports that showed specific anti T-cell therapies (cyclosporine, 6-thioguanine and the diptheria-IL-2 fusion toxin) were quite effective in psoriasis [5–7]. The consistent reduction in psoriatic lesions with targeted therapies directed at the T cell costimulatory molecules LFA-1 and CD28/CD80/CD86 further underscores the importance of T lymphocytes in psoriasis [8, 9].

Synovial Membrane

The cellular and molecular interactions taking place in the psoriatic synovial membrane are remarkably similar to the events promoting inflammation in the plaque. For example, in both skin and joints, infiltrating T lymphocytes enter deeper layers (dermis, subsynovium) and promote hyperproliferation of cells native to the particular tissue – keratinocytes in the skin and synovial lining cells in the joint. The fact that psoriatic arthritis can affect two different tissues within the same individual raises the possibility that memory T cells could potentially migrate to both sites via a tissue-specific homing mechanism. Studies addressing this question, however, demonstrated that memory T lymphocytes preferentially migrate to the skin but not the joints in psoriatic arthritis patients [10]. Interestingly, studies performed on T cells isolated from the skin and joints of psoriatic arthritis patients revealed limited expansion of T cell receptor (TCR) Vβ gene repertoire at both sites, suggesting the presence of an antigen-driven response [11, 12].

The strong association of psoriatic arthritis with major histocompatibility complex (MHC) Class I molecules suggests that CD8 T lymphocytes or NK cells may be pivotal in pathogenesis [13]. Immunohistologic studies on psoriatic synovial membranes, however, revealed a predominance of CD45RO+ memory T cells in the synovial lining mononuclear cell infiltrate

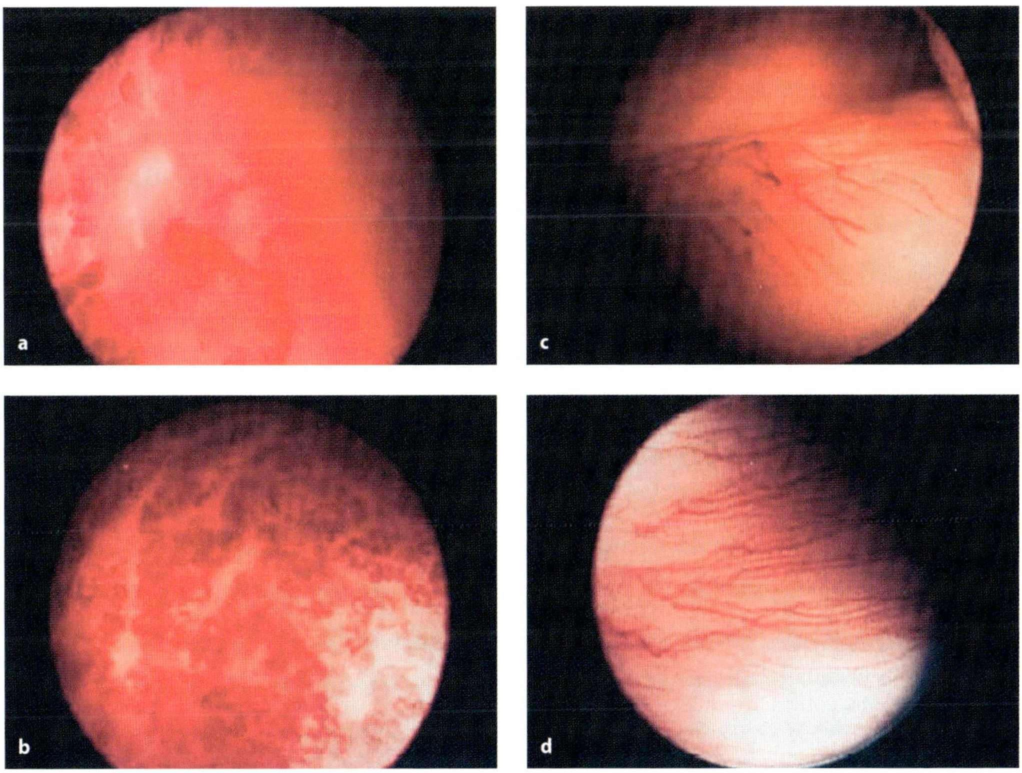

Fig. B1. Arthroscopic view of knees from patients with psoriatic **(a,b)** and rheumatoid **(c,d)** arthritis. Blood vessels in psoriatic tissues demonstrated highly tortuous appearance compared to the straight branching vessels in rheumatoid synovium. Adapted from [21] with permission

[14–16]. In contrast, the principal lymphocytes in synovial fluid are CD8 T cells, some of which demonstrate oligoclonal expansion of TCR B chains, a pattern characteristic of an antigen-driven response [17, 18].

A central question is whether there are characteristic histopathological features that can reliably distinguish psoriatic from rheumatoid synovial membranes. In one study, the degree of lymphocytic infiltration was similar in both groups, but psoriatic synovial tissues demonstrated significantly more vascularity and less synovial lining layer hyperplasia and monocyte/macrophage infiltration than rheumatoid specimens [16]. Expression of intercellular adhesion molecule (ICAM)-1 and vascular cell adhesion molecule (VCAM)-1 were similar in the two disorders but expression of endothelial leukocyte adhesion molecule (ELAM)-1 was reduced in psoriatic synovial tissues.

The increased vascularity characteristic of psoriatic synovium has been noted by many investigators [19, 20]. A particularly striking feature is the marked tortuosity and dilatation of blood vessels noted in psoriatic but not rheumatoid joints, when viewed through an arthroscope (Fig. B1) [21]. Similar changes have been observed in psoriatic skin [22]. Histopathologically, vessels were characterized by endothelial cell swelling accompanied by inflammatory cell infiltration and marked thickening of the vessel wall [20]. Fibrosis of the subsynovial tissue was also noted, especially in patients with chronic disease. Levels of the angiogenic factors vascular endothelial growth factor (VEGF) and angiopontin (ang)-2 were upregulated in psoriatic compared to rheumatoid synovium and treatment with methotrexate reduced tissue vascularity and VEGF levels [23].

Synovial explant tissues from psoriatic joints produce higher levels of the helper-T-lymphocyte (Th1) cytokines interleukin (IL)-2 and interferon-γ protein than explants similarly cultured from osteoarthritis and rheumatoid patients [24]. In contrast, while IL-4 and IL-5 were not identified in psoriatic explants, IL-10 was highly expressed in synovium but not skin from individual patients. This Th1 profile has been observed in both psoriasis and rheumatoid arthritis [25, 26]. Elevated levels of the cytokines IL-1β and tumor necrosis factor (TNF)-α were also released by psoriatic synovial explants. A similar pattern of cytokine production in psoriatic synovium was shown using immunohistochemical techniques [27]. Notably, staining for TNF was most striking in the synovial lining layer, with lower levels of expression noted in the subsynovium.

TNF-α is a multifunctional cytokine that promotes joint inflammation by multiple mechanisms [28]. Released predominantly by cells of the monocyte/macrophage lineage, TNF-α induces lymphocyte and neutrophil migration into the synovium, promotes release of matrix-degrading metalloproteinases, enhances the secretion of other pro-inflammatory cytokines (IL-1, IL-6, IL-8) and potentiates osteoclastic bone resorption [29]. TNF-α binds to two distinct but structurally similar receptors, p55 and p75. These receptors, located on the surface of many cells, can be cleaved to circulate as soluble molecules capable of attenuating the pro-inflammatory actions of TNF-α [30–33].

TNF levels are elevated in psoriatic skin as well as the synovium of patients with psoriatic arthritis [24]. Several lines of evidence support the concept that TNF-α is an important cytokine in the psoriatic joint. TNF-α transgenic mice exhibit extensive bone destruction similar to that observed in some PsA patients [34, 35]. As mentioned earlier, immunohistochemical studies demonstrated marked upregulation of TNF-α in the psoriatic synovial membrane [27]. Furthermore, histopathologic analysis of synovial specimens from spondyloarthropathy patients (four of eight with PsA) treated with the anti-TNF monoclonal antibody, infliximab, revealed decreased vascularity, synovial lining thickness, and mononuclear cell infiltration following therapy [36].

Enthesis

Unusual in rheumatoid arthritis, enthesopathy or inflammation at tendon or ligamentous insertion sites is a hallmark feature of psoriatic arthritis [37]. The most common enthesopathic clinical syndromes in psoriatic arthritis include plantar fasciitis, epicondylitis, and Achilles ten-

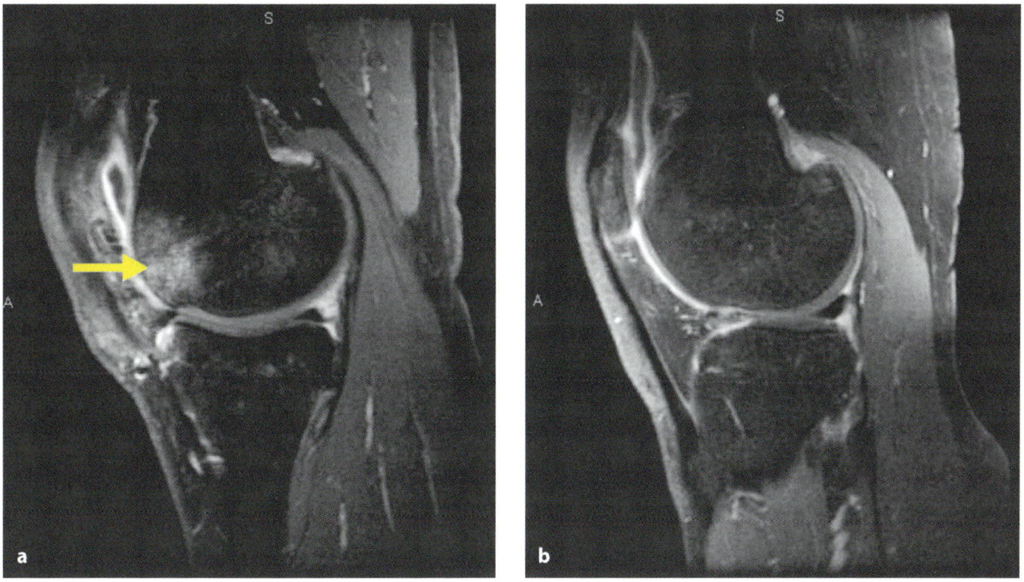

Fig. B2. Post-gadolinium T2-weighted fat suppressed MRI images of the knee in a patient with psoriatic arthritis before (**a**) and 12 months after starting etanercept (**b**). Note the bone marrow edema (*arrow*) in the femur that has almost completely resolved following treatment with a TNF-blocking agent

donitis. Most entheses are fibrocartilaginous insertions composed of type II collagen and aggrecan. They are highly vascular and richly innervated structures that absorb and dissipate mechanical stress [38]. Although the pathogenesis of enthesopathy is not well understood, fat-suppressed MRI studies reveal bone marrow edema adjacent to entheseal insertion sites [39] and biopsies show infiltration with CD-8 cells and macrophages in the underlying subchondral bone [40]. Of particular interest, treatment of spondyloarthritis patients (including PsA) with the anti-TNF agent etanercept reversed abnormal MRI signals in both the axial and peripheral skeleton adjacent to insertion sites, which suggests an important role for TNF-α in enthesitis [41]. Figure B2 shows resolution of bone marrow edema in a psoriatic joint following anti-TNF therapy.

Cartilage and Bone

Radiographs of psoriatic joints often reveal cartilage loss manifested as joint space narrowing. Markedly altered bone remodeling appears in the form of tuft resorption, large eccentric erosions, and pencil-in-cup deformities. In addition, there are often features of new bone formation, such as periostitis and bony ankylosis [48]. As in rheumatoid arthritis, matrix metalloproteinases (MMPs) and tissue inhibitors of MMPs (TIMPs) have been identified in the lining and sublining layers of psoriatic synovial membranes [42, 43]. In particular, immunohistochemical studies revealed that MMP-9 localized to blood vessel walls, while MMP-1, MMP-2, MMP-3, and both TIMPs-1 and 2 showed a cellular and interstitial staining pattern in the synovial lining. MMP-3 serum levels exhibited a marked, rapid decrease after successful anti-TNF therapy, which raises the possibility that MMP-3 may serve as a biomarker. Thus, the inflamed psoriatic joint contains proteases capable of degrading collagen and other core matrix molecules comprising cartilage.

With respect to bone, psoriatic joint biopsies demonstrate large multinucleated osteoclasts in deep resorption pits at the bone-pannus junction [44]. Osteoclastogenesis (differentiation of osteoclasts) is a contact-dependent pro-

III

cess directed by osteoblasts and stromal cells in the bone marrow [45]. These cells release two different signals necessary for differentiation of an osteoclast precursor (OCP) derived from the CD14+ monocyte population into an osteoclast. The first, macrophage-colony stimulating factor (M-CSF), triggers cellular proliferation and the second, receptor activator of NFκB ligand (RANKL), a member of the TNF superfamily, binds to RANK on the surface of OCP and osteoclasts promoting differentiation and cellular activation [46]. Since permissive quantities of M-CSF are constitutively expressed in the bone microenvironment, it has been proposed that the relative expression of RANKL and its natural antagonist osteoprotegerin (OPG) ultimately control osteoclastogenesis [47]. Interestingly, RANKL is also expressed by infiltrating T cells and synovial fibroblastoid cells in the synovial lining of inflamed joints [48].

In psoriatic synovial tissues, marked upregulation of RANKL protein and low expression of OPG was detected in the synovial lining. Osteoclasts were also noted in cutting cones traversing the subchondral bone, which indicates a bidirectional attack on the bone in psoriatic joints (Fig. B3). In addition, osteoclast precursors, derived from circulating CD14+ monocytes, were markedly elevated in the peripheral blood of PsA patients compared to healthy controls [44]. Treatment of PsA patients with anti-TNF agents significantly decreased the numbers of circulating osteoclast precursors, thus supporting a central role for TNF-α in the generation of this precursor population. The mechanisms responsible for new bone formation in the psoriatic joint are poorly understood. Bone morphogenic proteins (BMPs) and VEGF may be pivotal in this process, given that TGF-β, a member of this family, is strongly expressed in synovial tissues isolated from ankylosing spon-

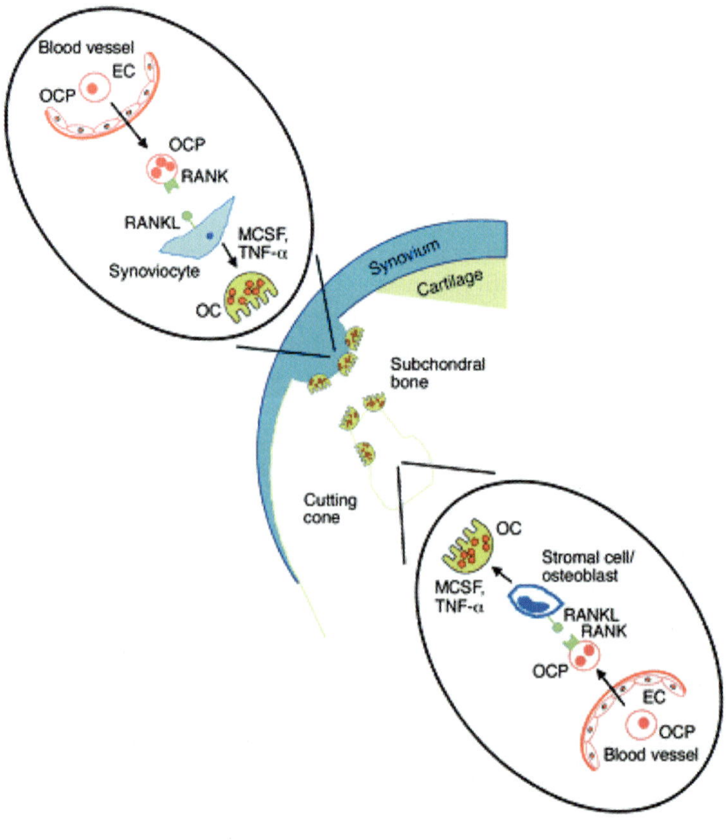

Fig. B3. Schematic model of osteolysis in the psoriatic joint. Extensive erosions observed in the PsA joint are mediated by a bidirectional attack on bone. In this model, circulating osteoclast precursors enter the synovium and are induced to become osteoclasts via RANKL expressed by synoviocytes (outside-in). In parallel, osteoclast precursors traverse endothelial cells in the subchondral bone and undergo osteoclastogenesis following RANKL stimulation from osteoblasts and stromal cells (inside-out). From [44], with permission dylitis patients, where new bone formation is a central component of the disease [49], and BMP-4 synergizes with VEGF to induce bone formation in animal models [50].

Environmental Factors

Compelling evidence suggests that trauma and infection play a prominent role in the etiologic pathway of PsA. The Koebner phenomenon, described as psoriatic lesions arising at sites of trauma, occurs in 24–52% of psoriasis patients [51, 52]. In joint disease, the development of PsA following trauma has been reported in the Toronto longitudinal observational cohort, where 50 of 203 (24.6%) patients reported a traumatic event prior to the diagnosis of PsA [53].

Some studies suggest involvement of bacterial agents in psoriasis and PsA. A strikingly high association between guttate psoriasis and preceding streptococcal pharyngitis and tonsillitis exists in children [54]. The link between gram-positive infection and PsA was suggested by high levels of circulating antibodies to microbial peptidoglycans and elevated levels of group A streptococcus 16 S RNA in the peripheral blood of PsA [55, 56]. These results promoted the concept that infection may trigger psoriasis. While the clinical data are intriguing, the finding that up to 30% of PsA synovial tissue-derived T cells proliferate following exposure to group A streptococci supports a superantigen mechanism of cell activation [57]. Both streptococcal and staphylococcal superantigens promote inflammation and upregulation of keratinocyte TNF in non-involved psoriatic skin, but not in other inflammatory dermatoses, pointing to the potential importance of this novel immune pathway in psoriasis [58].

Human Immunodeficiency Virus (HIV) infection has been associated with unusually severe forms of psoriasis and psoriatic arthritis [59]. Early studies in the United States noted a temporal proximity of psoriatic arthritis and psoriasis to the development of Acquired Immunodeficiency Syndrome (AIDS). The rapid progression of skin and joint disease in patients with progressive loss of CD4+ cells favored a role for CD8+ cytotoxic lymphocytes in the psoriatic pathology [60]. A dramatic increase in psoriatic arthritis has been reported among HIV infected patients in sub-Saharan Africa [61]. In Zambia, psoriatic arthritis is typically polyarticular, progressive, and more common in the lower limbs [62]. Unlike earlier reports, joint disease in these patients improved with the onset of AIDS. Thus, the mechanisms that foster skin and joint inflammation in HIV-infected patients remain an enigma. It is conceivable, however, that the HIV virus or a concomitant infection could trigger psoriatic plaque formation or synovitis in genetically susceptible individuals.

3 Animal Models

The absence of a reliable animal model has hindered research in psoriatic arthritis. Recently, however, it was reported that transgenic mice lacking endogenous MHC Class II molecules spontaneously developed extensive resorption of distal phalangeal bones, along with hyperkeratosis, parakeratosis, pitting, and frequent loss of nails (Fig. B4) [63]. These mice did not manifest arthritis in other peripheral joints or in the axial skeleton. Moreover, the skin findings were localized to the affected toes. Of note, joint involvement has not been described in any of the psoriasis rodent models [64–66].

Two other models that spontaneously develop arthritis have been described in rodents transgenic for HLA-B27 Class I molecules. The HLA-B27/β_2 rat developed gut lesions, peripheral arthritis, psoriasiform skin lesions, alopecia, and nail lesions; however, no thickening or shortening of the distal joints was reported. When these transgenic rats were raised in a germ-free environment, they developed characteristic skin lesions but no gut or joint inflammation. Likewise, paw swelling, joint ankyloses, nail changes, and hair loss developed in transgenic mice lacking β_2 microglobulin [67]. In these mice, the disease frequency was highly influenced by non-MHC background genes. While these models do not fully mimic the phenotype observed in humans with psoriatic arthritis, they suggest that alteration of MHC expression combined with microbial interactions

III

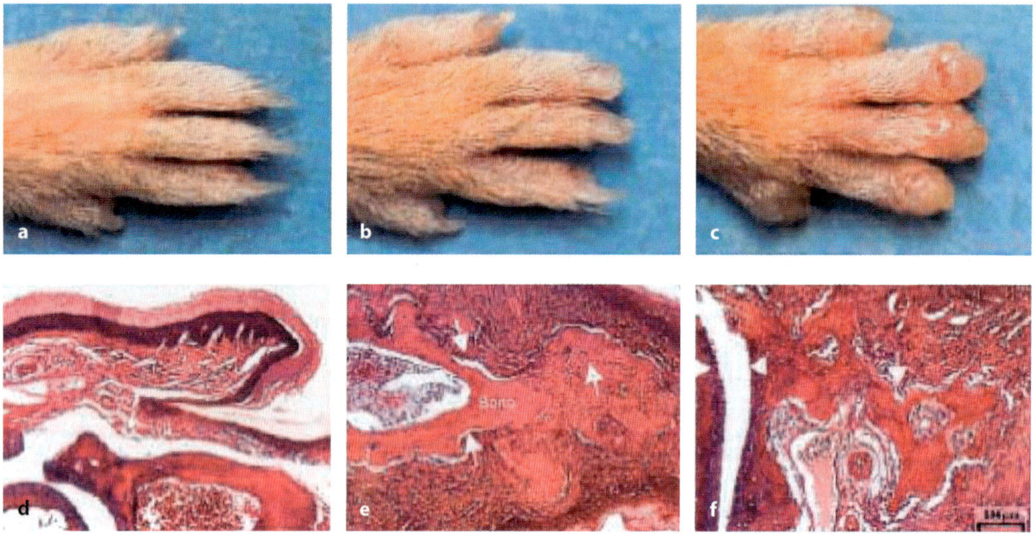

Fig. B4a–f. Gross appearance of toes and corresponding histopathologic findings in spontaneous psoriatic-arthritis toe disease in HLA-DR4.Ab° transgenic mice. These mice have deficient endogenous class II MHC expression. Disease progression in a single paw at 6 - months (**a**), 8 months (**b**) and 12 months (**c**). The earliest changes are elevation and thickening of the nails followed by dactylitis. The digit acquires a drumstick-like appearance. Histopathologic changes at 6 months (**d**), 8 months (**e**) and 12 months (**f**). The *arrows* point to sites of bone resorption that are replaced by an osteofibrotic granulomatous tissue. Adapted from [63] with permission

may play a critical role in the pathogenesis of skin and joint disease.

Spondyloarthropathies have been identified in a variety of primate and non-primate species. In baboons, radiographic studies revealed that the prevalence of spondyloarthritis reaches 30% [68]. The distribution of erosive disease and axial joint involvement in Old World primates is quite characteristic of that noted in human psoriatic arthritis [69]. Thus, these primates may be a more appropriate animal model for deciphering mechanisms of disease in psoriatic arthritis.

4 Conclusion

Collectively, the evidence suggests that trauma or infection in a genetically susceptible individual triggers psoriatic arthritis and that the initial inciting event probably occurs in the skin, which triggers activation of T lymphocytes. In some patients with psoriasis, local events in the joint promote angiogenesis followed by influx of T lymphocytes, increased expression of TNF-α and IL-1β, and an elevated ratio of RANKL to OPG. Circulating osteoclast precursors enter the joint after binding to activated endothelial cells and undergo osteoclastogenesis and resorb bone. The events responsible for new bone formation remain unknown although studies in animal models suggest that TGF-β and VEGF may be important in this process. In addition, metalloproteinases released by synovial lining cells degrade cartilage and foster blood vessel remodeling. Presumably, perpetual release of pro-inflammatory cytokines, particularly TNF, leads to persistent synovitis, enthesitis, and progressive matrix degradation. The events that drive the chronic release of these pro-inflammatory cytokines have not been elucidated.

References

1. Gladman DD (2002) Current concepts in psoriatic arthritis. Curr Opin Rheumatol 14:361–366
2. Mease PJ (2003) Current treatment of psoriatic arthritis. Rheum Dis Clin N Am 29:495–511
3. Krueger GG, et al. (1984) Psoriasis. J Am Acad Dermatol 11:937–947
4. Wrone-Smith T, Nickoloff BJ (1996) Dermal injection of immunocytes induces psoriasis [comment]. J Clin Invest 98:1878–1887
5. Ellis CN, et al. (1991) Cyclosporine for plaque-type psoriasis. Results of a multidose, double-blind trial [see comment]. N Engl J Med 324:277–284
6. Murphy FP, et al. (1999) Clinical clearing of psoriasis by 6-thioguanine correlates with cutaneous T-cell depletion via apoptosis: evidence for selective effects on activated T lymphocytes. Arch Dermatol 135:1495–1502
7. Gottlieb SL, et al. (1995) Response of psoriasis to a lymphocyte-selective toxin (DAB389IL-2) suggests a primary immune, but not keratinocyte, pathogenic basis. Nature Med 1:442–447
8. Lebwohl M, et al. (2003) An international, randomized, double-blind, placebo-controlled phase 3 trial of intramuscular alefacept in patients with chronic plaque psoriasis [see comment]. Arch Dermatol 139:719–727
9. Abrams JR, et al. (1999) CTLA4Ig-mediated blockade of T-cell costimulation in patients with psoriasis vulgaris. J Clin Invest 103:1243–1252
10. Pitzalis C, et al. (1996) Cutaneous lymphocyte antigen-positive T lymphocytes preferentially migrate to the skin but not to the joint in psoriatic arthritis. Arthritis Rheum 39:137–145
11. Tassiulas I, et al. (1999) Clonal characteristics of T cell infiltrates in skin and synovium of patients with psoriatic arthritis. Hum Immunol 60:479–491
12. Borgato L, et al. (2002) The T cell receptor repertoire in psoriatic synovitis is restricted and T lymphocytes expressing the same TCR are present in joint and skin lesions. J Rheumatol 29:1914–1919
13. Winchester R (2003) Psoriatic arthritis, dermatology in general medicine. In: Freedberg IM, Eisen AZ, Wolff K, Austen KF, Goldsmith LA, Katz SI (eds) McGraw-Hill, New York, pp 428–429
14. Fyrand O (1979) Immunological studies on synovial joint membranes in psoriatic arthritis. Acta Derm Venereol Suppl 87:15–20
15. Smith MD, et al. (1992) Immunohistochemical analysis of synovial membranes from inflammatory and non-inflammatory arthritides: scarcity of CD5 positive B cells and IL2 receptor bearing T cells. Pathology 24:19–26
16. Veale D, et al. (1993) Reduced synovial membrane macrophage numbers, ELAM-1 expression, and lining layer hyperplasia in psoriatic arthritis as compared with rheumatoid arthritis. Arthritis Rheum 36:893–900
17. Costello PJ, et al. (2001) Psoriatic arthritis joint fluids are characterized by CD8 and CD4 T cell clonal expansions appear antigen driven. J Immunol 166:2878–2886
18. Curran SA, et al. (2004) Nucleotide sequencing of psoriatic arthritis tissue before and during methotrexate administration reveals a complex inflammatory T cell infiltrate with very few clones exhibiting features that suggest they drive the inflammatory process by recognizing autoantigens. J Immunol 172:1935–1944
19. Fassbender HG, Fassbender R (1992) Synovial characteristics of seronegative spondarthritides. Clin Investigator 70:706
20. Espinoza LR, et al. (1982) Vascular changes in psoriatic synovium. A light and electron microscopic study. Arthritis Rheum 25:677–684
21. Reece RJ, et al. (1999) Distinct vascular patterns of early synovitis in psoriatic, reactive, and rheumatoid arthritis. Arthritis Rheum 42:1481–1484
22. Dupont E, et al. (1998) Antiangiogenic properties of a novel shark cartilage extract: potential role in the treatment of psoriasis. J Cutan Med Surg 2: 146–152
23. Fearon U, et al. (2003) Angiopoietins, growth factors, and vascular morphology in early arthritis. J Rheumatol 30:260–268
24. Ritchlin C, et al. (1998) Patterns of cytokine production in psoriatic synovium. J Rheumatol 25: 1544–1552
25. Austin LM, et al. (1999) The majority of epidermal T cells in psoriasis vulgaris lesions can produce type 1 cytokines, interferon-gamma, interleukin-2, and tumor necrosis factor-alpha, defining TC1 (cytotoxic T lymphocyte) and TH1 effector populations: a type 1 differentiation bias is also measured in circulating blood T cells in psoriatic patients. J Invest Dermatol 113:752–759
26. Vervoordeldonk MJ, Tak PP (2002) Cytokines in rheumatoid arthritis. Curr Rheumatol Rep 4: 208–217
27. Danning CL, et al. (2000) Macrophage-derived cytokine and nuclear factor kappaB p65 expression in synovial membrane and skin of patients with psoriatic arthritis. Arthritis Rheum 43:1244–1256
28. Vilcek J, Lee TH (1991) Tumor necrosis factor. New insights into the molecular mechanisms of its multiple actions. J Biol Chem 266:7313–7316
29. Bazzoni F, Beutler B (1996) The tumor necrosis factor ligand and receptor families. N Engl J Med 334: 1717–1725
30. Brennan FM, Feldmann M (1992) Cytokines in autoimmunity. Curr Opin Immunol 4:754–759
31. Saxne T, et al. (1988) Detection of tumor necrosis factor alpha but not tumor necrosis factor beta in rheumatoid arthritis synovial fluid and serum. Arthritis Rheum 31:1041–1045
32. Smith CA, et al. (1990) A receptor for tumor necrosis factor defines an unusual family of cellular and viral proteins. Science 248:1019–1023

33. Mohler KM, et al. (1993) Soluble tumor necrosis factor (TNF) receptors are effective therapeutic agents in lethal endotoxemia and function simultaneously as both TNF carriers and TNF antagonists. J Immunol 151:1548–1561
34. Sfikakis PP, Kollias G (2003) Tumor necrosis factor biology in experimental and clinical arthritis. Curr Opin Rheumatol 15:380–386
35. Redlich K, et al. (2004) Overexpression of tumor necrosis factor causes bilateral sacroiliitis. Arthritis Rheum 50:1001–1005
36. Baeten D, et al. (2001) Immunomodulatory effects of anti-tumor necrosis factor alpha therapy on synovium in spondylarthropathy: histologic findings in eight patients from an open-label pilot study [comment]. Arthritis Rheum 44:186–195
37. Moll JM, Wright V (1973) Psoriatic arthritis. Semin Arthritis Rheum 3:55–78
38. Benjamin M, McGonagle D (2001) The anatomical basis for disease localisation in seronegative spondyloarthropathy at entheses and related sites. J Anat 199:503–526
39. McGonagle D, et al. (1998) Characteristic magnetic resonance imaging entheseal changes of knee synovitis in spondylarthropathy [comment]. Arthritis Rheum 41:694–700
40. Laloux L, et al. (2001) Immunohistological study of entheses in spondyloarthropathies: comparison in rheumatoid arthritis and osteoarthritis. Ann Rheum Dis 60:316–321
41. Marzo-Ortega H, et al. (2001) Efficacy of etanercept in the treatment of the entheseal pathology in resistant spondylarthropathy: a clinical and magnetic resonance imaging study [comment]. Arthritis Rheum 44:2112–2117
42. Ribbens C, et al. (2002) Increased matrix metalloproteinase-3 serum levels in rheumatic diseases: relationship with synovitis and steroid treatment. Ann Rheum Dis 61:161–166
43. Vandooren B, et al. (2004) Matrix metalloproteinases and their inhibitors are involved in peripheral synovitis and downregulated by TNF blockade in spondyloarthropathy. Arthritis Rheum (in press)
44. Ritchlin CT, et al. (2003) Mechanisms of TNF-alpha- and RANKL-mediated osteoclastogenesis and bone resorption in psoriatic arthritis. J Clin Invest 111: 821–831
45. Suda T, et al. (1999) Modulation of osteoclast differentiation and function by the new members of the tumor necrosis factor receptor and ligand families. Endocr Rev 20:345–357
46. Lacey DL, et al. (1998) Osteoprotegerin ligand is a cytokine that regulates osteoclast differentiation and activation. Cell 93:165–176
47. Hofbauer LC, Heufelder AE (2001) The role of osteoprotegerin and receptor activator of nuclear factor kappaB ligand in the pathogenesis and treatment of rheumatoid arthritis. Arthritis Rheum 44:253–259
48. Udagawa N, et al. (2002) The molecular mechanism of osteoclastogenesis in rheumatoid arthritis. Arthritis Res 4:281–289
49. Braun J, et al. (1995) Use of immunohistologic and in situ hybridization techniques in the examination of sacroiliac joint biopsy specimens from patients with ankylosing spondylitis. Arthritis Rheum 38: 499–505
50. Peng H, et al. (2002) Synergistic enhancement of bone formation and healing by stem cell-expressed VEGF and bone morphogenetic protein-4. J Clin Invest 110:751–759
51. Stankler L (1969) An experimental investigation on the site of skin damage inducing the Koebner reaction in psoriasis. Br J Dermatol 81:534–535
52. Melski JW, Bernhard JD, Stern RS (1983) The Koebner (isomorphic) response in psoriasis. Associations with early age at onset and multiple previous therapies. Arch Dermatol 119:655–659
53. Langevitz P, Buskila D, Gladman DD (1990) Psoriatic arthritis precipitated by physical trauma. J Rheumatol 17:695–697
54. Rasmussen JE (2000) The relationship between infection with group A beta hemolytic streptococci and the development of psoriasis. Pediatr Infect Dis J 19:153–154
55. Rahman MU, et al. (1990) High levels of antipeptidoglycan antibodies in psoriatic and other seronegative arthritides. J Rheumatol 17:621–655
56. Vasey FB, et al. (1982) Possible involvement of group A streptococci in the pathogenesis of psoriatic arthritis. J Rheumatol 9:719–722
57. Leung DY, et al. (1995) Evidence for a streptococcal superantigen-driven process in acute guttate psoriasis. J Clin Invest 96:2106–2112
58. Travers JB, et al. (1999) Epidermal HLA-DR and the enhancement of cutaneous reactivity to superantigenic toxins in psoriasis [comment]. J Clin Invest 104:1181–1189
59. Arnett FC, Reveille JD, Duvic M (1991) Psoriasis and psoriatic arthritis associated with human immunodeficiency virus infection. Rheum Dis Clin North Am 17:59–78
60. Brancato L, et al. (1989) Aspects of the spectrum, prevalence and disease susceptibility determinants of Reiter's syndrome and related disorders associated with HIV infection. Rheumatol Int 9:137–141
61. Mijiyawa M, Oniankitan O, Khan MA (2000) Spondyloarthropathies in sub-Saharan Africa. Curr Opin Rheumatol 12:281–286
62. Njobvu P, McGill P (2000) Psoriatic arthritis and human immunodeficiency virus infection in Zambia. J Rheumatol 27:1699–1702
63. Bardos T, et al. (2002) Mice lacking endogenous major histocompatibility complex class II develop arthritis resembling psoriatic arthritis at an advanced age. Arthritis Rheum 46:2465–2475
64. Nickoloff BJ (2000) The search for pathogenic T cells and the genetic basis of psoriasis using a severe combined immunodeficient mouse model. Cutis 65:110–114
65. Nickoloff BJ, Wrone-Smith T (1999) Injection of pre-psoriatic skin with CD4+ T cells induces psoriasis. Am J Pathol 155:145–158

66. Hong K, et al. (1999) IL-12, independently of IFN-gamma, plays a crucial role in the pathogenesis of a murine psoriasis-like skin disorder. J Immunol 162: 7480–7491
67. Khare SD, Luthra HS, David CS (1995) Spontaneous inflammatory arthritis in HLA-B27 transgenic mice lacking beta 2-microglobulin: a model of human spondyloarthropathies. J Exp Med 182:1153–1158
68. Rothschild BM, Woods RJ (1989) Spondyloarthropathy in gorillas. Semin Arthritis Rheum 18:267–276
69. Rothschild BM, Woods RJ (1992) Erosive arthritis and spondyloarthropathy in Old World primates. Am J Phys Anthropol 88:389–400

Epidemiology IV

A Psoriasis

Christine C. Jacobson,
Alexa B. Kimball

Contents

1 Introduction

Psoriasis is a chronic, relapsing inflammatory skin disease affecting between 1% and 3% of the world's population [45]. Recent studies have attempted to better characterize the prevalence of psoriasis, and have also established genetic ties to the development of psoriasis. Epidemiologic studies on psoriasis involve unique challenges, as psoriasis type, disease severity and lesional locations fluctuate over time, and remissions are not uncommon. Psoriasis is associated with multiple comorbidities [61], including arthritis, Crohn's disease, obesity, hypertension and diabetes, whereas other diseases, such as atopic dermatitis and allergies have been found to be less common in psoriatics.

2 Incidence and Prevalence

The worldwide prevalence of psoriasis ranges from between 1% and 3%, although differences in prevalence rates for various countries, geographical regions, racial and ethnic groups exist and are at times pronounced. Population-based studies have demonstrated a range of psoriasis incidence from 0% up to 11.8% (Table A1). It is generally accepted that psoriasis affects males and females equally [14, 31, 102], although some studies show a slight female predominance [74]. Between 4.5 and 5.5 million Americans are affected with psoriasis [102, 103]; of those approximately 1.5 million adults have moderate to severe disease [103]. Roughly 260,000 new cases are diagnosed annually in the United States [35].

Table A1. Prevalence rates for different groups

Population	Reference(s)	Prevalence
Samoa	[100]	0%
South American Andes	[24]	0%
China	[59, 118, 143]	0.35–1.67%
Sri Lanka	[48]	0.4%
Norway	[11, 31]	1.1–1.4%
Yugoslavia	[2]	1.18%
Norwegian Lapps	[31]	1.4%
Spain	[2]	1.4%
Sweden	[58]	1.4%
UK	[104, 114]	1.48–1.6%
US	[103]	2.1%
Denmark	[14]	2.8% (after correction)
Faroe Islands	[87]	2.84%
Arctic-Kasach'ye	[29]	11.8%

IV

Variable factors such as genetics, climate, hygiene (e.g., regularity of bathing), and physical conditions can influence the prevalence rates of psoriasis [127]. Antecedent infection [28, 47], emotional stress [110], and low humidity have been linked to psoriasis exacerbations or initial diagnoses [100, 107]. Drugs also can precipitate or exacerbate psoriasis, including beta-blockers [1], lithium, systemic steroids, and antimalarials. Sunlight, on the other hand, will improve most patients' psoriasis [107]. Childhood psoriasis is often precipitated by an upper respiratory infection, notably with *Streptococcus* sp. [107]. Generalized pustular psoriasis can be provoked by premenstrual hormonal changes, by pregnancy, by high dose estrogen therapy and/or by cessation of oral or strong topical steroids [5, 95, 115, 141].

Genetics have been the most studied causal factor in psoriasis. Population studies, family studies, pedigree analyses and twin studies have proven a complicated genetic influence that is polygenic, multifactorial, and variably penetrant. In about one-third of cases, psoriasis is inherited [102]. Epidemiologic studies show that between 4.4% and 41% of psoriasis patients report a positive family history of the disease [34, 37, 48, 70, 71, 78, 104, 140]. The inheritance of a susceptibility gene is neither sufficient nor necessary for psoriasis. Children with one psoriatic parent have a 10–25% chance of developing the disease, while those with two psoriatic parents have a 50% chance [103, 136].

As reviewed earlier in this text, genetic studies have uncovered a psoriasis susceptibility locus, PSORS1, which may account for 35–50% of genetic susceptibility [10, 131]. While population studies have demonstrated that HLA Cw6 and HLA-DR7 have among strong associations with the development of psoriasis [19, 51, 129], the identity of PSORS1 is still in question. Possibilities include HLA-Cw6, HCR, and CDSN (corneodesmosin), or that polymorphisms in each are required in order to manifest psoriasis [18]. Additionally, in some families predisposed to psoriasis, there is a linkage with a genetic locus on the distal end of chromosome 17q [130]. Psoriatic arthritis may also have a genetic basis; a recent study has demonstrated that a locus at 16q may be involved in the paternal transmission of psoriatic arthritis [69]. Some authors speculate that variable patient responses to psoriasis treatments are related to genetics, as well.

Table A2. Types of psoriasis

Type of psoriasis	References	Incidence
Chronic plaque	[8, 37, 71, 78]	65–86%
Arthritis	[8, 34, 103]	10–34%
Guttate	[8, 37, 71, 78]	2.8–22%
Erythrodermic	[37, 71, 78]	0.8–4.1%
Inverse	[37, 78]	3–4%
Localized pustular	[37, 71, 78]	0.5–4%
Generalized pustular	[8, 37, 71, 78]	0.9–2%

Psoriasis varies in its cutaneous manifestations and sites of involvement. The most frequent type is chronic plaque psoriasis, representing between 65–86% of psoriatics [8, 37, 71, 78]. Other common types include guttate, erythrodermic, pustular and inverse psoriasis (Table A2). There is a wide prevalence range of guttate psoriasis reported; this variation may be due to environmental or genetic differences, or due to definitional differences in the diagnosis, as psoriasis patients can have a mixed plaque and guttate presentation. More rare manifestations include light-sensitive psoriasis and HIV-induced psoriasis [50]. In children, plaque psoriasis (34–69%) and guttate psoriasis (6.4–44%) are the most common [93, 101, 107] while generalized pustular psoriasis [25], pustular psoriasis of the palms and soles, erythroderma [3], and psoriatic arthritis [3, 34] are relatively rare. Up to 70% of patients that present with a guttate eruption of psoriasis will develop chronic plaque psoriasis [90, 138].

The most frequent sites of involvement include the scalp, elbows, trunk, and lower extremities [32, 34, 58, 71, 87, 140] (Table A3). Less common areas of involvement include the palmoplantar surfaces and flexural areas (psoriasis inversus). In children, the most frequent sites of involvement are the scalp (82%) and face (43%) [107]. Nail changes are present in 13–15% of children [3, 75, 107].

Nail psoriasis and psoriatic arthritis are being increasingly recognized in patients with

Table A3. Distribution of psoriasis

Body region	References	Percent of psoriatics with involvement
Scalp	[32, 34, 48, 71, 104,]	35–54%
Lower extremities	[32, 34, 71]	34–65%
Upper extremities	[32, 34, 71]	26–52%
Trunk	[32, 34, 71]	57–68%
Nails	[32, 37, 48, 71, 78, 104]	4.3–50%
Face	[32, 34, 71]	16–28%

psoriasis, although they are likely present in the minority. Nail involvement has been reported in anywhere from 13% to 50% of patients [37, 71, 78, 145], and with age may increase to between 80% and 90% [145]. Psoriasis of the nails is associated with a more severe course and the development of psoriatic arthritis [6, 37, 116, 123].

3 Natural History

Psoriasis can present anytime after birth through the final years of life. Roughly 60% of psoriasis sufferers develop the disease before the age of thirty, 35% before the age of twenty and 14% before the age of ten [21, 27, 32, 60, 65]. The average age of onset ranges from 25–33 [32, 34, 48, 103, 104], although it may differ from region to region; in Scandinavia, 45% of psoriatics present with disease before the age of 16 [87]. Women tend to develop psoriasis at an earlier age than men (20–37 years old versus 29–41 years old, respectively) [32, 34, 37, 48, 71, 78], as do those with a family history of the disease [32, 48, 60].

Age of onset has been described as having two peaks, the largest between the second and early third decades, and a smaller one between the mid-fifth and sixth decades [10, 17, 48, 60, 71, 121, 126]. This finding led to studies which demonstrated two distinct forms of non-pustular psoriasis: an early-onset type (Type I), HLA-Cw6 associated with strong family linkage and a tendency to become generalized; and a late-onset type (Type II) which is sporadic and usually milder [37, 60]. Type I psoriatics have a peak age of onset from the teens to the early 20s, while those with Type II disease have peak onset from their mid-40s through the 50s. Type I disease is characterized by more widespread and recurrent disease, a history of affected parents (Type I: Type II: 44%: 0%), and a significantly higher frequency of HLA Cw6 (85% vs. 15%) and DR7 (70% vs. 30%) [23]. Studies of psoriasis patients' HLA-Cw6 status confirm that HLA-Cw6 positivity is correlated with an earlier age of onset, more extensive disease, a higher incidence of Koebner's phenomenon, and a guttate-type initial presentation [46].

Studies vary significantly on the frequency of disease remissions for psoriatics, ranging from 0.4% to 55% [32, 87, 100, 104, 140]. Some remissions appear to be spontaneous, while others are treatment induced. The length of remission varies considerably but long term remissions are rare, with studies reporting between 1% and 3% having 5-year disease-free intervals [16, 88]. One study found an average remission of 6 months [16]. Fortunately, the overall prognosis for patients with psoriasis is relatively good. While quality of life can be greatly impacted [26, 38, 77, 137], very few people actually die from psoriasis.

4 Classification of Disease Subgroups

Definitions of disease severity in psoriasis are continually being revised, but currently used categories include mild, moderate, and severe. These definitions are important because they influence the range of treatments offered to patients. They impact clinical trial enrollment, determine FDA-defined drug indications, and can lead to denial of reimbursement for new drugs. Currently, there is an emerging consensus as to what constitutes mild, moderate, or severe disease, but the situation is complex because in any given patient, the disease severity will fluctuate over time.

Severity grading systems, which have been developed for use in clinical trials, generally include scores for both body surface area involvement and plaque severity [30, 56, 73, 99, 122,

134]. Physical components of plaque severity vary, but often involve erythema, induration and scale. Other important considerations may include areas of involvement, symptoms of pruritus, pain in the lesions, remission length, and the presence of arthritis. There is growing consensus that assessments of disease severity are incomplete without evaluating quality-of-life, and some have argued that severe impairment of quality of life could alone be a criterion for systemic therapy use [76].

Using body surface area involvement as a way to define severity has been accepted by drug developers and regulatory agencies. The National Psoriasis Foundation defines mild disease as less than 2% body surface area (BSA) involvement, moderate disease as between 3% and 10% BSA, and severe disease as over 10% [103]. Although traditionally 20% BSA was the benchmark for enrollment in clinical trials testing systemic agents, recent clinical trials have used 10% body surface area involvement instead [79, 80, 82] and the FDA appears to have also accepted 10% BSA as a marker of severe disease [76].

Some researchers use the patient's Psoriasis Area and Severity Index (PASI) as a measure of psoriasis severity. Developed in 1978, the PASI is the most frequently used clinical psoriasis severity scale and is currently considered the gold standard [4, 39, 40, 132]. PASIs – which range from 0 to 72 – are calculated using a formula including variables of plaque erythema, induration and scale, and body surface area involvement. A review of several journal articles reveals that the average PASI scores of patients enrolled in "moderate-to-severe" [7, 72, 111, 120, 147] and "severe" [37, 43, 68, 128] psoriasis trials extend from 16 to 30.5, although patients with PASIs as low as an 8 still qualify for some moderate-to-severe psoriasis trials [62].

Based on body surface area, 33% of psoriatics have moderate to severe disease, although the percent would increase if some of those on systemic medications were to stop treatment [103]. Psoriasis patients seen in dermatology clinics likely have more severe disease than the general psoriasis population. One study of 1754 dermatology patients demonstrated that 21% had mild disease (PASI score of 0–3), 49% had moderate disease (PASI score of >3–15), and 30% had severe disease (PASI score of >15) [37].

5 Comorbidities

Patients diagnosed with psoriasis tend to have concurrent comorbidities, both physical and psychosocial. Psoriatic arthritis is the most common comorbidity, diagnosed in 6–34% of psoriatics [8, 77, 102, 103, 116, 119, 123, 144, 146], and it follows the onset of psoriasis between 68–80% of the time [8, 15]. Of psoriatics with psoriatic arthritis, studies have shown that psoriasis skin findings predate the onset of arthritis in 65–68%, is synchronous in 8–16%, and antedates arthritis in 19–26% [8, 34, 116]. It affects both sexes equally and is characterized by several possible patterns of joint involvement.

Epidemiological research has shown that hypertension, heart failure, and diabetes are significantly more common in patients with psoriasis than in control dermatology patients (observed/expected, O/E, ratios of 1.9, 1.83, and 1.47 respectively) [61]. Diabetes in psoriatics is especially seen in females [61], although the high prevalence of obesity in this population may be a confounding factor. Celiac disease may also be higher in psoriasis patients than in controls [109].

Psoriasis and Crohn's disease are concomitant diagnoses in individuals at a higher rate than would be expected if the two diseases were independent of each other. In various case-control studies, between 1–2% of controls were diagnosed with psoriasis, while between 7–11% of those with Crohn's disease were found to have the disease [66, 81, 92, 142]. Family studies have demonstrated that family members of those diagnosed with either Crohn's or psoriasis have an increased incidence of the other disease; specifically, one study showed that 10% of patients with Crohn's disease had a first degree relative with psoriasis while the same was true of only 2.9% of controls [81]. There are both genetic [52, 67, 96, 97] and pathologic [13, 94, 105, 135] connections between these two diseases, although no definitive link has been discovered yet.

Cancer risk also appears to be elevated, at least in severe psoriatics. Psoriasis patients who had used systemic therapies have a higher incidence of non-melanoma skin cancers and lymphoproliferative diseases than those with milder psoriasis or controls, although psoriatics with mild disease also had a slightly increased incidence [89]. Another study demonstrated that psoriasis patients over the age of 65 had almost a threefold increase in lymphoma [44]. Older studies have contradictory evidence regarding the relationship between psoriasis and lymphoproliferative diseases [9, 41, 55, 83, 124]. Systemic PUVA- and climatotherapy-treated patients are at increased risk for nonmelanoma skin cancers [42, 84, 86, 125], and this risk remains increased for up to 15 years after stopping PUVA [106]. Bath PUVA is not associated with an increased risk of either non-melanoma skin cancers or melanoma [53, 54, 85].

Other forms of cancer are also more prevalent in psoriatics than controls. A population-based series of 9773 patients hospitalized for their psoriasis demonstrated an increased risk of cancers of the oral cavity and pharynx; esophagus; liver; pancreas; lung; skin (squamous cell carcinoma); bladder; kidney; female breast; male genital cancers; and mycosis fungoides in men when compared to standardized incidence ratios [9]. A Swedish population based study found a significant association between psoriasis and both male breast cancer (O/E: 6.90) and female kidney cancer (O/E: 2.79) [83]. A third study demonstrated psoriatics have an elevated risk for SCC (O/E: 4.1), BCC (O/E: 2.2), cancer of the lung (O/E: 1.5), oral cavity (O/E: 2.3), larynx (O/E: 2.4) and pharynx (O/E: 4.1) in men; and cancer of the lung (O/E: 1.6), colon (O/E: 1.4) and "unspecified sites" (O/E: 2.5) in women [41]. It is unclear if the increased incidence of these malignancies is secondary to potentially carcinogenic and immunosuppressive agents used in psoriasis treatments (i.e., coal tar, PUVA, methotrexate, cyclosporine, etc), due to behavioral characteristics more prevalent in psoriatics (i.e., alcoholism, smoking) or whether some genetic predisposition exists.

Conversely, in most studies, psoriasis patients are less likely to be diagnosed with Th2-associated diseases such as atopic dermatitis, allergic asthma, urticaria and contact dermatitis (O/E ratios of 0.02, 0.07, 0.17 and 0.34 respectively) [22]. There is also a decreased risk of melanoma [9].

Certain psychosocial comorbidities are associated with psoriasis as well. Epidemiologic research has determined an increased rate of obesity in psoriatics (O/E ratio 2.05), which is especially common in women [61]. Comorbid depressive illness is relatively common among psoriasis patients, and the relationship between psoriasis and depression may be reciprocal. Studies have found notably higher degrees of depression in psoriatic patients than in controls [27, 57], and in one study of moderate-to-severe psoriatics, 46% of 35 study patients claimed they were "often" or "always" depressed due to their condition [137]. Researchers have found that higher levels of depression are present in patients who have a greater percentage of their skin affected by psoriasis [117]. One study found that there was a higher prevalence of suicidal ideation among the psoriasis patients in their study in comparison to the general population [49]. Suicidal ideation appears to be most common in those who rate their psoriasis as severe [49].

There is also an increased incidence of alcoholism and alcohol misuse in psoriasis patients, which may be related to the emotional burden of having a stigmatizing disease [11, 33, 112, 139]. Conversely, alcohol use is related to a higher incidence and greater severity of psoriasis [20, 63, 64], while alcohol-related disorders – such as alcoholic liver cirrhosis – can also exacerbate psoriasis or prevent the expected response to prescribed therapy [33]. Abstinence alone can induce psoriasis remission and restarting drinking can be associated with disease relapse [63, 133].

Cigarette smoking is more common in psoriasis patients than controls [11, 91, 98, 113], and has been noted by some researchers to contribute to the development of pustular psoriasis [108]. However, smoking is also common among alcohol misusers [63, 64] and prior studies on smoking and psoriasis did not account for the occurrence of both drinking and smoking; therefore, psoriasis outbreaks reported in these studies may be secondary to alcohol use and not smoking [63, 64]. Higgins and du Vivier report that in studies inclusive of confounding variables [63, 64], it appeared that smoking is not an independent risk factor for psoriasis.

6 Conclusion

Much is known about the epidemiology of psoriasis, and there is a high level of consistency in observations made worldwide. Less understood is whether associated findings including the comorbidities are linked to the disease itself, to effects of psoriasis treatments, to behavioral characteristics of psoriasis patients, or to some interplay between these variables. Further research may be helpful in determining whether there are aspects of psoriasis that are preventable, and whether a given patient's responsiveness to therapy can be predicted. Additionally, definitions of psoriasis severity are in the process of being refined, which has important implications for improving epidemiologic studies, clinical trial design, and treatment recommendations.

References

1. Arntzen N, Kavli G, Volden G (1984) Psoriasis provoked by beta-blocking agents. Acta Derm Venereol (Stockh) 64:346–348
2. Arzensek J, Kansky A, Kavcic C, Pejovnik-Pustinek A, Sturbej S (1984) Epidemiology of psoriasis in the Celje area. Acta Derm Venereol (Stockh) Suppl 113:106–108
3. Asboe-Hansen G (1971) Psoriasis in childhood. In: Farber EM, Cox AJ (eds) Psoriasis. Proceedings of the international symposium. Stanford University Press, Stanford, CA, p 53
4. Ashcroft DM (1999) Clinical measures of disease severity and outcome in psoriasis: a critical appraisal of their quality. Br J Dermatol 141:185–191
5. Baker H, Ryan TJ (1968) Generalized pustular psoriasis: a clinical and epidemiological study of 104 cases. Br J Dermatol 80:771–793
6. Baker H, Golding DN, Thompson N (1964) The nails in psoriatic arthritis. Br J Dermatol 76:549–554
7. Balagon MV, Tan PL, Prestidge R, et al. (2001) Improvement in psoriasis after intradermal administration of dilapidated, deglycolipidated *Mycobacterium vaccae* (PVAC): results of an open label trial. Clin Exp Dermatol 26:233–241
8. Biondi Oriente C, Scarpa R, Pucino A, Oriente P (1989) Psoriasis and psoriatic arthritis. Dermatological and rheumatological co-operative clinical report. Acta Derm Venereol Suppl 146:69–71
9. Boffetta P, Gridley G, Lindelof B (2001) Cancer risk in a population-based cohort of patients hospitalized for psoriasis in Sweden. J Invest Dermatol 117:1531–1537
10. Bowcock AM, Barker JN (2003) Genetics of psoriasis: the potential impact on new therapies. J Am Acad Dermatol Suppl 49:S51–56
11. Braathen LR, Botten G, Bjerkedal T (1989a) Prevalence of psoriasis in Norway. Acta Derm Venereol Suppl 142:5–8
12. Braathen LR, Botten G, Bjerkedal T (1989b) Psoriatics in Norway. A questionnaire study on health status, contact with paramedical professions, and alcohol and tobacco consumption. Acta Derm Venereol Suppl 142:9–12
13. Braegger C, Nicholls S, Murch S, Stephens S, MacDonald T (1992) Tumor necrosis factor alpha in stool as a marker of intestinal inflammation. Lancet 339:89–91
14. Brandrup E, Green A (1981) The prevalence of psoriasis in Denmark. Acta Derm Venereol (Stockh) 61:344–346
15. Brockbank J, Gladman D (2002) Diagnosis and management of psoriatic arthritis. Drugs 62:2447–2457
16. Buntin DM, Skinner RB, Rosenberg EW (1983) Onset of psoriasis at age 108. J Am Acad Dermatol 9:276–277
17. Burch PRJ, Rowell NR (1965) Psoriasis: aetiological aspects. Acta Derm Venereol (Stockh) 45:366–380
18. Capon F, Toal IK, Evans JC, et al. (2003) Haplotype identity of distantly related populations implicates corneodesmosin in psoriasis susceptibility. J Med Genet 40:447–452
19. Chang YT, Tsai SF, Lee DD, et al. (2003) A study of candidate genes for psoriasis near HLA-C in Chinese patients with psoriasis. Br J Dermatol 148:418–423
20. Chaput JC, Poynard T, Naveau S, Penso D, Durrmeyer O, Suplisson D (1985) Psoriasis, alcohol and liver disease. Br Med J 291:25
21. Christophers E (2000) What does epidemiology tell us about disease mechanisms in psoriasis. Clin Exp Dermatol 25:164
22. Christophers E (2001) Psoriasis – epidemiology and clinical spectrum. Clin Exp Dermatol 26:314–320
23. Christophers E, Henseler T (1990) Psoriasis Type I and II are subtypes of nonpustular psoriasis. In:

Roenigk HH, Maibach HI (eds) Psoriasis, 2nd edn. Marcel Dekker, New York, pp 15–21
24. Convit J (1963) Investigation of the incidence of psoriasis among Latin American Indians. In: Proceedings of the 12th International Congress of Dermatology, Washington 1962. International Congress Series No. 55, Excerpta Medica Foundation, Amsterdam
25. Crow KD, Hargreaves GK (1968) Infantile pustular psoriasis. Trans St. John's Hosp Dermatol Soc 54: 42
26. De Arruda LHF, De Moraes APF (2001) The impact of psoriasis on quality of life. Br J Dermatol 144: Suppl 58 : 33–36
27. Devrimici-Ozguven H, Kundakci N, Kumbasar K, Boyvat A (2000) The depression, anxiety, life satisfaction and affective expression levels in psoriasis patients. J Eur Acad Dermatol Venereol 14 : 267–271
28. Duvic M (1991) Papulosquamous disorders associated with human immunodeficiency virus infection. Dermatol Clin 9 : 523–530
29. Eckes L, Ananthakrishnan R, Walter H (1975) Zur geographischen Verteilung der Psoriasis. Hautarzt 26 : 563–567
30. Exum ML, Rapp SR, Feldman SR, et al. (1996) Measuring severity of psoriasis: methodological issues. J Dermatol Treat 7 : 119–124
31. Falk ES, Vandbakk Y (1993) Prevalence of psoriasis in a Norwegian Lapp population. Acta Derm Venereol 182 : 6–9
32. Farber E, Nall LM (1974) The natural history of psoriasis in 5600 patients. Dermatologica 148: 1–18
33. Farber EM, Nall L (1994) Psoriasis and alcoholism. Cutis 53 : 21–27
34. Farber EM, Bright RD, Nall ML (1968) Psoriasis. A questionnaire survey of 2,144 patients. Arch Dermatol 98 : 248
35. Feldman SR, Fleischer AB, Reboussin DM, et al. (1997) The economic impact of psoriasis increases with psoriasis severity. J Am Acad Dermatol 37: 564–569
36. Ferrandiz C, Bordas X, Garcia Patos V, Puig S, Pujol R, Smandia A (2001) Prevalence of psoriasis in Spain (Epiderma project: phase I). J Eur Acad Dermatol 15 : 20–23
37. Ferrandiz C, Pujol RM, Garcia-Patos V, Bordas X, Smandia JA (2002) Psoriasis of early and late onset: a clinical and epidemiological study from Spain. J Am Acad Dermatol 46: 867–873
38. Finlay AY, Coles EC (1995) The effect of severe psoriasis on the quality of life of 369 patients. Br J Dermatol 132 : 236–244
39. Food and Drug Administration (1998) Dermatologic and ophthalmic drugs advisory committee 49th meeting (minutes from meeting). March 20, 1998
40. Fredriksson T, Pettersson U (1978) Severe psoriasis: oral therapy with a new retinoid. Dermatologica 157 : 238–244
41. Frentz G, Olsen JH (1999) Malignant tumors and psoriasis: a follow-up study. Br J Dermatol 140: 237–242
42. Frentz G, Olsen JH, Avrach WW (1999) Malignant tumours and psoriasis: climatotherapy at the Dead Sea. Br J Dermatol 141 : 1088–1091
43. Geilen CC, Arnold M, Orfanos CE (2001) Mycophenolate mofetil as a systemic antipsoriatic agent: positive experience in 11 patients. Br J Dermatol 144 : 583–586
44. Gelfand JM, Berlin J, Van Voorhees A, Margolis DJ (2003) Lymphoma rates are low but increased in patients with psoriasis – results from a population based cohort study in the United Kingdom. Arch Dermatol 139 : 1425–1429
45. Greaves MW, Weinstein GD (1995) Treatment of psoriasis. N Engl J Med 332 : 581–588
46. Gudjonsson JE, Karason A, Antonsdottir AA, et al. (2002) HLA-Cw6-positive and HLA-Cw6-negative patients with psoriasis vulgaris have distinct clinical features. J Invest Dermatol 118 : 362–365
47. Gudjonsson JE, Thorarinsson AM, Sigurgeirsson B, Kristinsson KG, Valdmiarsson H (2003) Streptococcal throat infections and exacerbation of chronic plaque psoriasis: a prospective study. Br J Dermatol 149 : 530–534
48. Gunawardena DA, Gunawardena KA, Vasanthanathan NS, Gunawardena JA (1978) Psoriasis in Sri Lanka – a computer analysis of 1366 cases. Br J Dermatol 98 : 85–96
49. Gupta MA, Gupta AK (1998) Depression and suicidal ideation in dermatology patients with acne, alopecia areata, atopic dermatitis and psoriasis. Br J Dermatol 139 : 846–850
50. Habif TP (1996) Psoriasis and other papulosquamous disorders. In: Clinical dermatology: a color guide to diagnosis and therapy, 3rd edn. Mosby-Year Book, St. Louis, pp 190–235
51. Hammon MG, Reeve CE, Sargent AV, et al. (1977) Psoriasis. In: Bodmer WF, et al. (eds) Histocompatibility testing 1977. Munksgaard, Copenhagen, pp 230–231
52. Hampe J, Schreiber S, Shaw SH, et al. (1999) A genome wide analysis provides evidence for novel linkages in inflammatory bowel disease in a large European cohort. Am J Hum Genet 64: 808–816
53. Hannuksela M, Karvonen J (1984) Topical trioxsalen PUVA therapy. Acta Derm Venereol (Stockh) Suppl 113 : 135–138
54. Hannuksela-Svahn A, Sigurgeirsson B, Pukkala E, et al. (1999) Trioxsalen bath PUVA did not increase the risk of squamous cell skin carcinoma and cutaneous malignant melanoma in a joint analysis of 944 Swedish and Finnish patients with psoriasis. Br J Dermatol 141 : 497–501
55. Hannuksela-Svahn A, Pukkala E, Laara E, Poikolainen K, Karvonen J (2001) Psoriasis, its treatment, and cancer in a cohort of Finnish patients. J Invest Dermatol 117 : 1531–1537

56. Harari M, Shani J, Hristakieva E, et al. (2000) Clinical evaluation of a more rapid and sensitive Psoriasis Assessment Severity Score (PASS), and its comparison with the classic method of Psoriasis Area and Severity Index (PASI), before and after climatotherapy at the Dead Sea. Int J Dermatol 39: 913–918
57. Hardy GE, Cotterill JA (1982) A study of depression and obsessionality in dysmorphophobic and psoriatic patients. Br J Psychiatry 140:19–22
58. Hellgren L (1967) Psoriasis: the prevalence in sex, age, and occupational groups in total populations in Sweden. Morphology, inheritance and association with other skin and rheumatic diseases. Almqvist and Wiskell, Stockholm
59. Henan Dermatoses Survey Group (1982) An analysis of 487 cases of psoriasis in 100,000 natural population of Henan rural district. Chinese J Dermatol 15:83–84
60. Henseler T, Christophers E (1985) Psoriasis of early and late onset: characterization of two types of psoriasis vulgaris. J Am Acad Dermatol 13: 340–346
61. Henseler T, Christophers E (1995) Disease concomitance in psoriasis. J Am Acad Dermatol 32: 982–986
62. Heydendael VMR, Spuls PI, Opmeer BC, et al. (2003) Methotrexate versus cyclosporine in moderate-to-severe chronic plaque psoriasis. N Eng J Med 349:658–665
63. Higgins EM, du Vivier AW (1994a) Alcohol abuse and treatment resistance in skin disease. J Am Acad Dermatol 30:1048
64. Higgins EM, du Vivier AW (1994b) Cutaneous disease and alcohol misuse. Br Med Bull 50:85–98
65. Holgate MC (1975) The age-of-onset of psoriasis and the relationship to parental psoriasis. Br J Dermatol 92:443–448
66. Hughes S, Williams SE, Turnberg LA (1983) Crohn's disease and psoriasis. N Engl J Med 308:101
67. Hugot J, Laurent-Puig P, Gower-Rousseau C, et al. (1996) Mapping of a susceptibility locus for Crohn's disease on chromosome 16. Nature 379: 821–823
68. Inaoki M, Sato S, Shimada Y, et al. (2000) Decreased expression levels of L-selectin on subsets of leucocytes and increased serum L-selectin in severe psoriasis. Clin Exp Immunol 122:484–492
69. Karason A, Gudjonsson JE, Upmanyu R, et al. (2003) A susceptibility gene for psoriatic arthritis maps to chromosome 16q: evidence for imprinting. Am J Hum Genet 72:125–131
70. Kavli G, Forde OH, Arnessen E, Stenvold SE (1985) Psoriasis: familial predisposition and environmental factors. Br Med J (Clin Res Ed) 291: 999–1000
71. Kawada A, Tezuka T, Nakamizo Y, et al. (2003) A survey of psoriasis patients in Japan from 1982 to 2001. J Dermatol Sci 31:59–64
72. Kimball AB, Kawamura T, Tejura K, et al. (2002) Clinical and immunologic assessment of patients with psoriasis in a randomized, double-blind, placebo-controlled trial using recombinant human interleukin 10. Arch Dermatol 138:1341–1346
73. Kirby B, Fortune DG, Bhushan M, et al. (2000) The Salford Psoriasis Index: an holistic measure of psoriasis severity. Br J Dermatol 142:728–732
74. Kononen M, Torppa J, Lassus A (1986) An epidemiological survey of psoriasis in the Greater Helsinki Area. Acta Derm Venereol 124:1–10
75. Krueger GG, Duvic M (1994) Epidemiology of psoriasis: clinical issues. J Invest Dermatol Suppl 102: 14–18
76. Krueger GG, Feldman SR, Camisa C, et al. (2000) Two considerations for patients with psoriasis and their clinicians: What defines mild, moderate and severe psoriasis? What constitutes a clinically significant improvement when treating psoriasis? J Am Acad Dermatol 43:281–285
77. Krueger G, Koo J, Lebwohl M, Menter A, Stern R, Rolstad T (2001) The impact of psoriasis on quality of life. Results of a 1998 National Psoriasis Foundation patient-membership survey. Arch Dermatol 137:280–284
78. Kundakci N, Tursen U, Babiker MOA, Gurgey E (2002) The evaluation of the sociodemographic and clinical features of Turkish psoriasis patients. Int J Dermatol 41:220–224
79. Lebwohl M, Christophers E, Langley R, Ortonne JP, Roberts J, Griffiths CEM (2003a) An international, randomized, double-blind, placebo-controlled phase 3 trial of intramuscular alefacept in patients with chronic plaque psoriasis. Arch Dermatol 139: 719–727
80. Lebwohl M, Tyring SK, Hamilton TK, et al. (2003b) A novel targeted T-cell modulator, efalizumab, for plaque psoriasis. N Eng J Med 349:2004–2013
81. Lee F, Bellary S, Francis C (1990) Increased occurrence of psoriasis in patients with Crohn's disease and their relatives. Am J Gastroenterol 85:962–963
82. Leonardi CL, Powers JL, Matheson RT, et al. (2003) Etanercept as monotherapy in patients with psoriasis. N Engl J Med 349:2014–2022
83. Lindelof B, Eklund G, Liden S, Stern RS (1990) The prevalence of malignant tumors in patients with psoriasis. J Am Acad Dermatol 22:1056–1060
84. Lindelof B, Sigurgeirsson B, Tegner E, et al. (1991) PUVA and cancer: a large scale epidemiological study. Lancet 338: 91–93
85. Lindelof B, Sigurgeirsson B, Tegner E, Larko O, Berne B (1992) Comparison of the carcinogenic potential of trioxsalen bath PUVA and oral methoxsalen PUVA. Arch Dermatol 128:1341–1344
86. Lindelof B, Sigurgeirson B, Tegner E, et al. (1999) PUVA and cancer risk: the Swedish follow-up study. Br J Dermatol 141:108–112
87. Lomholt G (1963) Psoriasis: Prevalence, spontaneous course and genetics. A census study on the prevalence of skin diseases in the Faroe Islands. GEC Gad, Copenhagen
88. MacLennan A, Hellier FF (1961) The treatment time in psoriasis. Br J Dermatol 73:439–444

89. Margolis D, Bilker W, Hennessy S, Vittorio C, Santanna J, Strom BL (2001) The risk of malignancy associated with psoriasis. Arch Dermatol 137: 778–783
90. Martin BA, Chalmers RJ, Telfer NR (1996) How great is the risk of further psoriasis following a single episode of acute guttate psoriasis? Arch Dermatol 132:717–718
91. Mills CM, Srivastava ED, Harvey IM, Swift GL, Newcombe RG, Holt PJ, Rhodes J (1992) Smoking habits in psoriasis: a case controlled study. Br J Dermatol 127:18–21
92. Moll JMA, Haslock I, Macrae MB, et al. (1974) Associations between ankylosing spondylitis, psoriatic arthritis, Reiter's disease, the intestinal arthropathies and Behçet's syndrome. Medicine 53: 343–362
93. Morris A, Rogers M, Fischer G, Williams K (2001) Childhood psoriasis: a clinical review of 1262 cases. Pediatr Dermatol 18:188–198
94. Murch S, Braegger C, Walker-Smith J, MacDonald T (1993) Location of tumor necrosis factor-alpha by immunohistochemistry in chronic inflammatory bowel disease. Gut 34:1705–1709
95. Murphy FR, Stolman LP (1979) Generalized pustular psoriasis. Arch Dermatol 115:1215–1216
96. Nair R, Henseler T, Jenisch S, Stuart P, Bichakjian C, Lenk W (1997) Evidence for 2 psoriasis susceptibility loci (HLA and 17q) and 2 novel candidate regions (16q and 20p) by genome-wide scan. Hum Mol Genet 6:1349–1356
97. Nair RP, Stuart P, Henseler T, et al. (2000) Localization of psoriasis-susceptibility locus PSOR1 to a 60-kb interval telomeric to HLA-C. Am J Hum Genet 66:1833–1844
98. Naldi L, Parazzini F, Brevi A, et al. (1992) Family history, smoking habits, alcohol consumption and risk of psoriasis. Br J Dermatol 127:212–217
99. Naldi L, Svensson A, Diepgen T, et al. (2003) Randomized clinical trials for psoriasis 1977–2000; the EDEN survey. J Invest Dermatol 120:738–741
100. Nall ML, Farber EM (1977) World epidemiology in psoriasis. In: Farber EM, Cox AJ (eds) Psoriasis: Proceedings of the Second International Symposium. Yorke Medical Books, New York, pp 331–333
101. Nanda A, Kaur S, Kaur I, Kumar B (1990) Childhood psoriasis: an epidemiologic survey of 112 patients. Pediatr Dermatol 7:19–21
102. National Institute of Arthritis and Musculoskeletal and Skin Diseases Data (2002) Accessed Dec 5, 2003; last updated January 2002. Available from: URL: http://www.niams.nih.gov/hi/topics/psoriasis/psoriafs.htm
103. National Psoriasis Foundation Data (2003) Accessed Dec 5, 2003; last updated 2003. Available from: URL: http://www.psoriasis.org/facts/psoriasis
104. Nevitt GJ, Hutchinson PE (1996) Psoriasis in the community: prevalence, severity and patients' beliefs and attitudes towards the disease. Br J Dermatol 135:533–537
105. Nickoloff B, Karabin G, Barker J, et al. (1991) Cellular localization of interleukin-8 and its inducer, tumor necrosis factor-alpha in psoriasis. Am J Pathol 138:129–140
106. Nijsten TEC, Stern RS (2003) The increased risk of skin cancer is persistent after discontinuation of psoralen + ultraviolet A: a cohort study. J Invest Dermatol 121:252–258
107. Nyfors A, Lemholt K (1975) Psoriasis in children. Br J Dermatol 92:437–442
108. O'Doherty CJ, Macintyre C (1985) Palmoplantar pustulosis and smoking. BMJ 291:861–864
109. Ojetti V, Sanchez JA, Guerriero C, Fossati B, Capizzi R, De Simone C, et al. (2003) High prevalence of celiac disease in psoriasis. Am J Gastroenterol 98: 2574–2575
110. Paljan D, Kansky A, Cividini-Stranic E (1984) Psychosomatic factors influencing the course of psoriasis. Acta Derm Venereol (Stockh) Suppl 113: 121–122
111. Papp K, Bissonnette R, Krueger JG, et al. (2001) The treatment of moderate to severe psoriasis with a new anti-CD11a monoclonal antibody. J Am Acad Dermatol 45:665–674
112. Poikolainen K, Reunala T, Karvonen J, Lauharanta J, Karkkainen P (1990) Alcohol intake: a risk factor for psoriasis in young and middle aged men? BMJ 300:780–783
113. Poikolainen K, Reunala T, Karvonen J (1994) Smoking, alcohol and life events related to psoriasis among women. Br J Dermatol 130:473–477
114. Rea JN, Newhouse ML, Halil T (1976) Skin disease in Lambeth: a community study of prevalence and use of medical care. Br J Prev Soc Med 30: 107–114
115. Ryan TJ, Baker H (1969) Systemic corticosteroids and folic acid antagonists in the treatment of generalized pustular psoriasis. Evaluation and prognosis based on the study of 104 cases. Br J Dermatol 81:134–145
116. Scarpa R, Oriente P, Pucino A, et al. (1984) Psoriatic arthritis in psoriatic patients. Br J Rheum 23: 246–250
117. Scharloo M, Kaptein AA, Weinman J, Bergman W, Vermeer BJ, Rooijmans HGM (2000) Patients' illness perceptions and coping as predictors of functional status in psoriasis: a 1-year follow-up. Br J Dermatol 142:899–907
118. Shao CG, Zhang FW, Wang KC (1987) The distribution of psoriasis. A nationwide screening in the People's Republic of China, 1984. In: Farber EM, Nall L, Morhenn V, Jacobs PH (eds) Psoriasis. Proceedings of the Fourth International Symposium, Elsevier, New York, pp 398–399
119. Shbeeb M, Uramoto KM, Gibson LE, et al. (2000) The epidemiology of psoriatic arthritis in Olmsted County, Minnesota, USA, 1982–1991. J Rheumatol 27:1247–1250
120. Sigmundsdottir H, Gudjonsson JE, Jonsdottir I, et al. (2001) The frequency of CLA+ CD8+ T cells in the blood of psoriasis patients correlates closely

with the severity of their disease. Clin Exp Immunol 126:365–369
121. Smith AE, Kassab JY, Payne RCME, Beer WE (1993) Bimodality in age of onset of psoriasis, in both patients and their relatives. Dermatology 186: 181–186
122. Snellman E, Lauharanta J, Revnanen A, et al. (1993) Effect of heliotherapy on skin in psoriasis: a 6-month follow up study. Br J Dermatol 128:172–177
123. Stern RS (1985) The epidemiology of joint complaints in patients with psoriasis. J Rheumatol 12: 315–320
124. Stern RS, Vakeva LH (1997) Noncutaneous malignant tumors in the PUVA follow-up study: 1975–1996. J Invest Dermatol 108:897–900
125. Stern RS, Liebman EJ, Vakeva L (1998) Oral psoralen and ultraviolet A light (PUVA) treatment of psoriasis and persistent risk of non-melanoma skin cancer. PUVA follow-up study. J Natl Cancer Inst 90:1278–1284
126. Swanbeck G, Inerot A, Martinsson T, et al. (1995) Age of onset and different types of psoriasis. Br J Dermatol 133:768–773
127. Tagami H (1997) Triggering factors. Clin Dermatol 15:677–685
128. Thaci D, Brautigam M, Kaufmann R, et al. (2002) Body-weight independent dosing of cyclosporine micro-emulsion and three times weekly maintenance regimen in severe psoriasis. Dermatology 205:383–388
129. Tiwari JL, Lowe NJ, Abramovits J, et al. (1982) Association of psoriasis with HLA-DR7. Br J Dermatol 106:227–230
130. Tomfohrde J, Silverman A, Barnes R, et al. (1994) Gene for familial psoriasis susceptibility mapped to the distal end of chromosome 17Q. Science 264: 1141–1145
131. Trembath RC, Clough RL, Rosbotham JL, et al. (1997) Identification of a major susceptibility locus on chromosome 6p and evidence for further disease loci revealed by a two stage genome-wide search in psoriasis. Hum Mol Genet 6:813–820
132. Van de Kerkhof PCM (1997) The PASI and alternative approaches for the assessment of severity: persisting areas of confusion. Br J Dermatol 137: 661–662
133. Vincenti GE, Blunden SM (1987) Psoriasis and alcohol abuse. J R Army Med Corps 133:77–78
134. Wainwright NJ, Dawe RS, Ferguson J (1998) Narrowband ultraviolet B (TL-01) phototherapy for psoriasis: which incremental regimen? Br J Dermatol 139:410–414
135. Wakefield P, James W, Sallaska C, Meltzer M (1991) Tumor necrosis factor. J Am Acad Dermatol 24: 675–685
136. Watson W, Cann HM, Farber EM, Nall ML (1972) The genetics of psoriasis. Arch Dermatol 105: 197–207
137. Weiss SC, Kimball AB, Liewehr DJ, Blauvelt A, Turner ML, Emanuel EJ (2002) Quantifying the harmful effect of psoriasis on health-related quality of life. J Am Acad Dermatol 47:512–518
138. Williams RC, McKenzie AW, Roger JH, Joysey VC (1976) HL-A antigens in patients with guttate psoriasis. Br J Dermatol 95:163–167
139. Wolf R, Wolf D, Ruocco V (1999) Alcohol intake and psoriasis. Clin Dermatol 17:423–430
140. Yasuda T, Ishikawa E, Mori S (1971) Psoriasis in the Japanese. In: Farber EM, Cox AJ (eds) Psoriasis: proceedings of an international symposium. Stanford University Press, Stanford, CA, pp 25–34
141. Yasuda T, Ito M, Mizuno A, et al. (1976) Internal factors and pustular psoriasis. In: Farber EM, Cox AJ (eds) Psoriasis. Proceedings of the Second International Symposium. Yorke Medical Books, New York, pp 140–145
142. Yates VM, Watkinson G, Kelman A (1982) Further evidence of an association between psoriasis, Crohn's disease and ulcerative colitis. Br J Dermatol 106:323–330
143. Yip SY (1984) The prevalence of psoriasis in the Mongoloid race. J Am Acad Dermatol 10:965–968
144. Zachariae H, Zachariae R, Blomquist K, et al. (2002) Quality of life and prevalence of arthritis reported by 5,795 members of the Nordic Psoriasis Associations. Data from the Nordic Quality of Life Study. Acta Derm Venereol 82:108–113
145. Zaias N (1969) Psoriasis of the nail. A clinical pathological study. Arch Dermatol 99:567–579
146. Zanolli MD, Wikle JS (1992) Joint complaints in psoriasis patients. Int J Dermatol 31:488–491
147. Zonneveld IM, Meinardi MM, Karlsmark T, et al. (1997) Ranitidine does not affect psoriasis: a multicenter, double-blind, placebo-controlled study. J Am Acad Dermatol 36:932–934

B Psoriatic Arthritis

Dafna D. Gladman

Contents

1 Introduction

Psoriatic arthritis (PsA) is an inflammatory arthritis associated with psoriasis, usually seronegative for rheumatoid factor [1]. It affects women and men at a similar rate, and the peak age of onset is around 36 years, although it may occur in childhood or older age. The arthritis usually follows the diagnosis of psoriasis by about 10 years. However, in 15% of the patients the arthritis and psoriasis begin simultaneously, and in an additional 15% the arthritis precedes the psoriasis by as long as 15 years [2]. The arthritis is described as inflammatory in nature, since it presents with pain and stiffness that is typically aggravated by rest and improves with activity, and manifests tenderness and swelling in the affected joints. Almost half the patients with PsA may have an inflammatory arthritis of the back as well, manifesting with pain and stiffness, particularly in the low back. Other typical features include enthesitis (inflammation at tendon insertion into bone) and dactylitis (inflammation of the whole digit).

Psoriatic arthritis was defined as an entity separate from rheumatoid arthritis (RA), which is the prototypical inflammatory arthritis, in the late 1950s based on work by the late Professor Verna Wright of Leeds, England. It was recognized as a specific entity by the American College of Rheumatology in 1964 [3]. While some still question whether PsA is a unique entity or the co-occurrence of an inflammatory arthritis with psoriasis, the epidemiological evidence showing that there is an increased frequency of inflammatory arthritis among patients with psoriasis and an increased frequency of psoriasis among patients with inflammatory arthritis, as well as the unique features of the disease, support its recognition as a unique entity [4].

2 Prevalence of PsA

The exact prevalence of PsA is unknown. Few epidemiological studies have been carried out (Table B1). Prevalence estimates have varied from 0.04% in the Faroe Islands, to 0.1% in the Mayo Clinic, to 1.2% in a Swedish study [5, 6]. A recent study from Greece estimated the prevalence for PsA at 0.05% [7]. However, like previous studies this study was based on physician diagnosis. One difficulty in estimating prevalence of PsA is the fact that the diagnosis may be missed [8]. Rheumatologists may miss the diagnosis of PsA when they fail to diagnose the presence of psoriasis in an individual presenting with an inflammatory arthritis. This occurs particularly in patients whose psoriasis is hidden in areas such the umbilicus, anal cleft, or behind the ears. At the same time, dermatologists may miss the presence of PsA, since patients with PsA may not complain of pain. Indeed, patients with PsA demonstrate less tenderness than patients with RA, whether on the most affected joint, fibromyalgia tender points or control sites [9]. Thus patients with PsA may present with joint destruction without previous complaints of pain. Similarly, the presence of sacroiliitis may be missed if radiographs are not obtained. The reported incidence rate of PsA has also varied from 3–8/100,000 [5, 10, 11]. In view of the diagnostic pitfalls described

Table B1. Clinical patterns in large series (>100 patients)

Feature	Roberts (1976) [42]	Kammer (1979) [43]	Gladman (1987) [2]	Scarpa (1989) [13]	Torre-Alonse (1991) [44]	Veale (1994) [23]	Jones (1994) [45]	Kane (2003) [46]
No. of patients	168	100	220	138	180	100	100	129
M/F	67/101	47/53	104/116	71/67	99/81	59/41	43/57	68/62
Age of onset (years)	36–45	33–45	37	40	39	34	37.6	40
Oligoarthritis (%)	53	54	14	13	37	43	26	40
Polyarthritis (%)	54	25	40	33	35	33	63	60
Distal (%)	17	?	12	9	0	16	1	NA
Back alone (%)	5	21	2	44	7	4	6	0
Mutilans (%)	5	?	16	1	4	2	4	0
Sacroiliitis (%)	?	?	27	?	20	15	6	17
Joints before skin (%)	16	30	17	?	15	?	18	?

above, both prevalence and incidence rates estimated to date may be underestimated.

The reported prevalence of arthritis among psoriatic patients has varied from 5% to 42%. The most commonly quoted frequencies are 7–10%. These figures were derived from a study in Sweden in 1948, based on inpatients with polyarthritis [12]. This study was performed before the description of PsA was widely accepted. More recent studies suggest that the prevalence of PsA among patients with psoriasis is about 30% [13, 14, 15]. These studies include assessment of skin and joints by dermatologists and rheumatologists, thus providing more reliable figures. Scarpa et al. found that 30% of the patients attending a psoriasis clinic had PsA [13]. Zachariea found that 30% of the members of the Nordic Psoriasis Association suffered from PsA [14]. Alenius et al. identified 97 of 202 patients with psoriasis (48%) as having inflammatory arthritis [15]. They also tested a psoriatic arthritis screening questionnaire which only provided 60% specificity and sensitivity and is thus not yet ready for wide-spread use. They point out that inflammatory arthritis is much more common among patients with psoriasis than previously thought. While it was initially believed that arthritis was more common among patients with severe psoriasis, the relationship between skin and joint manifestations has not been confirmed [16, 17].

Since the prevalence of psoriasis in the general population is 1–3%, based on the likelihood that a third of the patients will have psoriatic arthritis, the prevalence of PsA has likely been largely underestimated and should be between 0.3% and 1%. There are several reasons why PsA may be underestimated. First, there are no validated widely accepted classification or diagnostic criteria for this disease [4]. Second, as pointed out above, because of the lower level of tenderness, as well as the hidden psoriasis, the diagnosis of PsA may be missed by physicians and patients. Therefore, patients with psoriasis should be specifically questioned about joint pain, swelling, stiffness, and presence of joint deformities, as well as back pain, to determine whether they may have PsA.

3 Classification of PsA

PsA has been classified among the spondyloarthropathies because of the high frequency of spondyloarthritis, the presence of extra-articular features common to the spondyloarthropathies, and the association with HLA-B27 [1]. Moll and Wright described five clinical patterns in PsA: a distal pattern where the distal interphalangeal joints are involved; an oligoarticular pattern where four or less joints are affected; a polyarticular pattern, which may be indistinguishable from RA; a spondyloarthritis, affecting the sacroiliac joints as well as the apophyseal joints of the back; and arthritis mutilans, a severely deforming form of arthritis [1].

In the initial description of the clinical patterns of PsA, the oligoarticular pattern was the most common, occurring in 70% of the patients. The distal pattern and arthritis mutilans, though considered more specific for PsA, were uncommon, occurring in less than 5% each. However, subsequent studies have varied in terms of the relative frequency of the different patterns, with some authors not recognizing isolated distal joint disease and several noting that the polyarthritis was much more common [4]. This is likely due to the fact that with time there may be a change in pattern in patients with PsA, such that by the time patients had been followed for 10 years more than 50% have polyarticular disease [4, 18]. Although more than 40% of patients with PsA have evidence of inflammatory back disease, few patients have an isolated spondyloarthritis. The spondyloarthritis may be missed if radiographs are not obtained at the time of patient assessment, since patients with PsA may have asymptomatic back disease [19]. Arthritis mutilans may develop quickly in a patient with PsA without evidence of prior inflammation. Although these patterns were not meant to serve as either diagnostic or classification criteria, many clinicians and investigators have used them to diagnose patients or to define patients for clinical trials.

Because of the difficulties in using the patterns described by Moll and Wright, several attempts at providing better classification of patients with psoriasis and arthritis have been proposed. Gladman et al. devised a classification system based on the Moll and Wright patterns but set up such that each group was mutually exclusive [2]. They identified seven categories, including isolated DIP joint disease, oligoarticular pattern, polyarticular pattern, isolated spondyloarthritis, distal pattern with spondyloarthritis, oligoarticular pattern with spondyloarthritis and polyarticular pattern with spondyloarthritis. Since arthritis mutilans could occur in each of the settings, it was not considered a specific pattern, but could be identified by the presence of flail or ankylosed joints clinically or radiologically.

Seleznick et al. attempted to classify patients with psoriasis and an inflammatory arthritis in an objective manner [20]. They applied cluster analysis, a method which allows grouping of patients with similar sets of observations, to two cohorts of patients with PsA. There were 48 patients from the Stanford Clinic in the United States, and 218 patients from Leeds, England. Despite the fact that there were differences between the two groups, with the Stanford group showing more erosive disease, arthritis mutilans, DIP involvement and sacroiliitis, the analysis was done on the combined cohort of 266 patients. Thirteen clusters were identified primarily by articular manifestations, five of which included fewer than ten patients each. This analysis was not particularly helpful as it did not distinguish between patients with PsA and those with other types of inflammatory arthritis that may be associated with psoriasis.

A similar approach was more recently taken by Koó et al., who performed a hierarchical cluster analysis of data on 100 patients with psoriasis and inflammatory arthritis [21]. Their analysis identified 7 clusters: a distal form which included 8 patients with polyarthritis with DIP involvement and nail dystrophy in all and frequent dactylitis; an erythrodermal group of 8 patients who were not dissimilar to the first group, but had a history of erythroderma; a pustular group of 3 patients; oligoarticular group of 18 patients who had sacroiliitis and spondylitis as well as serious skin disease; RA-like arthritis I in 5 patients with mild psoriasis, symmetrical polyarthritis with dactylitis, positive rheumatoid factor and no evidence of

IV

spondylitis; RA-like arthritis II was defined in two rheumatoid factor positive patients, and likely represented patients with RA; a polyarticular group of 56 patients with asymmetric polyarthritis and mild psoriasis, a third of whom had evidence of spondylitis. This analysis was not particularly helpful as it did not distinguish specific groups of patients with mutually exclusive. Thus, the two cluster analyses did not identify mutually exclusive groups of patients and did not improve on the classification provided by Moll and Wright.

Helliwell et al. suggested that patients with psoriatic arthritis be classified as having a peripheral arthropathy, a spondyloarthropathy, and those with extra-articular osseous manifestations, such as the group with synovitis, acne, pustulosis, hyperostosis, and osteitis (the SAPHO syndrome) [22]. This classification may be too simplistic for psoriatic arthritis. Veale et al. also proposed reducing the number of classes of PsA to three: asymmetric oligoarthritis, symmetric polyarthritis, and spondyloarthritis [23]. However, it would be difficult to fit those patients who have an asymmetric polyarthritis, as well as those with a symmetric oligoarthritis, into this classification. Kane et al. recently highlighted the difficulty in defining patterns in patients with PsA who have been treated with disease modifying drugs [24]. They found that while the majority of their patients fit into the Veale classification of symmetric polyarthritis at presentation, at follow-up, following institution of drug therapy, most patients became oligoarticular. They suggest that the use of the clinical patterns in established disease is difficult [24]. Despite the fact that the clinical patterns described above are not diagnostic, they are relevant early in the course of the disease, and they do help differentiate PsA from other conditions.

Other attempts to classify psoriatic arthritis have been published. Bennet proposed provisional criteria for the diagnosis of psoriatic arthritis [25]. These included a mandatory criterion, namely the presence of psoriasis in association with pain and soft tissue swelling and/or limitation of motion in at least one joint observed by a physician for 6 weeks or longer, and the presence of six of ten supportive criteria (Table B2). These criteria have not been formally tested.

Table B2. Bennet criteria for psoriatic arthritis [25]

Mandatory criterion:

Psoriasis in association with pain and soft tissue swelling and/or limitation of motion in at least one joint observed by a physician for ≥6 weeks

Minor criteria:

1. Pain and soft tissue swelling and/or limitation of motion in ≥1 joint
2. An inflammatory arthritis in the DIP joints (excluding Heberden's or Bouchard's nodes)
3. Sausage fingers or toes
4. Asymmetric distribution of the arthritis in the hands and feet
5. Absence of rheumatoid nodules
6. Negative rheumatoid factor
7. Inflammatory synovial fluid with a normal or increased complement levels and an absence of infection or crystals
8. Synovial biopsy showing synovial lining hypertrophy with a predominantly mononuclear cell infiltrate
9. Peripheral radiographs showing an erosive arthritis of small joints with a relative lack of osteoporosis (excluding erosive osteoarthritis)
10. Axial radiographs showing one or more of: sacroiliitis, syndesmophytes or paravertebral calcifications

Vasey and Espinoza [26] proposed a classification comprised of just three criteria. The first was the presence of psoriasis. The second was the presence of peripheral arthritis, defined as the presence of pain and soft tissue swelling with or without limitation of motion in the DIP joints for at least 4 weeks; similar clinical features in other peripheral joints in an asymmetric distribution, including dactylitis; symmetric peripheral arthritis in the absence of rheumatoid factor or rheumatoid nodules; or radiological changes of pencil-in-cup, whittling of terminal phalanges, fluffy periostitis and bony ankylosis. The third criterion was spinal involvement, with spinal pain and stiffness, restriction of motion of the spine and radiological changes of sacroiliitis, either grade 2 symmetric or grade 3 or 4 asymmetric sacroiliitis.

This classification scheme has not been validated.

The European Spondyloarthropathy Study Group proposed preliminary criteria for the classification of spondyloarthropathy [27]. These criteria were developed for the spondyloarthropathies and were based on statistical analysis and clinical reasoning of 25 clinical features analysed in 403 patients considered to have a spondyloarthropathy, and 674 control patients with other rheumatic diseases. The resultant criteria include: the presence of inflammatory spinal pain or synovitis in the presence of one of the following: family history of a spondyloarthropathy, psoriasis, inflammatory bowel disease, alternating buttock pain, enthesopathy, acute diarrhea, urethritis, and radiological evidence of sacroiliitis. While the criteria were sensitive in identifying 100% of patients with inflammatory bowel disease, they had a sensitivity of 93.6% for ankylosing spondylitis, and only 81.6% in psoriatic arthritis. In a subsequent test of these criteria in Alaskan Eskimo population the sensitivity was 88.5% and specificity 89.3%. There was only one patient with psoriatic arthritis in that population. The ESSG criteria were found to be only 65% sensitive for psoriatic arthritis [28].

Fournier et al. conducted a retrospective case-control study of 260 patients, of whom 100 had psoriatic arthritis, 80 had ankylosing spondylitis and 80 had rheumatoid arthritis [29]. Data were obtained from chart review. Based on an initial bivariate chi square analysis, 11 variables were identified and used in both discriminant and logistic regression analyses. The results of both analyses yielded the same 9 variables, each receiving weights based on coefficients: psoriasis antedating or concomitant with joint disease (6 points); family history of psoriasis (3 points, to be counted only if the first criterion was not met); arthritis of a DIP joint (3 points); inflammatory involvement of the cervical or thoracic spine (3 points); asymmetric monoarthritis or oligarthritis (1 point); buttock pain, heel pain, spontaneous anterior chest wall pain or diffuse inflammatory pain in the entheses (2 points); radiological digit criteria (5 points); HLA antigen B16 or B17 (6 points); a negative rheumatoid factor (4 points). Based on receiver operative curves the logistic regression suggested that achieving 11 points provided sensitivity of 95% and specificity of 98%, while the discriminant analysis identified 13 points with a sensitivity of 95% and a specificity of 93%. These criteria have yet to be validated in another set of patients.

An international group, CASPAR (ClASsification of Psoriatic ARthritis), under the leadership of Dr. Philip Helliwell of Leeds, England, has been collecting PsA patients and controls to establish classification and diagnostic criteria. The CASPAR study will be able to compare these classification criteria and develop widely accepted classification criteria. Once these are available, proper epidemiological studies of incidence and prevalence may be performed.

4 Differentiating PsA from Other Inflammatory Forms of Arthritis

PsA needs to be differentiated from RA, the prototypical inflammatory arthritis. This is particularly important since patients with rheumatoid arthritis may have concomitant psoriasis. There are clinical and radiological differences between PsA and RA (Table B3). RA affects women much more commonly than men. PsA affects both genders equally. Clinically, the joint distribution is different, particularly in early disease. RA tends to be a symmetrical arthritis, affecting small, medium and large joints bilaterally. It tends to spare the distal interphalangeal joints. PsA tends to be asymmetric, and tends to affect all the joints in one digit, in a "ray" distribution, rather than the same groups of joints on both sides. Joints affected by PsA may present with a reddish purplish color, which is unusual in RA [30]. As noted above, patients with PsA have less tenderness than patients with RA on their most affected joint, on fibromyalgia tender points and on control points [9]. About 40–50% of patients with PsA have a spondyloarthritis in addition to their peripheral arthritis. With the exception of cervical involvement, the spine is generally spared in RA.

Table B3. Differentiating psoriatic arthritis from rheumatoid arthritis

Features	Psoriatic arthritis	Rheumatoid arthritis
Gender distribution M:F	1:1.1	1:3
Age at onset	36–40	30–50
Joint distribution	Asymmetric	Symmetric
Distal joint involvement	Common	Uncommon
Pattern of involvement	All joints of one digit "ray"	All joints of the same level
Spinal involvement	Common	Rare
Rheumatoid nodules	Never	Common
Nail lesions	Common	Uncommon
Psoriasis	Almost always	Uncommon
HLA associations	HLA-B*27, B*17, C*0602	HLA-DRB1*04

PsA is differentiated from the other spondyloarthropathies by the presence of marked inflammatory arthritis, and the presence of psoriasis and nail lesions. The spondyloarthritis of PsA is not as severe as AS with regard to symptoms of back pain and stiffness, as well as radiological features. In PsA there is often an asymmetric sacroiliitis, and asymmetric syndesmophytes which often skip vertebrae and are not associated with as much limitation of movement in the back [31].

5 Disease Severity in PsA

While the initial description of PsA by Moll and Wright suggested that the disease was mostly oligoarticular, and thus less severe than RA, and a more recent study from the Mayo clinic supported the concept of PsA as mild disease [32], other studies suggest that the majority of patients have polyarticular involvement. Polyarticular presentation has been shown to be associated with worse outcome, both in terms of clinical damage and radiological damage [33, 34]. It is clear that as patients are followed for prolonged periods of time they tend to progress to polyarticular disease [18, 35]. This observation is important since patients with PsA had not been treated aggressively until the early 1980s.

Both clinical and genetic factors predict progression of clinical damage [33, 36]. Clinical damage has been defined by the presence of deformities, flail joints, and ankylosis. For this analysis, states of damage based on the number of joints involved were identified as follows: state 1: no damaged joints; state 2: one to four damaged joints; state 3: five to nine damaged joints; and state 4: ten or more damaged joints. In a study of 305 PsA patients with fewer than 10 damaged joints at presentation to clinic, 5 or more swollen joints and a high previous medication level at presentation predicted progression of joint damage through the states of the damage, whereas a low erythrocyte sedimentation rate (ESR) was protective of progression of damage [33]. When HLA antigens present in these patients were added to this model, HLA-B22 was found to be protective. The presence of HLA-B27 in association with HLA-DR7, HLA-B39 and HLA-DQw3 in the absence of HLA-DR7 were predictive of progression of damage [37].

In a subsequent study that included variables that changed over time, the presence of an actively inflamed joint (tenderness, stress pain, and/or swelling) at any visit was shown to increase the risk of progression of joint damage on a subsequent clinic visit by 4% [38]. Functional status and a higher degree of damage detected at each visit also predicted further progression of joint damage. Importantly, this study suggests that a patient with 20 tender joints (comparable to the typical baseline number in drug trials) has an 80% risk of progression of clinical damage within a 6-month trial. Although a recent study failed to identify the importance of HLA-B27 in prognosis of PsA, that study included a small number of patients who were not followed prospectively [34].

6 Mortality in PsA

PsA has been associated with increased mortality compared with the general population. A study of 428 patients followed in a PsA clinic showed that there was an increased mortality risk of 1.62 overall, 1.59 for women and 1.65 for men [39]. While the causes of death are similar to the general population, predictors for early mortality included severe disease at presentation, as defined by a higher damage score count and a higher medication level at presentation to clinic [40].

7 Remission in PsA

Not all patients with PsA fare poorly. Among patients followed prospectively in a longitudinal observational cohort of 514 patients with PsA, 69 (17.6%) patients achieved remission, defined as the absence of actively inflamed joints for a period of 12 months [41]. The period of remission lasted 2.6 years on the average. Thirty-six (52%) of the patients went on the flare after this period of remission, and six patients achieved a complete remission, with no actively inflamed or damaged joints and taking no medications. Male patients and patients with fewer affected joints at presentation had a higher likelihood of achieving remission.

8 Conclusion

Psoriatic arthritis has been defined as an inflammatory arthritis associated with psoriasis. Its exact prevalence is unknown, and current estimates of prevalence and incidence are likely under estimated. While many patients with PsA do well, there is a group of patients who have severe disease, with progression of damage and increased mortality. An international effort currently underway should provide classification criteria, which can then be applied to epidemiological studies to further assess prevalence and outcome in this disease.

References

1. Wright V, Moll JMH (1976) Psoriatic arthritis. In: Seronegative polyarthritis. North Holland, Amsterdam, pp 169–223
2. Gladman DD, Shuckett R, Russell ML, Thorne JC, Schachter RK (1987) Psoriatic arthritis – clinical and laboratory analysis of 220 patients. Q J Med 62: 127–141
3. Blumberg BS, Bunim JJ, Calkins E, Pirani CL, Zvaifler NJ (1964) ARA nomenclature and classification of arthritis and rheumatism (tentative). Arthritis Rheum 7: 93–97
4. Gladman DD (1995) Psoriatic arthritis. In: Classification and assessment of rheumatic disease, part 1. In: Silman AJ, Symmons DPM (eds) Baillière's clinical rheumatology. International practice and research. Baillière's Tindall, London, pp 319–329
5. Bruce IN (2003) Psoriatic arthritis clinical features. In: Hochberg M, Silman A, Smolen J, Weinblatt M, Weiseman M (eds) Rheumatology. Mosby, St. Louis, pp 1241–1253
6. Hellgren L (1969) Association between rheumatoid arthritis and psoriasis in total populations. Acta Rheumatol Scand 15: 316–326
7. Alamanos Y, Papadopoulos NG, Voulgari PV, Siozos C, Psychos DN, Tympanidou M, Drosos AA (2003) Epidemiology of psoriatic arthritis in northwest Greece, 1982–2001. J Rheumatol 30: 2641–2644
8. Gorter S, van der Heijde DM, van der LS, Houben H, Rethans JJ, Scherpbier AJ, van der Vleuten CP (2002) Psoriatic arthritis: performance of rheumatologists in daily practice. Ann Rheum Dis 61: 219–224
9. Buskila D, Langevitz P, Gladman DD, Urowitz S, Smythe H (1992) Patients with rheumatoid arthritis are more tender than those with psoriatic arthritis. J Rheumatol 19: 1115–1119
10. Savolainen E, Kaipiainen-Seppanen O, Kroger L, Luosujarvi R (2003) Total incidence and distribution of inflammatory joint diseases in a defined population: results from the Kuopio 2000 arthritis survey. J Rheumatol 30: 2460–2468

11. Soderlin MK, Borjesson O, Kautiainen H, Skogh T, Leirisalo-Repo M (2002) Annual incidence of inflammatory joint diseases in a population based study in southern Sweden. Ann Rheum Dis 61: 911–915
12. Leczinsky CG (1948) The incidence of arthropathy in a ten-year series of psoriasis cases. Acta Derm Venereol 28:483–487
13. Scarpa R, Oriente P, Pucino A, Torella M, Vignone L, Riccio A, Biondi Oriente C (1984) Psoriatic arthritis in psoriatic patients. Br J Rheumatol 23:246–250
14. Zachariae H (2003) Prevalence of joint disease in patients with psoriasis: implications for therapy. Am J Clin Dermatol 4:441–447
15. Alenius GM, Stenberg B, Stenlund H, Lundblad M, Dahlqvist SR (2002) Inflammatory joint manifestations are prevalent in psoriasis: prevalence study of joint and axial involvement in psoriatic patients, and evaluation of a psoriatic and arthritic questionnaire. J Rheumatol 29:2577–2582
16. Cohen MR, Reda DJ, Clegg DO (1999) Baseline relationships between psoriasis and psoriatic arthritis: analysis of 221 patients with active psoriatic arthritis. J Rheumatol 26:1752–1756
17. Elkayam O, Ophir J, Yaron M, Caspi D (2000) Psoriatic arthritis: interrelationships between skin and joint manifestations related to onset, course and distribution. Clin Rheumatol 19:301–305
18. McHugh NJ, Balachrishnan C, Jones SM (2003) Progression of peripheral joint disease in psoriatic arthritis: a 5-yr prospective study. Rheumatology (Oxford) 42:778–783
19. Khan M, Schentag C, Gladman DD (2003) Clinical and radiological changes during psoriatic arthritis disease progression. J Rheumatol 30:1022–1026
20. Seleznick M, Feigenbaum P, Wright V, Fries J (1985) Psoriatic arthritis subsets: a cluster analysis. In: Brooks PM, York JR (eds) Rheumatology. Elsevier Science, Amsterdam, pp 309–312
21. Koó É, Nagy Z, Seszták M, Ujfalussy I, Merétey K, Böhm U, Forgács S, Szilágyi M, Czirják L, Farkas V (2001) Subsets in psoriatic arthritis formed by cluster analysis. Clin Rheum 20:36–43
22. Helliwell P, Marchesoni A, Peters M, Barker M, Wright V (1991) A re-evaluation of the osteoarticular manifestations of psoriasis. Br J Rheumatol 30: 339–345
23. Veale D, Rogers S, Fitzerald O (1994) Classification of clinical subsets in psoriatic arthritis. Br J Rheumatol 33:133–138
24. Kane D, Stafford L, Bresnihan B, FitzGerald O (2003) A classification study of clinical subsets in an inception cohort of early psoriatic peripheral arthritis – 'DIP or not DIP revisited'. Rheumatology (Oxford) 42:1469–1476
25. Bennet RM (1979) Psoriatic arthritis. In: McCarty DJ (ed) Arthritis and related conditions. Lea & Febiger, Philadelphia, p 645
26. Vasey F, Espinoza LR (1984) Psoriatic arthropathy. In: Calin A (ed) Spondyloarthropathies. Grune and Stratton, Orlando, FL, pp 166–167
27. Dougados M, van der Linden S, Juhlin R, Huitfeldt B, Amor B, Calin A, Cats A, Dijkmans B, Olivieri I, Pasero G (1991) The European Spondylarthropathy Study Group preliminary criteria for the classification of spondylarthropathy. Arthritis Rheum 34: 1218–1227
28. Salvarani C, Lo Scocco G, Macchioni P, Cremonesi T, Rossi F, Mantovani W, Battistel B, Bisighini G, Portioli I (1995) Prevalence of psoriatic arthritis in Italian psoriatic patients. J Rheumatol 22:1499–1503
29. Fournie B, Crognier L, Arnaud C, Zabraniecki L, Lascaux-Lefebvre V, Marc V Ginesty E, Andrieu V, Dromer C, Fournie A (1999) Proposed classification criteria of psoriatic arthritis. A preliminary study in 260 patients. Rev Rheum Engl Ed 66:446–456
30. Jajic J (2001) Blue-coloured skin over involved joints in psoriatic arthritis. Clin Rheumatol 20: 304–305
31. Gladman DD, Brubacher B, Buskila D, Langevitz P, Farewell VT (1993) Differences in the expression of spondyloarthropathy: a comparison between ankylosing spondylitis and psoriatic arthritis. Genetic and gender effects. Clin Invest Med 16:1–7
32. Shbeeb M, Uramoto KM, Gibson LE, O'Fallon WM, Gabriel SE (2000) The epidemiology of psoriatic arthritis in Olmsted County, Minnesota, USA, 1982–1991. J Rheumatol 27:1247–1250
33. Gladman DD, Farewell VT, Nadeau C (1995) Clinical indicators of progression in psoriatic arthritis (PSA): multivariate relative risk model. J Rheumatol 22:675–679
34. Queiro-Silva R, Torre-Alonso JC, Tinture-Eguren T, Lopez-Lagunas I (2003) A polyarticular onset predicts erosive and deforming disease in psoriatic arthritis. Ann Rheum Dis 62:68–70
35. Gladman DD (1994) The natural history of psoriatic arthritis. In: Wright V, Helliwell P (eds) Psoriatic arthritis. Baillière's clinical rheumatology. International practice and research. Baillière's Tindall, London, pp 379–394
36. Gladman DD, Farewell VT (1995) The role of HLA antigens as indicators of progression in psoriatic arthritis (PsA): multivariate relative risk model. Arthritis Rheum 38:845–850
37. Gladman DD, Farewell VT, Kopciuk K, Cook RJ (1998) HLA antigens and progression in psoriatic arthritis. J Rheumatol 25:730–733
38. Gladman DD, Farewell VT (1999) Progression in psoriatic arthritis: Role of time varying clinical indicators. J Rheumatol 26:2409–2413
39. Wong K, Gladman DD, Husted J, Long J, Farewell VT (1997) Mortality studies in psoriatic arthritis. Results from a single centre. I. Risk and causes of death. Arthritis Rheum 40:1868–1872
40. Gladman DD, Farewell VT, Husted J, Wong K (1998) Mortality studies in psoriatic arthritis. Results from a single centre. II. Prognostic indicators for mortality. Arthritis Rheum 41:1103–1110
41. Gladman DD, Ng Tung Hing E, Schentag CT, Cook R (2001) Remission in psoriatic arthritis. J Rheumatol 28:1045–1048

42. Roberts MET, Wright V, Hill AGS, Mehra AC (1976) Psoriatic arthritis: A follow-up study. Ann Rheum Dis 35:206–219
43. Kammer GM, Soter NA, Gibson DJ, Schur PH (1979) Psoriatic arthritis. A clinical, immunologic and HLA study of 100 patients. Semin Arthritis Rheum 9:75–97
44. Torre-Alonso JC, Rodriguez-Perez A, Arribas-Castrillo JM, et al. (1991) Psoriatic arthritis (PA): a clinical, immunological and radiological study of 180 patients. Br J Rheumatol 30:245
45. Jones SM, Armas JB, Cohen MG, Lovell C, Evison G, McHugh NJ (1994) Psoriatic arthritis: outcome of disease subsets and relationship of joint disease to nail and skin disease. Br J Rheumatol 33:834
46. Kane D, Stafford L, Bresniham B, Fitzgerald O (2003) A prospective, clinical and radiological study of early psoriatic arthritis: an early synovitis clinic experience. Rheumatology 42:1460–1468

Clinical Presentation V

A Psoriasis

Jennifer Soung, Mark Lebwohl

Contents

1 Introduction

The clinical manifestations of psoriasis and its variants have been described for over two centuries. The diagnosis is typically made by the recognition of the classic and distinctive lesions – well-demarcated erythematous plaques with adherent silvery scales. The most frequent areas of involvement include the elbows, knees, lower back, and buttocks but the disease can involve any cutaneous surface. Therefore, the evaluation of psoriasis should include a careful examination for the presence of lesions involving other areas including the perineum, scalp, nails, intertriginous areas, and genitalia. The disease varies widely in severity and extent of involvement as some patients present with a few isolated plaques and others can have complete coverage of their body surface. Variations in the morphology of psoriasis have been classified into several clinical subtypes, which will be described in the following section in further detail. Because psoriasis is usually a chronic, relapsing disease, it is important to appreciate that the clinical appearance is rarely stagnant and the lesions continually evolve [16].

2 Types of Psoriasis

Plaque Psoriasis

More than 80% of patients who present with psoriasis have plaque psoriasis, also known as psoriasis vulgaris. The classic lesions are well circumscribed erythematous circular or ovoid plaques with adherent silvery scales (Fig. A1). Although psoriasis can affect any cutaneous surface, patients usually present as young adults with symmetric involvement of the extensor surfaces of the lower and upper extremities, gluteal cleft (Fig. A2), scalp and nailplates [13].

The lesions may begin as red, scaling papules that eventually evolve to form round-oval plaques, which can be easily differentiated from the surrounding normal skin. The plaques vary from a pink to red color and are usually covered by a thick silvery scale. The thickness of the scale can be quite variable depending on the site of involvement – extremely dense in the scalp and more dispersed in the intertriginous areas. The diameter of the lesions can range

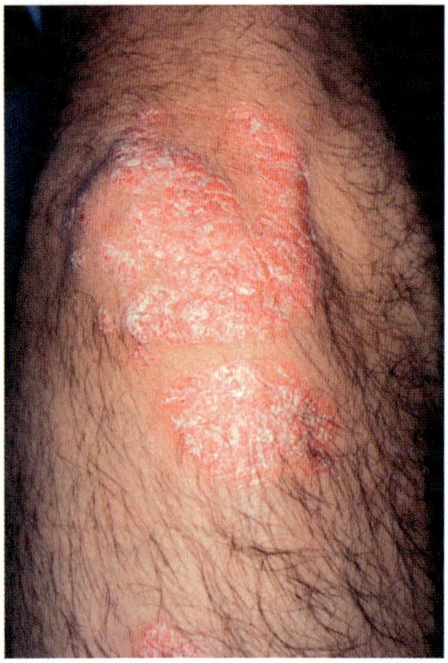

Fig. A1. Note the sharply demarcated erythematous scaling oval plaques that typically affect the extensor surfaces

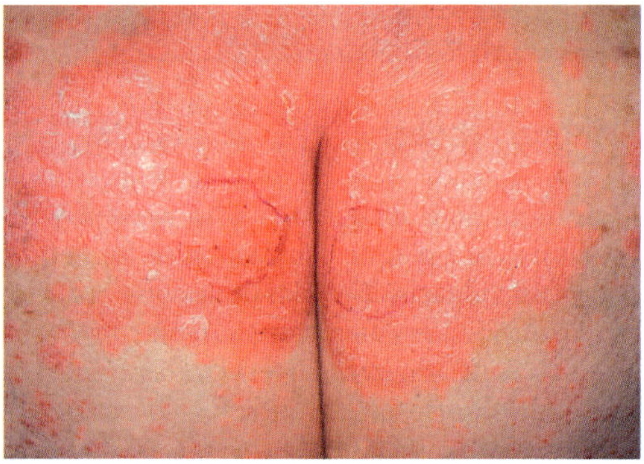

Fig. A2. Classic plaque psoriasis of the intergluteal cleft

from less than 1 cm to more than 10 cm. Small bleeding points may occur when the tightly adherent scales are removed from the surface of the plaque. This commonly noted clinical sign of psoriasis is called Auspitz sign and is neither sensitive nor specific for psoriasis [1].

Psoriasis is well known to develop at sites of physical trauma (scratching, sunburn or surgery), the isomorphic or Koebner's phenomenon [7]. The disease affects the extensor surfaces more than the flexor surfaces and usually spares the palms, soles and face. Although some patients are asymptomatic, approximately half of patients consider pruritus as the most distressing symptom [11].

Guttate Psoriasis

Guttate psoriasis refers to the acute onset of generalized multiple small papules. This morphology most commonly affects children, adolescents, and young adults with no previous history of psoriasis but may also occur as an acute exacerbation of pre-existing plaque psoriasis. In many instances, an episode of guttate psoriasis is a sign of the patient's predisposition to develop generalized plaque psoriasis. Often, a history of streptococcal infection precedes this eruption by 1 or 2 weeks [15, 19].

The lesions in guttate psoriasis are easily distinguished as a distinct form of psoriasis. They are small, usually less than 1 cm in diameter, uniformly erythematous or pink papules with slightly less scale and induration than chronic lesions of plaque psoriasis (Fig. A3).

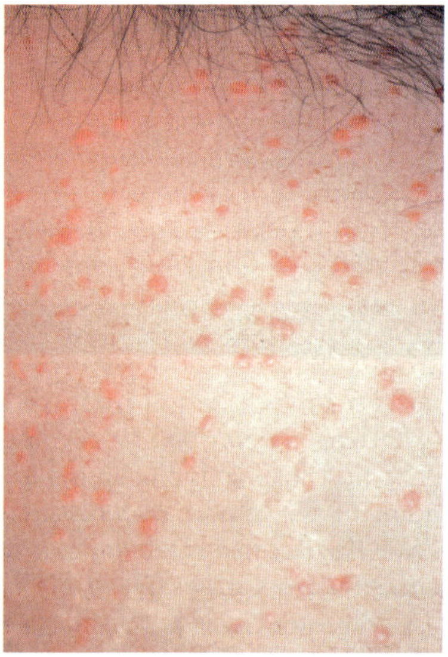

Fig. A3. Guttate psoriasis. Multiple uniform small (less than 1 cm in diameter) lesions with less scale and induration compared to psoriasis vulgaris. Numerous papules appear abruptly on the trunk and extremities following recent streptococcal infection

These lesions tend to enlarge rapidly while remaining as single lesions and are generally found in crops on the trunk, buttocks, hips and extremities. The appearance of the guttate form with many small lesions may resemble other cutaneous conditions like pityriasis rosea or secondary syphilis.

Pustular Psoriasis

Unlike most psoriatic patients, those with this rare form of psoriasis (also called *von Zumbusch psoriasis*) can be systemically ill. The disease typically occurs in patients who have antecedent nonpustular psoriasis or a genetic predisposition and have recently withdrawn from systemic corticosteroids.

Pustular psoriasis is the most severe form of psoriasis and can be life-threatening. In the generalized form, the trunk and extremities are covered with sterile pustules arising from the surface of large erythematous patches of skin (Fig. A4). The pustules on the affected skin eventually dry and peel. This condition results in a loss of the protective functions of the skin. In extremely ill patients, these pustules rapidly enlarge and become confluent, forming lakes of pus. Systemic symptoms include fever, diarrhea, arthralgias and chills.

Less severe and localized variants of pustular psoriasis can occur on the palms and soles. This form is also known as palmar-plantar pustulosis. Patients with this type of psoriasis are typically females 50–70 years of age. Palmar or plantar pustules develop which then turn dark brown and crust over creating a tender and diffusely eroded surface (Fig. A5). Although not life-threatening, this subtype can be particularly frustrating since affected patients have difficulty walking or using their hands. Patients with palmoplantar psoriasis experience greater functional and social disability than patients with psoriasis located elsewhere on the body [17]. A specific form of palmar plantar pustolosis is acrodermatitis continuea. These pustules are located on the fingertips or toes and are very painful and disabling. A final localized form of pustular psoriasis is often seen during an acute flare of psoriasis vulgaris as pustules on the surface of plaque type psoriasis.

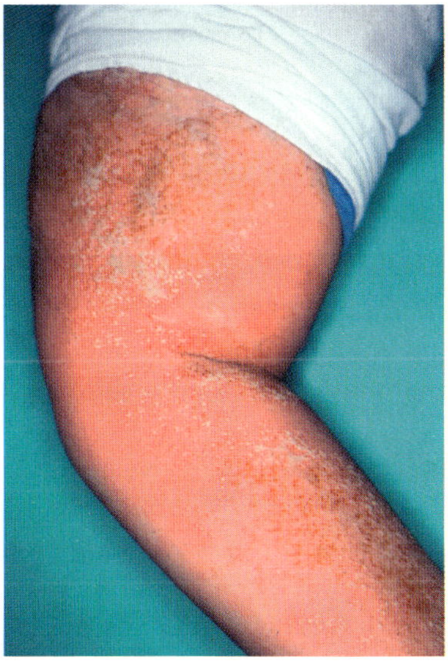

Fig. A4. Pustular psoriasis. Crops of sterile pustules arising on the surface of erythematous plaques cover the extremities

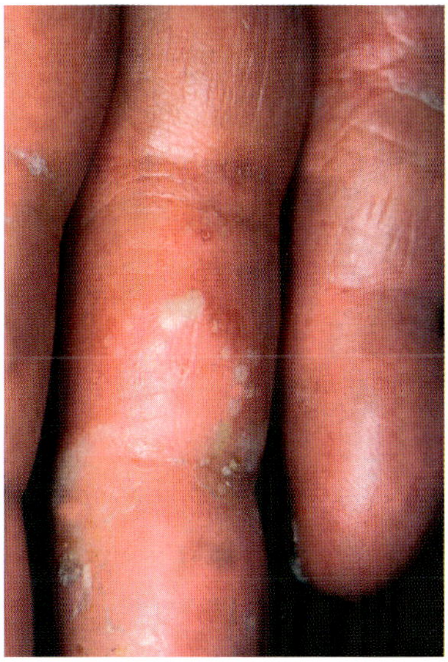

Fig. A5. Pustular psoriasis. Sterile yellow pustules on the digits

Inverse Psoriasis

This clinical subtype of psoriasis occurs in the flexural creases of the inguinal areas, submammary folds, gluteal fold, retroauricular fold, axillae, groin and genital regions. The presentation is the reverse of the classical presentation on extensor surfaces. Inverse psoriasis frequently occurs in patients who are obese.

Lesions of inverse psoriasis are smooth with no visible scaling, unlike classical plaque psoriasis (Fig. A6). These deep red, well-demarcated plaques frequently contain moist white debris and extend to and stop at the junction of the skin folds. Infection, friction and heat may induce psoriasis in these flexural creases, a manifestation of the Koebner phenomenon. In the absence of visible scaling, this variant can be easily misdiagnosed as a fungal infection or erythrasma (a chronic superficial infection of the intertriginous areas of the skin) [8].

Erythrodermic Psoriasis

Erythrodermic psoriasis is an acute, severe form of psoriasis characterized by generalized inflamed erythema and widespread scaling which affects more than 90% of the body surface area (Fig. A7). Like pustular psoriasis, the most common precipitating cause of erythrodermic form is withdrawal of systemic steroids and patients are usually systemically ill with fever, chills, rigors and arthralgias [2].

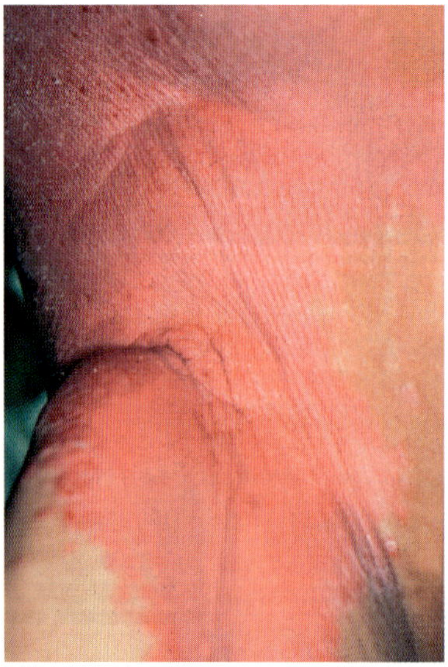

Fig. A6. Inverse psoriasis of the axilla. Note the absence of visible scales

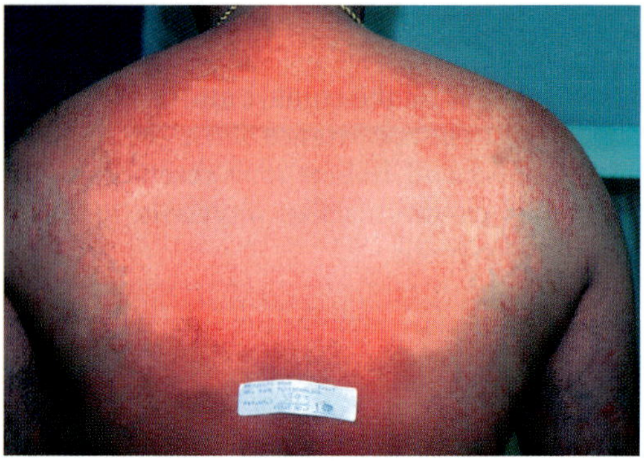

Fig. A7. Erythrodermic psoriasis. Note the inflamed red erythema of the plaque surface

Patients usually suffer from extensive desquamation and generalized inflamed erythema resulting in a loss of the protective function of the skin. Multiple medical complications can develop including loss of the skin's ability to protect against infection, to maintain electrolyte balance, and to control body temperature. Therefore, loss of this barrier function making death from sepsis a well-known complication of erythrodermic psoriasis [6].

3 Specific Locations of Psoriasis

Although psoriasis favors certain areas, there are several other locations that should be examined in patients in whom the diagnosis of psoriasis is suspected. Nail involvement is characteristic of psoriasis and aids in diagnosis when characteristic skin changes are equivocal or absent. Psoriatic nail changes may occur alone but rarely in the absence of other cutaneous disease. Nail changes can affect some or all of the fingernails or toenails and may extend to the entire nail including the proximal and lateral nail folds and the hyponychium.

The most common stigma of nail psoriasis is pitting – few to multiple tiny punched-out depressions on the nail plate surface. These pits result from psoriatic involvement of the nail matrix producing abnormal nail plate growth. Psoriasis of the nail bed can also cause separation of the nail from the nail matrix, referred to as onycholysis. These changes can then result in a nail losing its structural integrity and thick crumbling nails which can resemble a fungal infection (Fig. A8). In addition, a specific localized color change in the nail may occur that resembles the tan-brown color of new motor oil, the "oil drop sign" (Fig. A9). Nail involvement with psoriasis can be the most troublesome aspect for patients who relate significant quality of life issues [12].

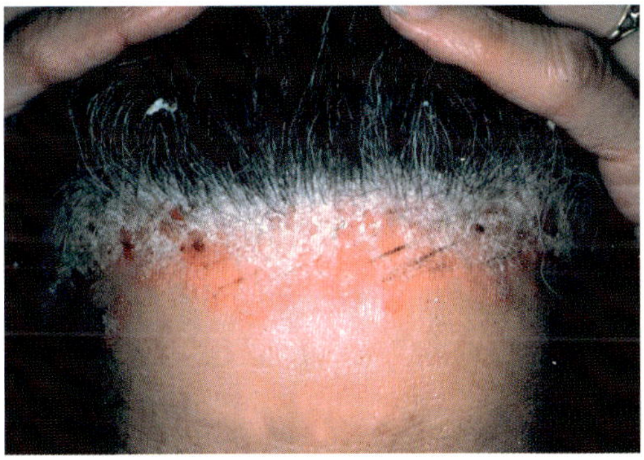

Fig. A8. Scalp psoriasis. Sharply defined plaques characterized by erythema and silvery scale

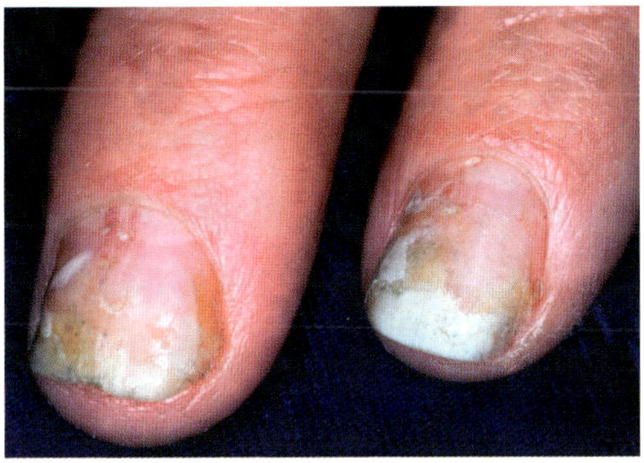

Fig. A9. Onycholysis of the nails. Psoriatic involvement of the nail matrix results in poorly formed nails

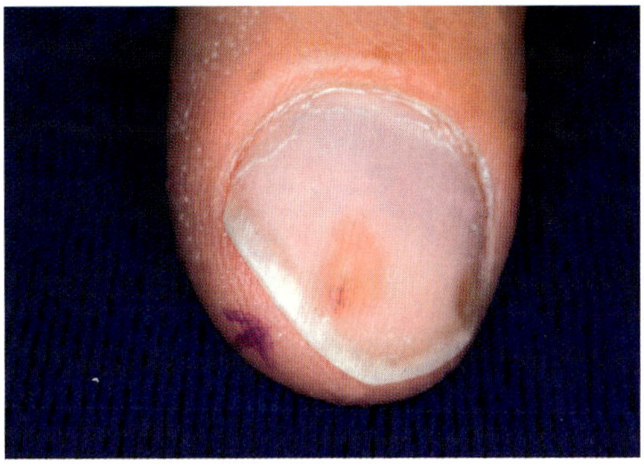

Fig. A10. Psoriasis of the nails. The "oil drop" sign

Psoriasis of the scalp is a common site of plaques similar to those of the skin except that the scale is more adherent (Fig. A10). Some individuals develop psoriasis on the palms and soles as the only sites involved or before other regions are affected. The patterns of presentation on the palms and soles can vary from superficial red plaques with thick brown scale to smooth, deep red plaques such as those found in the flexural areas. Uncommonly, psoriasis can also affect the oral mucosa [4].

4 Keratoderma Blennorrhagicum (Reiter's Syndrome)

Patients with Reiter's syndrome, a reactive immune response characterized by urethritis and/or cervicitis, peripheral arthritis of more than 1 month's duration, can develop psoriasiform skin lesions 1–2 months after the onset of arthritis. The distinctive lesions, known as keratoderma blennorrhagica, appear on the soles, toes, legs, scalp and hands. The psoriasiform plaque has distinctive circular scaly borders that develop from fusion of papulovesicular plaques with thickened yellow scale. Similar variants of psoriasis can be found on the penis (balanitis circinata).

5 Conclusion

Recognition of the variation in the clinical presentations of psoriasis is important for many reasons. First, some forms of psoriasis such as pustular or erythrodermic psoriasis can be life-threatening and must be managed aggressively. Second, different forms of psoriasis respond differently to different treatments. For example, mild topical corticosteroids or topical immunomodulators are highly effective in inverse psoriasis but much less effective on thick plaques of the elbows or knees. Similarly, guttate psoriasis often responds well to phototherapy with ultraviolet B, at times giving long remissions that are not as easily achieved with a typical patient who has generalized plaque psoriasis. Finally, as the genetic basis of psoriasis is better understood, it will be interesting to see if different forms of the disease correspond to variations in genetic susceptibility or to differences in gene expression. As we get closer to the identification of genetic defects in psoriasis, variations in the clinical manifestations of the disease may be easier to understand and lead to better therapeutic outcomes.

References

1. Bernhard JD (1990) Auspitz sign is not sensitive or specific for psoriasis. J Am Acad Dermatol 22: 1079–1081
2. Boyd AS, Menter A (1989) Erythrodermic psoriasis. J Am Acad Dermatol 21:985
3. Brockbank JE, Schentag C, Rosen C, Gladman DD (2001) Psoriatic arthritis (PsA) is common among patients with psoriasis and family medicine clinical attendees. Arthritis Rheum 44:S94
4. Bruce AJ (2003) Oral psoriasis. Dermatol Clin 21: 99–104
5. Christophers E, Kiene P (1995) Guttate and plaque psoriasis. Dermatol Clin 13:751–752
6. Green MS, Prystowsky JH, Cohen SR, Cohen JI, Lebwohl MG (1996) Infectious complications of erythrodermic psoriasis. J Am Acad Dermatol 34:911–914
7. Habif TP (1996) Clinical dermatology: Diagnosis and therapy. Mosby-Year Book, St. Louis, pp 190–201
8. Holdiness MR (2002) Erythrasma and common bacterial skin infections. Am Fam Physician 67:254
9. Jones SM, Armas JB, Cohen MG, Lovell CR, Evison G, McHugh NJ (1994) Psoriatic arthritis: outcome of disease subsets and relationship of joint disease to nail and skin disease. Br J Rheumatol 33:834
10. Kane D, Greaney T, Bresnihan B, Gibney R, FitzGerald O (1999) Ultrasonography in the diagnosis and management of psoriatic dactylitis. J Rheumatol 26:1746
11. Koo J (1996) Population-based epidemiologic study of psoriasis with emphasis on quality of life assessment. Dermatol Clin 14:485–496
12. Larko O (1995) Problem sites: scalp, palm and sole, and nails. Dermatol Clin 13:771–773
13. Lebwohl MG (2003) Psoriasis. Lancet 361:1197–1204
14. Moll JM, Wright V (1973) Psoriatic arthritis. Semin Arthritis Rheum 3:55–78
15. Naldi L (2001) Family history of psoriasis, stressful life events, and recent infectious disease are risk factors for a first episode of acute guttate psoriasis: results of a case-control study. J Am Acad Dermatol 44:433–438
16. Nevitt GJ, Hutchinson PE (1996) Psoriasis in the community: prevalence, severity and patients' beliefs and attitudes towards the disease. Br J Dermatol 135:533–537
17. Pettey AA, Balkrishnan R, Rapp SR, Fleischer AB, Feldman SR (2003) Patients with palmoplantar psoriasis have more physical disability and discomfort than patients with other forms of psoriasis: implications for clinical practice. J Am Acad Dermatol 49:271–275
18. Ruderman EM (2003) Evaluation and management of psoriatic arthritis: The role of biologic therapy. J Am Acad Dermatol 49:125–132
19. Telfer NR, Chalmers RJ, Whale K, Coleman G (1992) The role of streptococcal infection in the initiation of guttate psoriasis. Arch Dermatol 128:39
20. Winchester R (1995) Psoriatic arthritis. Dermatol Clin 13:779–784

B Psoriatic Arthritis

Philip S. Helliwell

Contents

1 Introduction

Until the late 1950s, arthritis occurring coincidentally with psoriasis was thought to be rheumatoid arthritis, although certain differences were acknowledged. The pioneering work of Wright and Baker clarified and defined these differences [1]. Wright described the frequent involvement of the distal interphalangeal joints (DIP) with erosion and absorption of the terminal phalanges and frequent reduction of bone stock in the other digits leading to a mutilating form of arthritis. Wright also described sacroiliitis and spondylitis occurring alone and in association with the peripheral arthritis. The distinction between rheumatoid arthritis and psoriatic arthritis was supported by the absence of rheumatoid factor in the blood of patients with psoriatic arthritis.

Wright and Moll first fully defined the concept of the seronegative spondyloarthropathies as a group of disorders sharing common clinical features, including (as a hallmark feature) sacroiliitis, a seronegative anodular asymmetrical peripheral oligoarthritis, a hyperkeratotic and sometimes pustular rash on the hands and soles (keratoderma blennorrhagica), peripheral and central enthesitis, anterior uveitis and familial aggregation [2]. The discovery of the high prevalence of HLA-B27 in ankylosing spondylitis and other diseases in this group provided confirmation of this concept [3]. Diseases within this group include ankylosing spondylitis, reactive arthritis, the arthritis of inflammatory bowel disease and psoriatic arthritis. Although psoriatic arthritis as a disease fit very well into the spondyloarthropathy group, a lack of validated classification criteria has hampered further clinical, immunological, and genetic research into this disorder [4].

2 Epidemiology

Precise figures for psoriatic arthritis in patients with psoriasis are not available. Most surveys have been carried out on populations of people with psoriasis seen in secondary care where the prevalence has been found to be as high as 39%, although prevalences of 5–8% for secondary care patients are more commonly described [5]. More recent figures are available from community surveys in England, where 14.4% of psoriasis patients had arthritis using a validated questionnaire; the adjusted prevalence rate for psoriatic arthritis in the community as a whole was 0.3% [6]. Further figures have come from the unique data available in Olmstead County, Minnesota, where Shbeeb and colleagues found a prevalence rate of 0.1% and an incidence rate of 6.59/100,000 [7]. These figures may not represent true community prevalence, as they were not based on primary care data.

Overall the sex ratio in psoriatic arthritis approximates 1:1 but will vary across the subgroups, so that male predominance occurs in the spondylitis predominant form, while females predominate in the most frequent subgroup, symmetrical polyarthritis.

The peak age of onset of psoriatic arthritis is similar to that found in rheumatoid arthritis (20–40 years). This is, in most cases, later than the onset of psoriasis, which appears for the most in young adults. This is reflected by the figures for onset of arthritis and psoriasis – psoriasis precedes arthritis in the majority of cases. However, a potential source of diagnostic confusion occurs when arthritis precedes psoriasis, as it does in 15–20% of cases [8–10].

In a minority of cases, psoriatic arthritis may also be first diagnosed at the extremes of life. The most recent criteria for classifying juvenile idiopathic arthritis include a specific subgroup for psoriatic arthritis yet use psoriasis as an exclusion for the group labelled 'enthesitis related arthritis' [11]. For this reason, certain modifications have been suggested to bring the enthesitis related and juvenile psoriatic groups together [12]. Additionally, there has been some interest in elderly onset psoriatic arthritis, which appears to differ only slightly from classical psoriatic arthritis, the most notable difference being the lower prevalence of axial disease in this cohort [13].

3 Clinical Subgroups

Wright and Moll originally described five subgroups reflecting the diverse clinical manifestations of this disorder:

- DIP predominant (5%)
- Asymmetrical oligoarthritis (70%)
- Symmetrical polyarthritis (15%)
- Predominant spondylitis (5%)
- Arthritis mutilans (5%)

The precise composition and relative frequency of these subgroups has since been the subject of some debate. Most of the published series in the last 20 years have reported that the symmetrical polyarthritis subgroup is the most frequent, at about 60%. The reason for this discrepancy is not entirely clear, although it is unlikely that the disease has changed since the original Moll and Wright description. It is more likely that Moll and Wright were using more specific, but unstated, criteria to identify their cases [14]. Secondly, disease involvement of both axial and peripheral sites is not disputed, but the utility and practicability of dividing the cases with predominant peripheral arthritis remains unclear [15, 16]. The situation is confounded by such factors as the precise method for ascertaining joint involvement – joint involvement may be much more extensive if tender as well as swollen joints are counted and if imaging modalities such as ultrasound are used. It must also be recognised that the disease pattern will change over time, both with evolution of the disease [9] and with treatment [17].

4 Clinical Features

Spondylitis

The spondylitis associated with psoriasis can take two forms. Although classical ankylosing spondylitis is seen in association with psoriasis, distinct features that differentiate psoriatic spondylitis from classical ankylosing spondylitis have been described and can be summarised as follows (and are illustrated in Fig. B1):

- Asymmetric sacroiliitis
- More frequent non-marginal 'chunky' syndesmophytes
- Less frequent marginal syndesmophytes
- Less frequent lumbar spine involvement

It may be more compelling to regard this issue as one of quantity rather than quality – the disease is merely less extensive in psoriatic arthritis, rather than a completely different disease process.

The prevalence of spondylitis depends to some extent on the method used to identify spinal involvement. Clinical maneuvers to test sacroiliac joint involvement are generally thought to be insensitive. Both Gladman [18] and Williamson et al. [19] have demonstrated a high prevalence of asymptomatic spinal involvement in psoriatic arthritis. Furthermore, Williamson et al. demonstrated the poor sensitivity (38%) and specificity (67%) of clinical tests for sacroiliac involvement. Gladman also

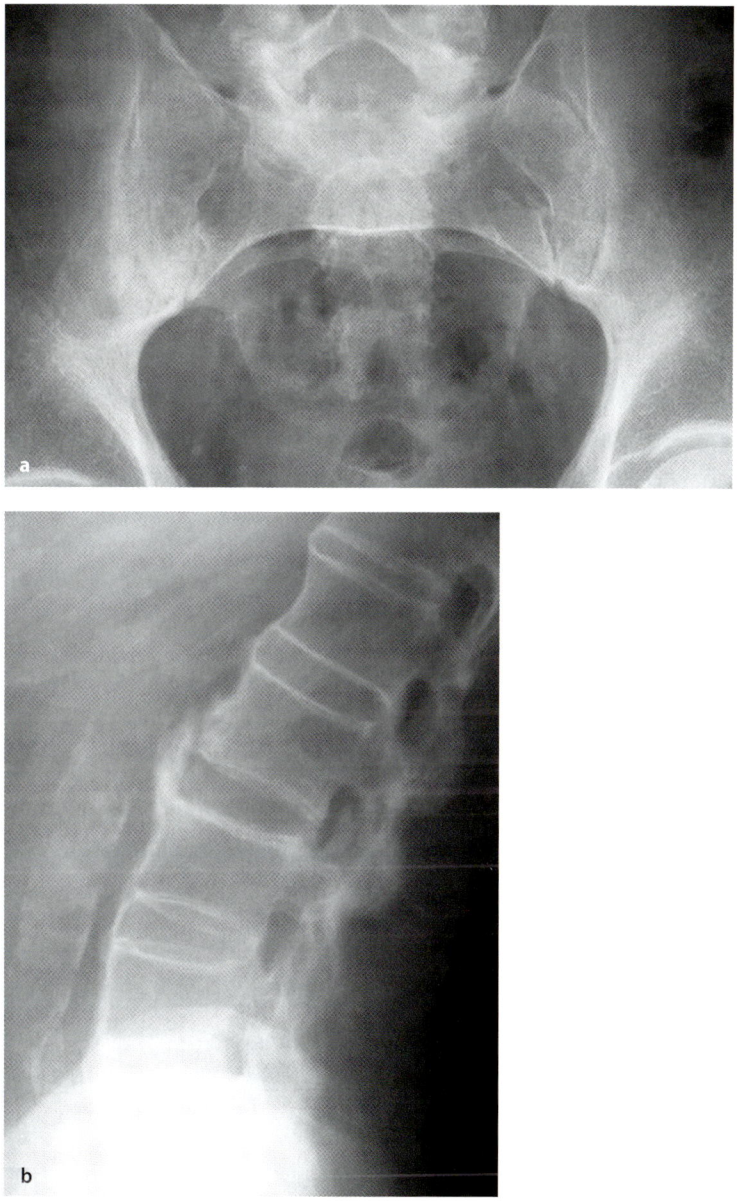

Fig. B1. **a** Asymmetric sacroiliitis (grade 3 right, grade 0 left). **b** Marginal and non-marginal syndesmophytes

confirmed that changes consistent with inflammatory spondylitis can occur in psoriatic arthritis in the absence of radiological sacroiliitis. This is an important observation in the context of the definition of spinal involvement in this disease, as the criteria for the diagnosis of ankylosing spondylitis require the presence of sacroiliitis [20].

Distal Interphalangeal Joint Involvement

DIP inflammation is a hallmark of this disease and is frequently seen in association with psoriasis of the nails (see Fig. B2). In the absence of psoriasis, clinical involvement of the DIP joints

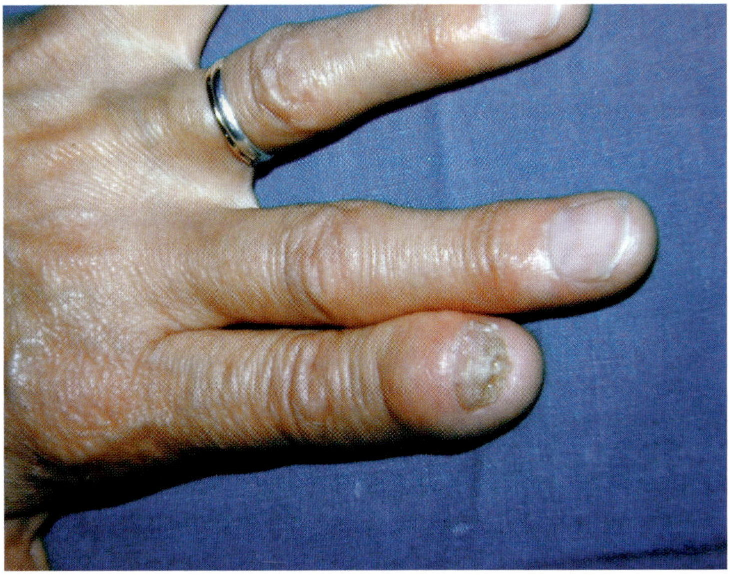

Fig. B2. Nail disease and distal interphalangeal joint involvement

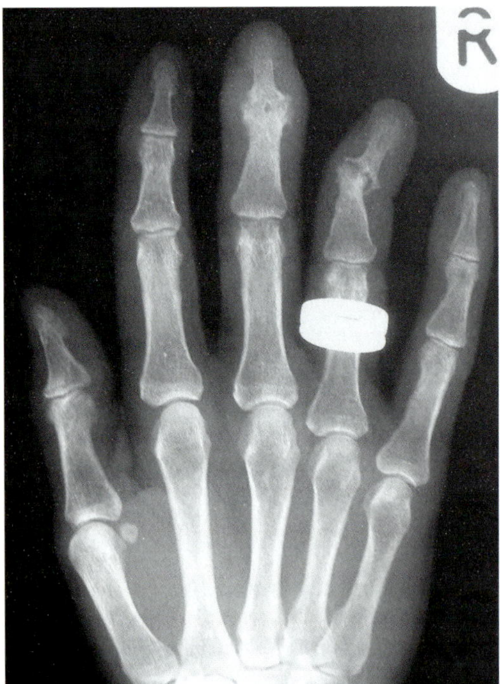

Fig. B3. Radiological features of distal interphalangeal psoriatic arthritis (distal interphalangeal erosions and ankylosis are demonstrated)

may be indistinguishable from inflammatory osteoarthritis. However, DIP inflammation may also present in such a way as to leave no doubt about the diagnosis, with characteristic involvement of the interphalangeal joints of the thumb and great toes (the eponymous Douglas digit) and of the DIP joints of the feet, rarely described in osteoarthritis. Further, involvement of the DIP joint is almost always associated with psoriatic nail changes. Despite this, isolated DIP joint involvement in psoriatic arthritis may be missed even by experienced observers [21]. If there is doubt clinically, radiological studies should help to separate inflammatory osteoarthritis from psoriatic arthritis as the latter, apart from producing characteristic differences at the joint (Fig. B3), may also produce typical changes in the terminal phalanx, including tuft erosion and osteolysis [22].

Asymmetric Oligoarthritis

Moll and Wright described this as the most common clinical presentation of psoriatic arthritis. The original description was of 'scattered DIP, PIP and MTP joints' in an asymmetric pattern [23]. Contemporary authors include a single large joint within this group [24]. Moll and Wright also included the occurrence of dactylitis in this group. The combination of heel pain (due to enthesitis), dactylitis and oligoarthritis is described as almost characteristic of psoriatic arthritis by some authors [25] (see Fig. B4).

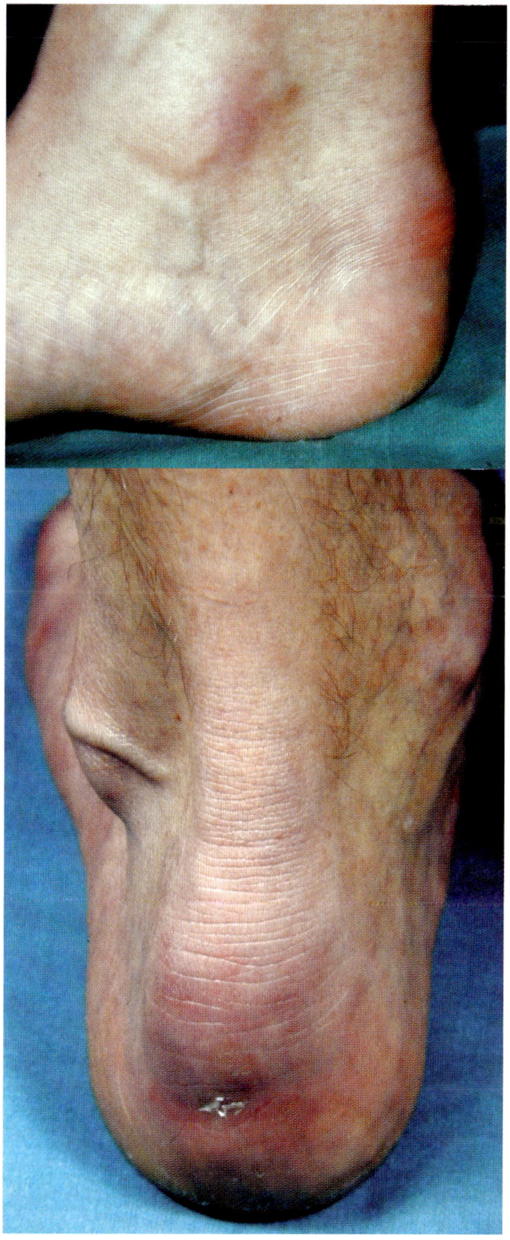

Fig. B4. Heel enthesopathy

Dactylitis

Dactylitis is one of the hallmark clinical features of psoriatic arthritis occurring in 16–48% of reported cases [8, 15, 26] (Fig. B5). Rothschild has defined dactylitis as *uniform swelling such that the soft tissues between the metacarpophalangeal and proximal interphalangeal, proximal and distal interphalangeal, and/or distal interphalangeal joint and digital tuft were diffusely swollen to the extent that the actual joint swelling could no longer be independently recognised* [27]. According to some authors dactylitis is predominantly due to swelling and inflammation in the flexor tendon sheaths [28] although other groups have recorded joint synovitis as well as tenosynovitis [29], and enthesitis may also contribute to the clinical picture. Chronic, non-tender diffuse dactylitic swelling occurs in psoriatic arthritis and may be less of an indicator of active disease than tenderness in the swollen digit. Rarely, unilateral limb edema is seen in psoriatic arthritis and, although there are clinical similarities with limb edema seen in rheumatoid arthritis, where an abnormality of lymphatic vessels has been described; this may be an extreme example of 'limb dactylitis'.

Enthesitis

McGonagle et al. rekindled interest in the enthesis as the major site of pathology underlying psoriatic arthritis [30]. There are literally hundreds of entheseal (the site of attachment of ligament and tendon to bone) sites. The most common sites in psoriatic arthritis are the calcaneum (both at the attachment of the Achilles tendon and at the attachment of the plantar fascia), the muscular and tendon attachments around the pelvis, the inferior aspect of the patella, and the elbow. Spondylitis may in fact be regarded as an example of multiple sites of enthesitis with syndesmophytes representing bony 'spurs'. The specificity of enthesitis in psoriatic arthritis remains to be determined, as one ultrasonographic study of calcaneal enthesitis demonstrated bony erosion at the enthesis more often in rheumatoid arthritis than psoriatic arthritis [31].

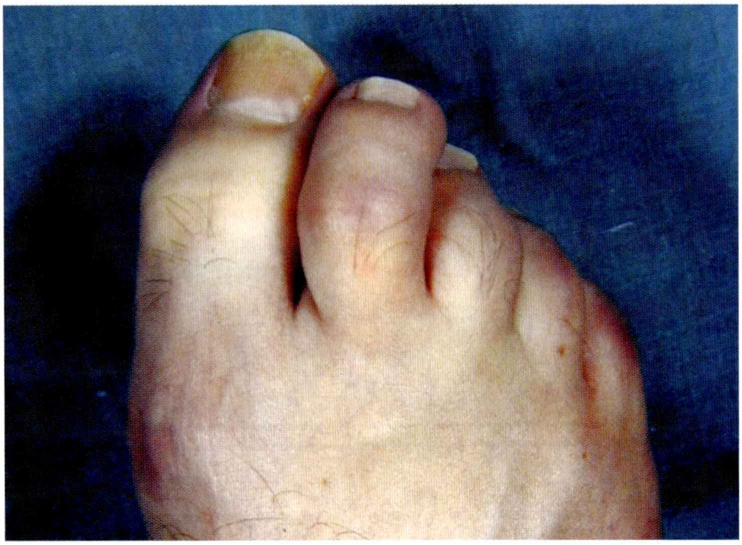

Fig. B5. Dactylitis of a toe

Other Clinical Features

In contrast to rheumatoid arthritis, it is unusual for psoriatic arthritis to cause systemic complications. Ocular involvement is perhaps the most frequent extra-articular feature after psoriasis. Both conjunctivitis (found in 20%) and uveitis (7%) have been described [32]. Uveitis is not unexpected, as psoriatic arthritis is a member of the spondyloarthropathy group, a hallmark of which is inflammation of the uveal tract, a clinical feature associated with the HLA-B27 antigen. Perhaps because HLA-B27 is less prevalent in psoriatic arthritis (about 20% overall) this recognized extra-articular feature of spondyloarthropathy is seen less frequently. Pulmonary involvement does not occur, and aortic valve disease is extremely uncommon.

There are numerous case reports of secondary amyloidosis affecting renal and gastrointestinal tissues in psoriatic arthritis, although it is not clear whether the skin or joint disease is responsible for this [33, 34].

The SAPHO syndrome is occasionally seen in association with PsA, and may even be a subgroup of this disease. SAPHO is an acronym for synovitis, acne (usually acne conglobata or fulminans), (palmoplantar) pustulosis, (sternoclavicular) hyperostosis and (sterile multifocal) osteomyelitis. There are wide regional variations in the prevalence of this condition, the more severe forms occurring in Japan and the Mediterranean littoral. However, in the United Kingdom, Helliwell et al. found a high prevalence of sternoclavicular abnormalities in psoriatic arthritis associated with psoriasis vulgaris leading them to include SAPHO as one of the osteoarticular manifestations of this disorder [15].

One variant of digital involvement in PsA has been termed 'psoriatic onycho-pachydermo-periostitis' [35]. This may occur in isolation, resulting in some diagnostic confusion, although solitary involvement of the great toe with underlying 'fluffy' periosteal new bone is characteristic. Both the underlying bone and the distal joint can be affected and there may be soft tissue swelling underneath the nail associated with severe discomfort – see Fig. B6.

Jajic has described an unusual blue discoloration of the digits in psoriatic arthritis [36]. The discoloration occurs over affected digits and may represent a form of acrocyanosis secondary to vascular changes in the underlying synovium. Macroscopically, the surface vessels of psoriatic synovium are distinct from those seen in rheumatoid arthritis, being more numerous and tortuous in psoriatic arthritis [37] (see Chap. IIIB). Further reports from other

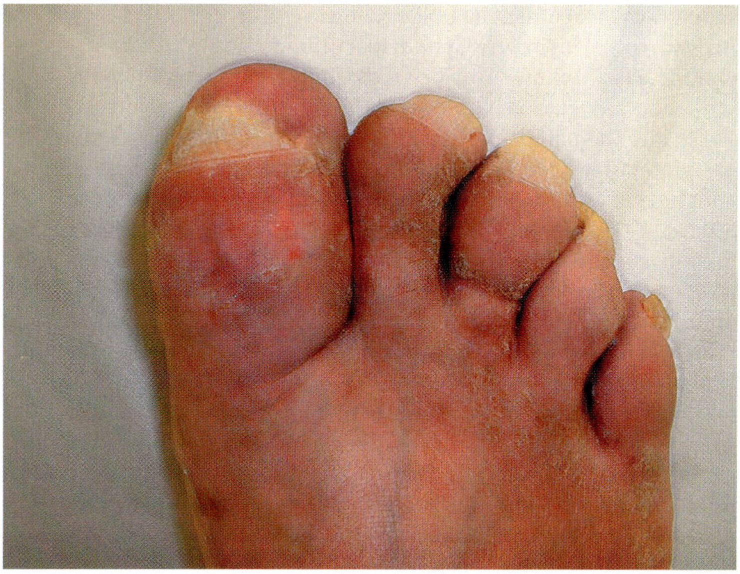

Fig. B6. Involvement of the interphalangeal joint of the great toe

centers, and elucidation of the mechanism of this blue discoloration, are awaited.

5 Relationship Between Skin and Joint Disease

Until recently, psoriatic arthritis was distinguished from other arthropathies, especially rheumatoid arthritis, by the presence of psoriasis and the absence of rheumatoid factor. However, as already mentioned, psoriasis can precede arthritis in a fair proportion of patients. Recognising the strong familial links, some criteria now include a family history of psoriasis in a first or second degree relative as evidence of the link to skin disease [11, 38].

There are further problems which can confound the clinician. Psoriasis may be present but hidden (such as in the natal cleft, under the breasts, around the umbilicus or in the hairline), or may be misdiagnosed or ignored (usually by rheumatologists) [21]. The psoriasis may only be evident in the nails; in fact, nail involvement is seen more frequently in psoriatic arthritis – 67% in the series by Jones et al. [9]. Further, psoriasis is a common skin disease, so it is likely that by chance alone some cases of other arthropathies (such as rheumatoid arthritis) will have coincidental psoriasis. Therefore, the finding of psoriasis and arthritis does not automatically mean that the disease is psoriatic arthritis, nor does the apparent absence of psoriasis rule out psoriatic arthritis as a diagnosis.

There is generally no association between the type of psoriasis and the clinical type of psoriatic arthritis, except perhaps in the case of palmoplantar pustulosis and the SAPHO syndrome, as mentioned above. However, involvement of the DIP joints is virtually never found unless there is associated psoriatic nail disease.

The relationship between the severity of the skin disease and the severity of the arthritis has been the subject of some debate. Early reports suggested psoriatic arthritis was more common in patients with severe psoriasis [5]. However, it seems more likely that a relationship between extent and severity, and linked flares, occurs only in those patients who have a simultaneous onset of skin and joint disease [39].

In the 1980s, reports suggested a link between psoriasis and HIV infection. Extensive skin disease was seen associated with the acquired immune deficiency syndrome, including widespread confluent patches and severe onychodystrophy. Subsequently, the association between HIV, AIDS, severe psoriasis and the spondyloarthropathies has been confirmed in African countries where spondyloarthropathy was virtually unknown prior to the outbreak [40]. The association has provided some insights into the pathogenesis of the disease and has emphasized the importance of the CD8+ lymphocyte in both the skin and the joint disorder [41]. Distinctive features of the arthropathy associated with HIV include severe enthesitis (particularly about the heel), dactylitis and rapidly progressive, lower limb, joint destruction. Axial involvement is seen less frequently. Under these circumstances, it may be difficult to distinguish cases of psoriatic arthritis from reactive arthritis as many of these patients are immunocompromised and may have unusual infections.

Initial reports suggested an association between skeletal hyperostosis and synthetic analogues of vitamin A used as treatment for both psoriasis and severe acne vulgaris [42, 43], although further studies suggested that with the therapeutic doses used for acne vulgaris hyperostosis is only rarely seen [44]. Skeletal hyperostosis always presents a diagnostic dilemma, as the non-marginal syndesmophytes seen classically in psoriatic spondylitis are radiologically very hard to distinguish from the new bone formation which occurs as part of diffuse idiopathic skeletal hyperostosis (DISH) and the new bone found in response to retinoids. Other radiological features may help, but in the absence of overt sacroiliitis the differential diagnosis becomes problematic.

6 Conclusion

The study of psoriatic arthritis presents a fascinating insight into the clinical manifestations of a disease in which the pathogenesis has both shared features with, and distinct differences from, those found in the other common inflammatory joint disorder – rheumatoid arthritis. Unfortunately, the clinical distinction between psoriatic arthritis and rheumatoid arthritis remains problematic in some cases. The problem is not with the classical presentation of PsA – with oligoarthritis, DIP involvement, calcaneal enthesitis and dactylitis – but with the group of patients who have seronegative polyarthritis and psoriasis. A positive test for rheumatoid factor may not be helpful, as this may be positive as a result of chronic inflammation. The more specific test for antibodies to cyclic citrullinated peptide may prove to be helpful [45] although no data are yet available.

Similarly, further data are required on the usefulness of MRI demonstrated enthesitis in relatively early disease, although the cost and availability of MRI is likely to remain a barrier to implementation of this test for some time yet. A similar argument is applied to synovial histology where the distinctive vascular pattern of psoriatic arthritis first reported by Reece and colleagues [37] has recently been reported to persist despite the institution of disease modifying therapy [46]. Clinical judgement remains the gold standard. The development of new therapies, particularly biologic therapies, has highlighted the need for validated classification criteria for psoriatic arthritis as well as for standardized outcome and response criteria for both skin and joint disease [4].

References

1. Wright V (1961) Psoriatic arthritis: a comparative study of rheumatoid arthritis and arthritis associated with psoriasis. Ann Rheum Dis 20:123
2. Wright V, Moll JMH (1976) Seronegative polyarthritis. North Holland, Amsterdam
3. Brewerton DA, Caffrey M, Hart FD, James DCO, Nicholls A, Sturrock RD (1973) Ankylosing spondylitis and HL-A27. Lancet 1:904–907
4. Taylor WJ, Helliwell PS (2000) Case definition of psoriatic arthritis. Lancet 356:2095
5. Leonard DG, O'Duffy JD, Rogers RS (1978) Prospective analysis of psoriatic arthritis in patients hospitalised for psoriasis. Proc Mayo Clin 53:511–518
6. Kay LJ, Parry-James JE, Walker DJ (1999) The prevalence of psoriasis and psoriatic arthritis in the pri-

mary care population in North East England. Ann Rheum Dis 58(Suppl 1):315
7. Shbeeb M, Uramoto KM, Gibson LE, O'Fallon WM, Gabriel SE (2000) The epidemiology of psoriatic arthritis in Olmsted County, Minnesota, USA 1982–1991. J Rheumatol 27:1247–1250
8. Gladman DD, Shuckett R, Russell ML, Thorne JC, Schachter RK (1987) Psoriatic arthritis (PSA) – an analysis of 220 patients. Q J Med 238:127–141
9. Jones SM, Armas JB, Cohen MG, Lovell CR, Evison G, McHugh NJ (1994) Psoriatic arthritis: outcome of disease subsets and relationship of joint disease to nail and skin disease. Br J Rheumatol 33:834–839
10. Biondi Oriente C, Scarpa R, Pucino A, Oriente P (1989) Psoriasis and psoriatic arthritis. Dermatological and rheumatological co-operative clinical report. Acta Derm Venereol Suppl 146:69–71
11. Petty RE, Southwood TR, Baum J, Bhettay E, Glass DN, Manners P, et al. (1998) Revision of the proposed classification for juvenile idiopathic arthritis: Durban 1997. J Rheumatol 25:1991–1994
12. Burgos-Vargas R, Rudwaleit M, Sieper J (2002) The place of juvenile onset spondyloarthropathies in the Durban 1997 ILAR classification criteria of juvenile idiopathic arthritis. International League of Associations for Rheumatology. J Rheumatol 29: 869–874
13. Lopez-Montilla MD, Gonzalez J, Martinez FG, Fernandez-Moreno JR, Collantes E (2002) Clinical features of late onset psoriatic arthritis. Exp Gerontol 37:441–443
14. Helliwell PS, Taylor WJ (2005) Classification and diagnostic criteria for psoriatic arthritis. Ann Rheum Dis (in press)
15. Helliwell P, Marchesoni A, Peters M, Barker M, Wright V (1991) A re-evaluation of the osteoarticular manifestations of psoriasis [see comments]. Br J Rheumatol 30:339–345
16. Veale D, Fitzgerald O (1992) Psoriatic arthritis – "DIP or not DIP? That is the question" [letter; comment]. Br J Rheumatol 31:430–431
17. Kane D, Stafford L, Bresnihan B, FitzGerald O (2003) A classification study of clinical subsets in an inception cohort of early psoriatic peripheral arthritis – 'DIP or not DIP revisited'. Rheumatology 42: 1469–1476
18. Khan M, Schentag C, Gladman DD (2003) Clinical and radiological changes during psoriatic arthritis disease progression. J Rheumatol 30:1022–1026
19. Williamson L, Dockerty JL, Dalbeth N, McNally E, Ostlere S, Wordsworth BP (2004) Clinical assessment of sacroiliitis and HLA-B27 are poor predictors of sacroiliitis diagnosed by magnetic resonance imaging in psoriatic arthritis. Rheumatology 43: 85–88
20. The HSG, Steven MM, Van der Linden SM, Cats A (1985) Evaluation of diagnostic criteria for ankylosing spondylitis: a comparison of the Rome, New York, and modified New York criteria in patients with a positive clinical history screening test for ankylosing spondylitis. Br J Rheum 24: 242–249
21. Gorter S, van der Heijde DMFM, van der Linden S, Houben H, Rethans J-J, Scerpbier AJJA, et al. (2002) Psoriatic arthritis: performance of rheumatologists in daily practice. Ann Rheum Dis 61:219–224
22. Avila R, Pugh DG, Slocumb CH, Winklemann RK (1960) Psoriatic arthritis: a roentgenological study. Radiology 75:691
23. Moll JMH, Wright V (1973) Psoriatic arthritis. Semin Arthr Rheum 3:51–78
24. Helliwell PS, Wright V (1998) Psoriatic arthritis: clinical features. In: Klippel JH, Dieppe PA (eds) Rheumatology. Mosby, London, pp 6.21.1–6.21.8
25. Eulry F, Diamano J, Launay D, Tabache F, Lechevalier D, Magnin J (2002) Sausage-like toe and heel pain: value for diagnosing and evaluating the severity of spondyloarthropathies defined by Amor's criteria. A retrospective study in 161 patients. Joint Bone Spine 69:574–579
26. Fournie B, Crognier L, Arnaud C, Zabraniecki L, Lascaux-Lefebvre V, Marc V, et al. (1999) Proposed classification criteria of psoriatic arthritis. Revue Rheumatisme (Engl Edn) 66:446–456
27. Rothschild BM, Pingitore C, Eaton M (1998) Dactylitis: implications for clinical practice. Semin Arthritis Rheum 28:41–47
28. Olivieri I, Barozzi L, Favaro L, Pierro A, De Matteis M, Borghi C, et al. (1996) Dactylitis in patients with seronegative spondylarthropathy. Assessment by ultrasonography and magnetic resonance imaging. Arthritis Rheum 39:1524–1528
29. Kane D, Greaney T, Bresnihan B, Gibney R, FitzGerald O (1999) Ultrasonography in the diagnosis and management of psoriatic dactylitis [comment]. J Rheumatol 26:1746–1751
30. McGonagle D, Gibbon W, Emery P (1998) Classification of inflammatory arthritis by enthesitis. Lancet 352:1137–1140
31. Falsetti P, Frediani B, Fioravanti A, Acciai C, Baldi F, Filippou G, et al. (2003) Sonographic study of calcaneal entheses in erosive osteoarthritis, nodal osteoarthritis, rheumatoid arthritis and psoriatic arthritis. Scand J Rheumatol 32:229–234
32. Lambert JR, Wright V (1976) Eye inflammation in psoriatic arthritis. Ann Rheum Dis 35:354–356
33. Mpofu S, Teh LS, Smith PJ, Moots RJ, Hawkins PN (2003) Cytostatic therapy for AA amyloidosis complicating psoriatic spondyloarthropathy. Rheumatology 42:362–366
34. Ujfalussy I, Bely M, Koo E, Sesztak M (2001) Systemic, secondary amyloidosis in a patient with psoriatic arthritis. Clin Exp Rheumatol 19:225
35. Boisseau-Garsaud AM, Beylot-Barry M, Doutre MS, Beylot C, Baran R (1996) Psoriatic onycho-pachydermo-periostitis. A variant of psoriatic distal interphalangeal arthritis? Arch Dermatol 132: 176–180
36. Jajic I (2001) Blue coloured skin in psoriatic arthritis. Clin Rheumatol 20:304–305

V

37. Reece RJ, Canete JD, Parsons WJ, Emery P, Veale DJ (1999) Distinct vascular patterns of early synovitis in psoriatic, reactive, and rheumatoid arthritis. Arthritis Rheum 42:1481–1484
38. Dougados M, van der Linden S, Juhlin R, Huitfeldt B, Amor B, Calin A (1991) The European Spondyloarthropathy Study Group preliminary criteria for the classification of spondyloarthropathy. Arthritis Rheum 34:1218–1227
39. Elkayam O, Ophir J, Yaron M, Caspi D (2000) Psoriatic arthritis: interrelationships between skin and joint manifestations related to onset, course and distribution. Clin Rheumatol 19:301–305
40. Njobvu P, McGill P, Kerr H, Ellis J, Pobee J (1998) Spondyloarthropathy and HIV infection in Zambia. J Rheumatol 25:1553–1559
41. Hohler T, Marker-Hermann E (2001) Psoriatic arthritis: clinical aspects, genetics, and the role of T cells. Curr Opin Rheumatol 13:273–279
42. Wendling D, Lamarque V, Portha P, Guidet M (1991) Hyperostose induite par l'etretinate. Rheumatologie 43:41–48
43. Kaplan G, Haettich B (1991) Rheumatological symptoms due to retinoids. Baillieres Clin Rheumatol 5: 77–97
44. Carey BM, Parkin GJS, Cunliffe WJ, Pritlove J (1988) Skeletal toxicity with isotretinoin therapy: a clinicoradiological evaluation. Br J Dermatol 119: 609–614
45. Lee DM, Schur PH (2003) Clinical utility of the anti-CCP assay in patients with rheumatic diseases. Ann Rheum Dis 62:870–874
46. Canete JD, Rodriguez JR, Salvador G, Gomez-Centeno A, Munoz-Gomez J, Sanmarti R (2003) Diagnostic usefulness of synovial vascular morphology in chronic arthritis. A systematic survey of 100 cases. Semin Arthritis Rheum 32:378–387

Diagnostic Evaluation VI

A Psoriasis

Bettina M. Prinz Vavricka,
Joan Guitart

Contents

1 Introduction

The diagnosis of psoriasis is often made upon clinical inspection of the skin. The clinical presentation often makes diagnostic testing and pathological examination of a biopsy from a plaque unnecessary. However, much of what is known about the pathophysiology of psoriasis comes from the pathological appearance of the disease. In this chapter, we will examine the pathological patterns seen in the skin of patients with psoriasis as well as laboratory abnormalities associated with clinical activity of the disease.

2 Laboratory Evaluation

The most common laboratory examination to confirm the clinical diagnosis of psoriasis is a skin biopsy using hematoxylin-eosin staining. However, additional staining with periodic acid-Schiff (PAS) is often done to exclude the possibility of dermatophyte infection, a condition that, like psoriasis, would have neutrophils found in the stratum corneum.

Other than skin biopsy, there are no specific laboratory abnormalities associated with psoriasis. Some patients, especially those with a generalized pustular or erythrodermic psoriasis, may develop some non-specific laboratory abnormalities associated with systemic inflammation that should be monitored. Specifically, decreased serum albumin is an important indicator of a negative nitrogen balance with chronic inflammation and protein loss in the skin. Increases in C-reactive protein, α2-macroglobulin and erythrocyte sedimentation rate (ESR) can also occur with severe forms of disease activity. In some cases increased serum IgA levels and IgA immune complexes have been reported, but the implications of this finding are unknown [20]. Patients with extensive psoriasis may have elevated serum uric acid levels, which will fluctuate in relation to the activity of the disease. These patients have an elevated risk of developing gouty arthritis, which could complicate the assessment and treatment of psoriatic arthritis. In general, the serum uric acid level normalizes once the active inflammatory process is under control [20, 83].

3 Pathological Evaluation of Psoriasis Vulgaris

The hallmark histological findings of psoriasis vulgaris, or plaque type psoriasis, are listed in Table A1. These observations are derived from an increased rate of proliferation of epidermal keratinocytes along with altered keratinocyte maturation. However, the pathological signals that drive the process are located in the dermis [8]. Just as the psoriatic plaques evolve clinically, the pathological findings will vary based on their stage of development. Pathological findings can be broken down into the early stage, the active stage, and the late stages of the plaques. Early and late plaque lesions may not show entirely diagnostic features and the pathological findings will need to be considered in the context of the clinical presentation.

Table A1. Pathologic findings in psoriasis vulgaris

- Uniform regular acanthosis
- Parakeratosis
- Papillomatosis
- Absence of granular layer
- Munro's abscesses (collection of neutrophil granulocytes)
- Atrophic epidermis above the tip of the dermal papilla, resulting in thinning of the suprapapillary plate
- Mitotic activity visible within keratinocytes
- Long and thin rete ridges
- Papillary edema
- Multiple tortuous and dilated capillaries in the papillae of the dermis
- Superficial infiltrate or inflammatory cells in the dermis with perivascular lymphocytes and some neutrophils

Early Stage

The early pathological changes of plaque psoriasis tend to be subtle and non-specific. There is slight epidermal hyperplasia with a limited amount of visible mitotic activity. The granular cell layer tends to be somewhat thinned. Subcorneal spongiform pustules may occasionally be present. The stratum corneum tends to show abnormal retention of the cellular nuclei (parakeratosis) with a few interspersed neutrophils. In early and more eruptive cases, the cornified layer may retain a normal basket-weave configuration. Other signs of an eruptive course include edema of the papillary dermis with a mononuclear and neutrophilic upper dermal infiltrate with exocytosis of some of these cells into the epidermis. Eventually elongation of the rete ridges develops. In the dermis, capillaries become dilated and tortuous with prominent endothelial cells. The perivascular infiltrate consists mostly of lymphocytes, monocytes and rare neutrophils. Margination of neutrophils can also be noted in the superficial vascular plexus. In general, dermal changes tend to appear before the characteristic epidermal changes can be observed.

Active Stage

Similar to the clinical presentation, the active stage of psoriatic plaques provides the classic findings of psoriasis. A typical biopsy from this stage is shown in Fig. A1. In this stage the epidermis shows hyperplasia with thin elongated rete ridges of approximately equal length. The proliferation of keratinocytes may increase about 10 times over the normal rate and can be seen with immunohistochemical staining for Ki-67, a marker of cell-cycle activity (Fig. A2a) [24]. These keratinocytes also mature abnormally, expressing keratins otherwise seen in wound healing including keratin-16 (Fig. A2b). The suprapapillar epidermis is thin, almost atrophic and mitotic figures can be appreciated one or two layers above the basal layer. Scattered neutrophils can be often seen within the epidermal layers. A collection of neutrophils

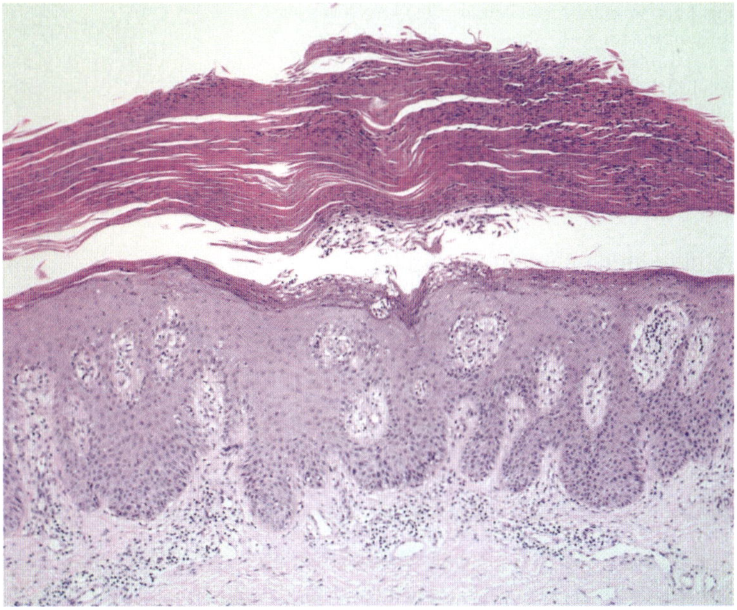

Fig. A1. Histopathological features of psoriasis vulgaris. Note the thickened stratum corneum with neutrophilic aggregates. The granular layer is thinned and there is marked elongation of the rete ridges. The capillaries of the dermal papillae are tortuous and dilated

within the spinous layer or spongiform pustule of Kogoj can frequently be found. Mild edema in between the keratinocytes (spongiosis) is common in the lower portion of the epidermis. The granular layer tends to be nearly absent. A prominent granular cell layer may only be seen at the opening of adnexal structures. The whole cornified layer is thickened and is firmly packed together (orthokeratosis) with confluent and prominent nuclear remnants (parakeratosis) as well as aggregates of neutrophils, the so-called Munro's microabscess (Fig. A3) [34]. Sometimes there are inclusions of serous exudates with or without hemorrhage within the thickened cornified layer. The changes in the dermis are similar to the early stage with dilated spiraled capillaries and edema of the papillary dermis. The dermal infiltrate consists of neutrophils, macrophages, lymphocytes, and mast cells. Migration of neutrophils from capillaries to the dermal papillae and to the epidermis through basement membrane gaps is one of the most valuable clues for the diagnosis of psoriasis.

Late Stage

Late lesions of psoriasis will show a trend towards normalization of the epidermal architecture. There is progressively less epidermal thickening while there is persistent compact orthokeratosis with less parakeratosis. The epidermis above the papillary plates is thin, and wedge-shaped hypergranulosis can be found. Dilated capillaries are still present in the dermal papillae. The perivascular and interstitial infiltrate consists of predominantly lymphocytes. Increases in the dermal fibrous tissue are generally absent with the exception of patients with chronic pruritus in whom lamellar fibroplasia parallel to the dermal epidermal junction can be found.

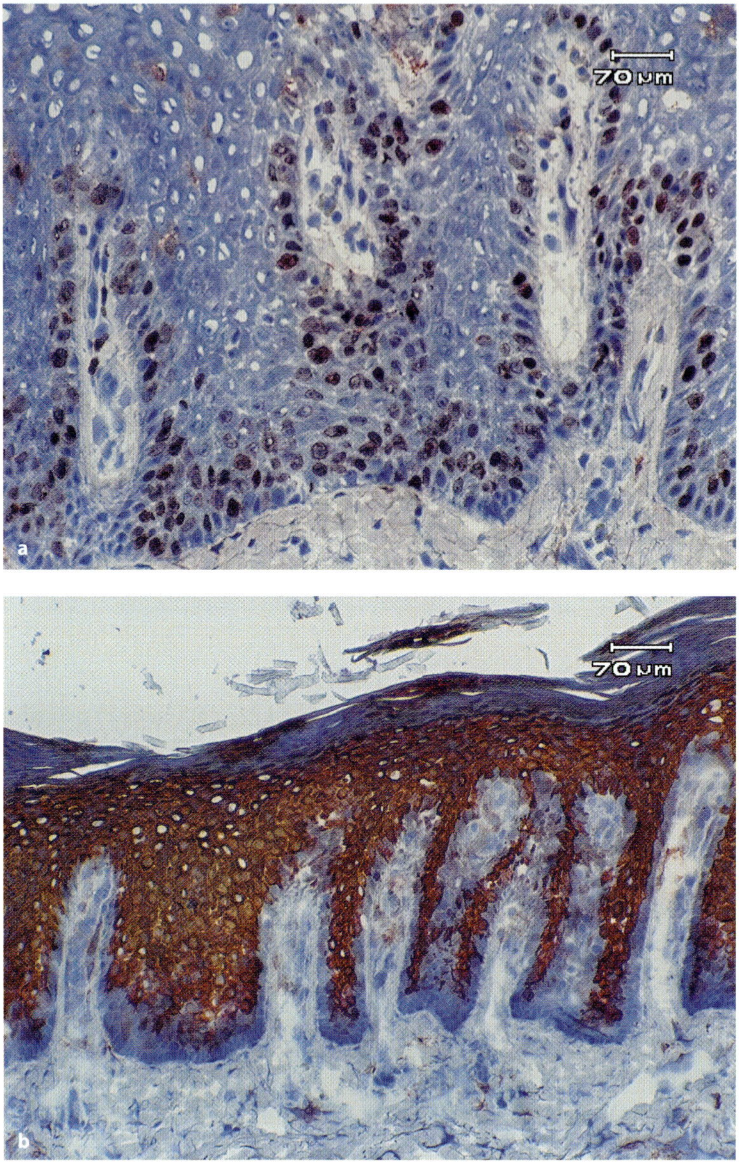

Fig. A2. **a** Immunohistochemical staining for Ki-67 showing a high proliferative index involving the basal and suprabasal keratinocytes in psoriasis. **b** Strong keratin 16 immunostaining in the spinous layer of a psoriatic plaque

4 Special Forms of Psoriasis

Guttate Psoriasis

The clinical appearance of guttate psoriasis is characterized by widely dispersed small red scaly plaques of 1–5 mm size. Guttate psoriasis affects mostly young people and is often preceded by a streptococcal pharyngitis [81, 91]. Histologically, a new onset of guttate lesions may not provide pathognomonic features. Such lesions often show spongiosis and a superficial mononuclear infiltrate without the typical findings of epidermal thickening or neutrophilic microabscesses found in well-established lesions. However, mounds of parakeratosis with spongiform neutrophilic pustules can be seen.

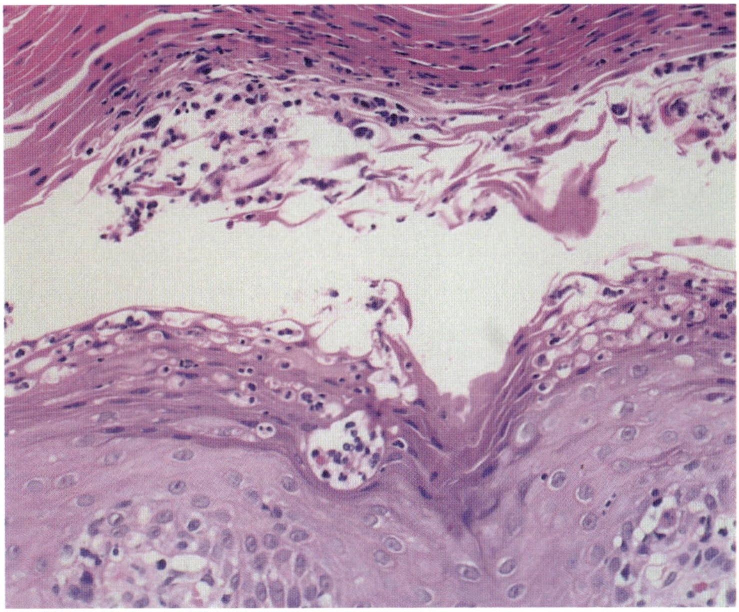

Fig. A3. H and E staining showing subcorneal collections of neutrophils called Munro's microabscesses

There is marked edema in the upper papillary dermis. The differential diagnosis of guttate psoriasis includes dermatophytosis, pityriasis rosea, and pityriasis lichenoides chronica.

Erythrodermic Psoriasis

Generalized exfolliative erythroderma with or without a pustular component is a rare presentation of psoriasis. In general, the psoriasiform pattern is preserved, but there is a near absence of parakeratosis, which is due to the constant shedding of scale or desquamation. The discohesiveness of corneocytes when compared to psoriasis vulgaris is an important sign of this variant. Extensive edema of the papillary dermis and some spongiosis mediated by lymphocytes is often noted. Serous exudates within the corneal layer are also common. The histological changes of erythrodermic psoriasis may be difficult to distinguish from other causes of erythroderma like atopic dermatitis or Sezary syndrome.

Pustular Psoriasis

Pustular psoriasis may be a systemic process with fever and chills (von Zumbusch or impetigo herpetiformis variants) or localized like acrodermatitis continua of Hallopeau, palmoplantar pustulosis and keratoderma blennorrhagicum of Reiter's syndrome [31, 46]. The histological presentation will depend on the site and timing of the biopsy and severity of the episode (Table A2). In the early stage there is a marked inflammatory infiltrate, predominantly of mononuclear cells with significant edema and spongiosis. A well-developed pustular eruption will show a macropustule with large

Table A2. Dermatopathological criteria of psoriasis pustulosa

- Parakeratosis
- Elongation of the rete ridges
- Perivascular mononucleous infiltrate in the upper dermis
- Spongiforme pustule (Kogoj)
- Minimal spongiform pustule in the lateral wall of a macro pustule

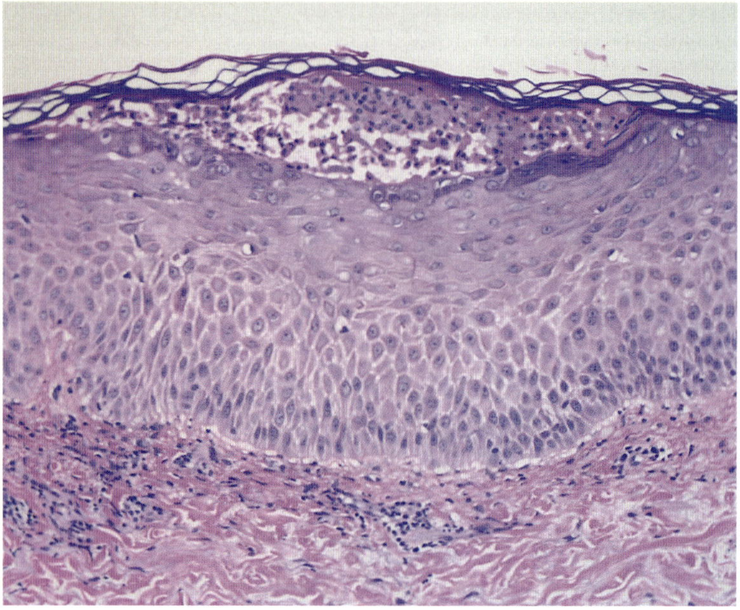

Fig. A4. Early lesion of pustular psoriasis, showing prominent exocytosis of neutrophils with subcorneal pustule formation

spongiotic intraepidermal or subcorneal space filled with aggregates of neutrophils and covered by a thick orthokeratotic stratum corneum (Fig. A4). Focal acantholysis, a separation of cells within the layers in the epidermis, may be noted as a result of enzymes released by neutrophils. The dermal changes are similar to psoriasis vulgaris with perhaps more edema and extravasated polymorphic neutrophils. Differential diagnosis of pustular psoriasis includes dermatophyte and candida fungal infection. Special stains for fungi should be performed in all cases. An acute pustular drug eruption can also resemble pustular psoriasis.

5 Histological Differential Diagnosis

Though psoriasis is generally a clinical diagnosis, the histologic appearance of biopsied lesions may suggest a number of other possible diagnoses. Most common among these is a chronic dermatitis with psoriasiform changes that can be found in patients with atopic dermatitis or other forms of eczema. Given the chronicity of both of these conditions, it may be difficult to distinguish from psoriasis both clinically and pathologically. The presence of dermal eosinophils rather than neutrophils may provide a valuable clue in favor of an eczematous process. Additionally, lichen simplex chronicus is the result of persistent scratching of a pruritic eczematous lesion. Prominent dermal fibrosis parallel to the dermal epidermal junction is a characteristic feature. Palmoplantar psoriasis and eczema also share common histological features often presenting with acanthosis, spongiosis and a dense lymphoid infiltrate with exocytosis. Unless other diagnostic clues like eosinophils or neutrophils in the infiltrate or other clinical clues like knee and elbow lesions for psoriasis are present, a definitive diagnosis may not be reached.

Chronic and severe lesions of seborrheic dermatitis may also reveal a histological pattern resembling psoriasis. A valuable histological clue is the presence of clusters of neutrophils in the stratum corneum adjacent to pilosebaceous ostia. Clinical judgment maybe needed to distinguish both entities. Furthermore overlap cases or sebopsoriasis will have features of both conditions.

Pityriasis rubra pilaris is also a psoriasiform papulosquamous condition that may present with a clinical picture similar to erythrodermic psoriasis. Histologically, it is characterized by icthyosiform keratin retention with plugging of the follicular infundibula. Vertical and horizontal areas with alternating hyperkeratosis and parakeratosis may be noted. Foci of acantholysis or detachment of adjacent keratinocytes has also been reported.

As mentioned above, differential diagnosis of psoriasis also includes some infectious diseases, especially dermatophyte and candida infection. A fungal stain should be performed whenever neutrophils are noted in the stratum corneum. Secondary syphilis may also resemble psoriasis under the microscope, but the notable presence of plasma cells in the infiltrate should provide a clue for this diagnostic possibility.

6 Clinicopathologic Correlation

The severity and timing of the biopsy procedure will influence the morphologic appearance under the microscope. If the disease develops quickly, the lesions become more guttate-like. If the course is even more accelerated and severe, pustules are formed. Clinically, a basket-weaved stratum corneum may be intact that corresponds to lesions that are not scaly [1]. As soon as the cornified layer is lost and parakeratosis is present, the characteristic scales appear. The erythema associated with psoriasis is caused by the dilated and tortuous vessels in the dermal papillae.

Auspitz's sign, classical clinical signs of psoriasis, can be explained by the histopathological features. Scratching of the scales results in the removal of the parakeratosis of the stratum corneum. Beneath the scale there is only a very thin suprapapillary plate above the papillary dermis. After removing this 'last membrane', Auspitz's sign with pinpoint bleeding develops due to trauma to the exposed dilated capillaries in the upper papillary dermis.

7 Pathology and Pathogenesis

While the pathological findings described above can give important clues as to the diagnosis of psoriasis, of equal importance are the clues to the pathogenic mechanisms of psoriasis given by the histology. Our understanding of ordered changes in local and infiltrating cell types can lead to a better understanding of the disease itself. Thus, any review of the pathology of psoriasis would be incomplete without a discussion of how these pathologic changes correlate to our understanding of the pathomechanisms of disease.

Angiogenesis and Adhesion Molecules

Some researchers have suggested that changes in the vasculature are the earliest morphological sign in the pathology of psoriasis [21, 33]. IL-8, TGF-α and endothelin-1 are released in plaques of psoriasis and are thought to play an important role in stimulating angiogenesis [21, 77]. Vascular endothelial growth factor (VEGF), a potent stimulus of angiogenesis, microvascular hyperpermeability, and endothelium-dependent vasodilation, is increasingly released by epidermal keratinocytes. Patients with psoriasis have high plasma levels of VEGF [96]. High endothelial venules play an important part in the recruitment of circulating lymphocytes [47]. The recruitment of lymphocytes into the papillary dermis is caused by various chemoattractants, such as platelet-activating factor and leukotriene B4 [35, 89]. As a consequence of the strong expression of diverse adhesion molecules by endothelial cells, these lymphocytes may bind and diapedese through the wall of the vessels into the papillary dermis [18]. Adhesion molecules of endothelial cells, like integrins and selectins (E-selectin), are expressed on the surface of the endothelium in psoriasis and are thought to be critical to this process [64]. The expression of the latter in the serum is correlated with the extent of psoriatic lesions [78]. Additional adhesion molecules found in increased amounts in psoriatic plaques are also known to be involved in the pathogenesis of disease. These include ICAM-1 (CD54), ICAM-2, and vascular cell adhesion molecule-I (VCAM-1), which belong to the immunoglobulin gene superfamily. The interaction between the integrins of blood derived cells and ICAM-1/VCAM-1 is important for recruitment of inflammatory cells [73]. These adhesion molecules might be induced by various pro-inflammatory cytokines, like IL-1, IL-2, IL-4, TNF-α, and IFN-γ [35, 62]. Conversely, these adhesion molecules can be reduced by UVB radiation [15]. Another cell adhesion molecule, cadherin, might be involved in the pathogenesis of psoriasis, especially in the hyperproliferation of keratinocytes. In psoriatic lesions T-cadherin was downregulated whereas P-cadherin was upregulated [97].

T Lymphocytes

As the process of neovascularization occurs, T lymphocytes migrate to the skin [87]. Lymphocytes are the first inflammatory cells to appear and their presence is accompanied by slight spongiosis [1]. In the dermis CD4+ cells are more abundant than CD8+ cells, while in the epidermis it is the opposite with mostly CD8 (+) T cells. Both subsets of T cells are activated in psoriatic-lesions expression HLA-DR and CD25 [86]. Intracellular staining of these cells suggests that psoriasis is a Th1 dominant disease based on the cytokine profile (IL-2 and IFN-γ) of the infiltrating cells [66]. In resolving lesions an influx of CD8(+) T cells occur, while the CD4(+) T cells decrease in number [3, 59, 65].

The Th-1-type cytokine network in chronic psoriatic plaques seems to be mediated in part by the nuclear factor-κB (NFκB) signaling pathway [11]. The role of T lymphocytes during the initiation stages of the disease is still controversial. Some groups have found that the presence of type I receptor for TNF-α is a required step. The pathogenesis of psoriasis may require interaction between keratinocytes and dermal cells that is probably mediated by TNF-α [12, 36]. Development of psoriatic lesions is associated with a strong increase in HLA-DR positive antigen presenting cells as well as heat shock protein (hsp) receptor CD91 expressing cells, a process that may be related to TNF-α and NFκB [25]. In psoriatic plaques CD 91 was strongly expressed by dermal dendritic cells as well as hsp 27, 60, and 70 in psoriatic epidermis [22].

Neutrophils

Chemoattraction of neutrophils within the epidermal compartment follows the influx of lymphocytes [1]. Like lymphocytes, neutrophils are recruited with the help of complement-split product C5a anaphylotoxin [79]. Other activating factors include IL-8, GRO-α (GRO/melanoma growth-stimulatory activity) and arachidonic acid metabolites, like leukotriene B_4 [71]. In nearly every stage of the disease, neutrophils are present in the epidermis and papillary dermis. Proinflammatory TNF-α facilitates the release of IL-8 from epidermal cells, which is both chemotactic and activating for neutrophils [30]. The azurophilic granules of neutrophils release human leukocytic elastase (HLE), a proteolytic enzyme involved with destruction of elastin, laminin and other collagenous fibers [94, 95]. The enzyme is also involved with keratinocyte discohesion. HLE activity, which is not expressed in normal skin, correlates with the stage of disease [48]. Elafin is an elastase inhibitor that can be found in the stratum spinosum of psoriatic lesions [52, 70, 93]. Inflammatory mediators such as Il-1β and TNF-α have been shown to be potent inducers of elafin [80].

Keratinocytes

The final step in the pathogenesis of psoriasis involves stimulation and proliferation of keratinocytes by various factors [91]. IFN-γ, which can be produced by lymphocytes and mast cells, leads to a growth stimulation of keratinocyte stem cells in psoriasis [2]. It has been suggested that psoriatic keratinocytes may have an aberrant sensitivity to IFN-γ resulting in a hyperproliferative response [88]. IL-8 and GRO-α, which are overexpressed in psoriasis, might also stimulate proliferation of keratinocytes [16, 42]. Other factors that may be involved in the exaggerated turnover of keratinocytes include IL-1, IL-3, IL-6, GM-CSF, TGF-α, EGF, amphiregulin, endothelin-1, and insulin growth factor [10, 57, 63, 90, 91]. As a counterpart TGF-β has an inhibitory effect on epithelial cell proliferation, and TNF-α [40].

Increased keratinocyte proliferation is associated with high expression of keratins K6, K16, and K17, which are present in the suprabasal layers in interfollicular psoriatic epidermis, but not in normal skin [43]. This is associated with downregulation of keratin K1 and K10 [58]. Keratin expression varies between the inner margin and outer margin of a psoriasis lesion. In the inner margin K6 positive cells were detected but not K10 cells. However, in the inner margin of a psoriatic lesion there is also a subpopulation of cells, which co-express K6 *and* K10 [53]. The decreased number of anti-apoptotic bcl-2 positive cells in the basal layer correlates with the increased rate of apoptosis [6]. An increased level of another serine protease, stratum corneum chymotryptic enzyme (SCCE), could be observed in psoriasis. SCCE is thought to play a role in desquamation of the skin by proteolyse of desmosomes in the stratum corneum [27].

8 Conclusion

The pathology findings from psoriasis can give important clues to both the clinical aspects and the pathophysiology of the disease. A clear understanding of the distinctions between earlier and later lesions of psoriasis vulgaris as well as special forms of psoriasis can help clinicians in identification and the clinical course for their patients. Likewise, more recent immunohistochemical findings have given important clues into the pathogenic processes and may provide the foremost clues for the development of new therapies.

References

1. Ackerman AB (1997) Psoriasis. In: Ackerman AB (ed) Histologic diagnosis of inflammatory skin diseases. An algorithmic method based on pattern analysis. Lippincott Williams and Wilkins, Baltimore, pp 663–673
2. Ackermann L, Harvima IT, Pelkonen J, Ritamaki-Salo V, Naukkarinen A, Harvima RJ, Horsmanheimo M (1999) Mast cells in psoriatic skin are strongly positive for interferon-gamma. Br J Dermatol 140: 624–633
3. Austin LM, Ozawa M, Kikuchi T, Walters IB, Krueger JG (1999) The majority of epidermal T cells in psoriasis vulgaris lesions can produce type 1 cytokines, interferon-gamma, interleukin-2, and tumor necrosis factor-alpha, defining TC1 (cytotoxic T lymphocyte) and TH1 effector populations: a type 1 differentiation bias is also measured in circulating blood T cells in psoriatic patients. J Invest Dermatol 113:752–759
4. Balendran N, Clough RL, Arguello JR, Barber R, Veal C, Jones AB, Rosbotham JL, Little AM, Madrigal A, Barker JN, Powis SH, Trembath RC (1999) Characterization of the major susceptibility region for psoriasis at chromosome 6p21.3. J Invest Dermatol 113: 322–328
5. Barker JN (2001) Genetic aspects of psoriasis. Clin Exp Dermatol 26:321–325
6. Bianchi L, Farrace MG, Nini G, Piacentini M (1994) Abnormal Bcl-2 and "tissue" transglutaminase expression in psoriatic skin. J Invest Dermatol 103: 829–833
7. Biondi Oriente C, Scarpa R, Pucino A, Oriente P (1989) Psoriasis and psoriatic arthritis. Dermatological and rheumatological co-operative clinical report. Acta Derm Venereol Suppl (Stockh) 146: 69–71
8. Boehncke WH, Sterry W, Hainzl A, Scheffold W, Kaufmann R (1994) Psoriasiform architecture of murine epidermis overlying human psoriatic dermis transplanted onto SCID mice. Arch Dermatol Res 286:325–330
9. Boisseau-Garsaud AM, Beylot-Barry M, Doutre MS, Beylot C, Baran R (1996) Psoriatic onycho-pachydermo-periostitis. A variant of psoriatic distal interphalangeal arthritis? Arch Dermatol 132: 176–180
10. Bos JD (1988) The pathomechanisms of psoriasis; the skin immune system and cyclosporin. Br J Dermatol 118:141–155
11. Bowcock AM, Shannon W, Du F, Duncan J, Cao K, Aftergut K, Catier J, Fernandez-Vina MA, Menter A (2001) Insights into psoriasis and other inflammatory diseases from large-scale gene expression studies. Hum Mol Genet 10:1793–1805
12. Boyman O, Hefti HP, Suter M, Nickoloff BJ, Nestle FO (2002) TBA-alpha-dependent induction of psoriasis in the absence of lymphocyte recruitment. Br J Dermatol 147:1047–1078
13. Braun-Falco O (1991) Psoriasis vulgaris. In: Braun-Falco O, Plewig G, Wolff HH, Winkelmann RK (eds) Dermatology. Springer, Berlin Heidelberg New York, pp 417–437
14. Burden AD (2000) Identifying a gene for psoriasis on chromosome 6 (Psors1). Br J Dermatol 143: 238–241

VI

15. Cai JP, Harris K, Falanga V, Taylor JR, Chin YH (1996) UVB therapy decreases the adhesive interaction between peripheral blood mononuclear cells and dermal microvascular endothelium, and regulates the differential expression of CD54, VCAM-1, and E-selectin in psoriatic plaques. Br J Dermatol 134:7–16
16. Champion RH (1986) Psoriasis. Br Med J (Clin Res Ed) 292:1693–1696
17. Cheng L, Zhang SZ, Xiao CY, Hou YP, Li L, Luo HC, Jiang HY, Zuo WQ (2000) The A5.1 allele of the major histocompatibility complex class I chain-related gene A is associated with psoriasis vulgaris in Chinese. Br J Dermatol 143:324–329
18. Chin YH, Falanga V, Taylor JR, Cai JP, Bax J (1990) Adherence of human helper/memory T-cell subsets to psoriatic dermal endothelium. J Invest Dermatol 94:413–417
19. Christophers E, Henseler T (1985) Characterization of disease patterns in nonpustular psoriasis. Semin Dermatol 4:271–275
20. Christophers E, Mrowietz U (1999) Psoriasis. In: Fitzpatrick TB, Eisen AZ, Wolff K (eds) Dermatology in general medicine, 5th edn. McGraw Hill, New York, pp 495–521
21. Creamer JD, Barker JN (1995) Vascular proliferation and angiogenic factors in psoriasis. Clin Exp Dermatol 20:6–9
22. Curry JL, Qin J-Z, Bonish B, Carrick R, Bacon P, Panella J, Robinson J, Nickoloff BJ (2003) Innate immune-related receptors in normal and psoriatic skin. Arch Pathol Lab Med 127:178–186
23. Daoud P, Mirc M, Tarazourte MF, Pollak M, Rousset A, Castaing H (2000) Neonatal hyperparathyroidism secondary to unknown maternal hypoparathyroidism. Arch Pediatr 7:45–48
24. Dover R, Wright NA (1993) Biology and function of epidermis and appendages. In: Fitzpatrick TB, Eisen AZ, Wolff K, Freedberg IM, Austen KF (eds) Dermatology in general medicine. McGraw-Hill, New York, p 159
25. Driessler F, Venstrom K, Sabat R, Asadullah K, Schottelius AJ (2004) Molecular mechanisms of interleukin-10-mediated inhibition of NF-κB activity: a role for p50. Clin Exp Immunol 135:64–73
26. Duffy DL, Spelman LS, Martin NG (1993) Psoriasis in Australian twins. J Am Acad Dermatol 29: 428–434
27. Ekholm E, Egelrud T (1999) Stratum corneum chymotryptic enzyme in psoriasis. Arch Dermatol Res 291:195–200
28. Elder JT, Nair RP, Voorhees JJ (1994) Epidemiology and the genetics of psoriasis. J Invest Dermatol 102: 24S–27S
29. Favre M, Majewski S, Noszczyk B, Maienfisch F, Pura A, Orth G, Jablonska S (2000) Antibodies to human papillomavirus type 5 are generated in epidermal repair processes. J Invest Dermatol 114:403–407
30. Gillitzer R, Ritter U, Spandau U, Goebeler M, Brocker EB (1996) Differential expression of GRO-alpha and IL-8 mRNA in psoriasis: a model for neutrophil migration and accumulation in vivo. J Invest Dermatol 107:778–782
31. Gillum PS, Golitz LE (1998) Psoriasiform dermatitis. In: Barnhill RL (ed) Textbook of dermatopathology. McGraw Hill, New York, pp 55–68
32. Gonzalez S, Martinez-Borra J, Del Rio JS, Santos-Juanes J, Lopez-Vazquez A, Blanco-Gelaz M, Lopez-Larrea C (2000) The OTF3 gene polymorphism confers susceptibility to psoriasis independent of the association of HLA-Cw*0602. J Invest Dermatol 115:824–828
33. Goodfield M, Macdonald Hull SM, Holland D, Roberts G, Wood E, Reid S (1994) Investigations of the 'active' edge of plaque psoriasis: vascular proliferation precedes changes in epidermal keratin. Br J Dermatol 131:808–813
34. Gordon M, Johnson WC (1967) Histopathology and histochemistry of psoriasis: I. The active lesion and clinically normal skin. Arch Dermatol 95:402–407
35. Griffiths CE (1994) Cutaneous leukocyte trafficking and psoriasis. Arch Dermatol 130:494–499
36. Haase I, Pasparakis M (2002) A new mouse model for psoriasis: evidence for a TNF-mediated, T cell-independent pathogenesis. Br J Dermatol 47:1047– 1078
37. Herbst RA, Hoch O, Kapp A, Weiss J (2000) Guttate psoriasis triggered by perianal streptococcal dermatitis in a four-year-old boy. J Am Acad Dermatol 42:885–887
38. Irimajiri J, Yamamoto T, Rimura K, Yokozeki H, Nishioka K (1998) Verruca vulgaris developing during cyclosporin therapy for psoriasis vulgaris. J Dermatol 25:688–690
39. Kere J (2002) PSORS1: towards gene identification. Br J Dermatol 147:1047–1078
40. Kono T, Tanii T, Furukawa M, Mizuno N, Taniguchi S, Ishii M, Hamada T (1990) Effects of human recombinant tumor necrosis factor-alpha (TNF-alpha) on the proliferative potential of human keratinocytes cultured in serum-free medium. J Dermatol 17:409–413
41. Krueger GG, Eyre RW (1984) Trigger factors in psoriasis. Dermatol Clin 2:373–381
42. Kulke R, Bornscheuer E, Schluter C, Bartels J, Rowert J, Sticherling M, Christophers E (1998) The CXC receptor 2 is overexpressed in psoriatic epidermis. J Invest Dermatol 110:90–94
43. Leigh IM, Navsaria H, Purkis PE, McKay IA, Bowden PE, Riddle PN (1995) Keratins (K16 and K17) as markers of keratinocyte hyperproliferation in psoriasis in vivo and in vitro. Br J Dermatol 133:501–511
44. Leung D, Walsh P, Giorno R, Norris D (1993) A potential role for superantigens in the pathogenesis of psoriasis. J Invest Dermatol 100:225–228
45. Leung DY, Gately M, Trumble A, Ferguson-Darnell B, Schlievert PM, Picker LJ (1995) Bacterial superantigens induce T cell expression of the skin-selective homing receptor, the cutaneous lymphocyte-associated antigen via stimulation of interleukin 12 production. J Exp Med 181:747–753

46. Linhart C, Wolter M, Kaufmann R (2003) Psoriasiforme entzündliche Dermatosen. In: Kerl H, Garbe C, Cerroni L, Wolff HH (eds) Histopathologie der Haut, 1st edn. Springer, Berlin Heidelberg New York, pp 145–150
47. Lowe PM, Lee ML, Jackson CJ, To SS, Cooper AJ, Schrieber L (1995) The endothelium in psoriasis. Br J Dermatol 132:497–505
48. Ludolph-Hauser D, Schubert C, Wiedow O (1999) Structural changes of human epidermis induced by human leukocyte-derived proteases. Exp Dermatol 8:46–52
49. Mahe E, Bodemer C, Descamps V, Mahe I, Crickx B, De Prost Y, Favre M (2003) High frequency of detection of human papillomaviruses associated with epidermodysplasia verruciformis in children with psoriasis. Br J Dermatol 149:819–825
50. Mallon E, Young D, Bunce M, Gotch FM, Easterbrook PJ, Newson R, Bunker CB (1998) HLA-Cw*0602 and HIV-associated psoriasis. Br J Dermatol 139:527–533
51. Mallon E, Bunce M, Savoie H, Rowe A, Newson R, Gotch F, Bunker CB (2000) HLA-C and guttate psoriasis. Br J Dermatol 143:1177–1182
52. Molhuizen HO, Schalkwijk J (1995) Structural, biochemical, and cell biological aspects of the serine proteinase inhibitor SKALP/elafin/ESI. Biol Chem Hoppe Seyler 376:1–7
53. Mommers JM, van Rossum MM, van Erp PE, van de Kerkhof PC (2000) Changes in keratin 6 and keratin 10 (co-)expression in lesional and symptomless skin of spreading psoriasis. Dermatology 201:15–20
54. Moynihan GD, Ruppe JP Jr (1985) Impetigo herpetiformis and hypoparathyroidism. Arch Dermatol 121:1330–1331
55. Nair RP, Stuart P, Henseler T, Jenisch S, Chia NV, Westphal E, Schork NJ, Kim J, Lim HW, Christophers E, Voorhees JJ, Elder JT (2000) Localization of psoriasis-susceptibility locus PSORS1 to a 60-kb interval telomeric to HLA-C. Am J Hum Genet 66: 1833–1844
56. Naldi L, Peli L, Parazzini F, Carrel CF, Psoriasis Study Group of the Italian Group for Epidemiological Research in Dermatology (2001) Family history of psoriasis, stressful life events, and recent infectious disease are risk factors for a first episode of acute guttate psoriasis: Results of a case-control study. J Am Acad Dermatol 44:433–438
57. Nanney LB, Yates RA, King LE Jr (1992) Modulation of epidermal growth factor receptors in psoriatic lesions during treatment with topicals EGF. J Invest Dermatol 98:296–301
58. Navarro JM, Casatorres J, Jorcano JL (1995) Elements controlling the expression and induction of the skin hyperproliferation-associated keratin K6. J Biol Chem 270:21362–21367
59. Nickoloff BJ (1999) The immunologic and genetic basis of psoriasis. Arch Dermatol 135:1104–1110
60. Nickoloff BJ, Wrone-Smith T (1998) Superantigens, autoantigens, and pathogenic T cells in psoriasis. J Invest Dermatol 110:459–460
61. Penas PF, Gomez M, Buezo GF, Rios L, Yanez-Mo M, Cabanas C, Sanchez-Madrid F, Garcia-Diez A (1998) Differential expression of activation epitopes of beta1 integrin in psoriasis and normal skin. J Invest Dermatol 111:19–24
62. Petzelbauer P, Pober JS, Keh A, Braverman IM (1994) Inducibility and expression of microvascular endothelial adhesion molecules in lesional, perilesional, and uninvolved skin of psoriatic patients. J Invest Dermatol 103:300–305
63. Piepkorn M (1996) Overexpression of amphiregulin, a major autocrine growth factor for cultured human keratinocytes, in hyperproliferative skin disease. Am J Dermatopathol 18:165–171
64. Plant D, Lear J, Marsland A, Worthington J, Griffiths CEM (2002) NOD2 single nucleotide polymorphisms do not confer susceptibility to chronic plaque psoriasis. Br J Dermatol 147:1047–1078
65. Prinz JC (1999) Which T cells cause psoriasis? Clin Exp Dermatol 24:291–295
66. Prinz JC (2001) Psoriasis vulgaris, a sterile antibacterial skin reaction, mediated by cross-reactive T-cells? An immunological view on the pathophysiology of psoriasis. Clin Exp Dermatol 26:326–332
67. Rajendran SS, Premalatha S, Yesudian P, Zahra A (1984) Psoriasis verruciformis. Int J Dermatol 23: 552–553
68. Russell TJ, Schultes LM, Kuban DJ (1972) Histocompatibility (HL-A) antigens associated with psoriasis. N Engl J Med 287:738–740
69. Sayama K, Midorikawa K, Hanakawa Y, Sugai M, Hashimoto K (1998) Superantigens production by *Staphylococcus aureus* in psoriasis. Dermatology 196:194–198
70. Schalkwijk J, Chang A, Janssen P, de Jongh GJ, Mier PD (1990) Skin-derived antileucoproteases (SKALPs): characterization of two new elastase inhibitors from psoriatic epidermis. Br J Dermatol 122:631–641
71. Schroder JM, Gregory H, Young J, Christophers E (1992) Neutrophil-activating proteins in psoriasis. J Invest Dermatol 98:241–247
72. Skov L, Baadsgaard O (2000) Bacterial superantigens and inflammatory skin diseases. Clin Exp Dermatol 25:57–61
73. Smith CH, Barker JNWN (1995) Cell trafficking and role of adhesion molecules in psoriasis. In: van de Kerkhof PCM, Bos JD (eds) Pathogenetic aspects of psoriasis. Elsevier, New York, pp 151–160
74. Snowden JA, Heaton DC (1997) Development of psoriasis after syngeneic bone marrow transplant from psoriatic donor: further evidence for adoptive autoimmunity. Br J Dermatol 137:130–132
75. Steffen C (2002) William John Munro and Munro's abscess, and Franz Kogoj and Kogoj's spongiform pustule. Am J Dermatopathol 24:364–368
76. Swanbeck G, Inerot A, Martinsson T, Wahlstrom J, Enerback C, Enlund F, Yhr M (1995) Age at onset and different types of psoriasis. Br J Dermatol 133: 768–773

77. Sweet WL, Smoller BR (1997) Differential proliferation of endothelial cells and keratinocytes in psoriasis and spongiotic dermatitis. J Cutan Pathol 24: 356–363
78. Szepietowski J, Wasik F, Bielicka E, Nockowski P, Noworolska A (1999) Soluble E-selectin serum levels correlate with disease activity in psoriasis patients. Clin Exp Dermatol 24:33–36
79. Takematsu H, Tagami H (1993) Quantification of chemotactic peptides (C5a anaphylatoxin and IL-8) in psoriatic lesional skin. Arch Dermatol 129:74–80
80. Tanaka N, Fujioka A, Tajima S, Ishibashi A, Hirose S (2000) Elafin is induced in epidermis in skin disorders with dermal neutrophilic infiltration: interleukin-1beta and tumor necrosis factor-alpha stimulate its secretion in vitro. Br J Dermatol 143:728–732
81. Telfer NR, Chalmers RJ, Whale K, Colman G (1992) The role of streptococcal infection in the initiation of guttate psoriasis. Arch Dermatol 128:39–42
82. Tiilikainen A, Lassus A, Karvonen J, Vartiainen P, Julin M (1980) Psoriasis and HLA-Cw6. Br J Dermatol 102:179–184
83. Travis L, Weinberg JM (2002) Medical background: Psoriasis. Drugs Today (Barc) 38:847–865
84. Valdimarsson H, Baker BS, Jonsdottir I, Powles A, Fry L (1995) Psoriasis: A T-cell-mediated autoimmune disease induced by streptococcal superantigens? Immunol Today 16:145–149
85. Van de Kerkhof PCM (1986) Clinical features. In: Mier PD, van der Kerkhof PCM (eds) Textbook of psoriasis. Churchill Livingstone, Edinburgh, pp 13–39
86. Van de Kerkhof PCM (2003) Psoriasis. In: Bolognia JL, Jorizzo JL, Rapini RP, Horn TD, Mancini AJ, Mascaro JM, Salasche SJ, Saurat JH, Stingl G (eds) Dermatology. Mosby, St. Louis, pp 125–149
87. Van de Kerkhof PCM, Gerritsen MJP, de Jong EMGJ (1996) Transition from symptomless to lesional psoriatic skin. Clin Exp Dermatol 21:325–329
88. Van der Fits L, Van der Wel LI, Boogaard MW, Laman JD, Versuchen MCM, Prens EP (2002) Type I and Type II interferon signalling are both activated in lesional psoriatic skin. Br J Dermatol 147:1047–1078
89. Wakita H, Takigawa M (1994) E-selectin and vascular cell adhesion molecule-1 are critical for initial trafficking of helper-inducer/memory T cells in psoriatic plaques. Arch Dermatol 130:457–463
90. Watts P, Stables GS, Akhurst RJ, MacKie RM (1994) Localization of transforming growth factor-alpha RNA and protein in the skin of psoriatic patients receiving therapy. Br J Dermatol 131:64–71
91. Weedon D (2002) The psoriasiform reaction pattern. In: Weedon D (ed) Skin pathology. Churchill Livingstone, London, pp 76–83
92. Weinstein GD, Van Scott EJ (1965) Autoradiographic analysis of turnover times of normal and psoriatic epidermis. J Invest Dermatol 45:257–262
93. Wiedow O, Schroder J-M, Gregory H, Young JA, Christophers E (1990) Elafin: An elastase-specific inhibitor of human skin. Purification, characterization, and complete amino acid sequence. J Biol Chem 265:14791–14795
94. Wiedow O, Wiese F, Streit V, Kalm C, Christophers E (1992) Lesional elastase activity in psoriasis, contact dermatitis, and atopic dermatitis. J Invest Dermatol 99:306–309
95. Wiedow O, Wiese F, Christophers E (1995) Lesional activity in psoriasis. Diagnostic and prognostic significance. Arch Dermatol Res 287:632–635
96. Young HS, Summers AM, Bhushan M, Brenchley PEC, Griffiths CE (2004) Single-nucleotide polymorphisms of vascular endothelial growth factor in psoriasis of early onset. J Invest Dermatol 122: 209–215
97. Zhou S, Matsuyoshi N, Takeuchi T, Ohtsuki Y, Miyachi Y (2003) Reciprocal altered expression of T-cadherin and P-cadherin in psoriasis vulgaris. Br J Dermatol 149:268–273
98. Zimmerman GM (1999) Alcohol and psoriasis. Arch Dermatol 135:1541–1542

B Psoriatic Arthritis

Soumya M. Reddy,
Clifton O. Bingham III

Contents

1 Introduction

Until recently, psoriatic arthritis (PsA) has not received the same attention as other inflammatory arthritides with regards to the development of formal outcome measures, in part due to the difficulty of studying such a heterogeneous disease. As a result, many of the treatments, as well as outcome measures, used in the evaluation of PsA have been borrowed from the study of rheumatoid arthritis (RA) and ankylosing spondylitis (AS). Indeed, there are currently very few instruments that are disease-specific for the evaluation of PsA. In this chapter we will review the existing indices that have been applied to PsA from other disease states and review those that have been further validated in this disease. Outcome measures specifically designed for the evaluation of PsA will also be reviewed. The need for disease-specific measures is highlighted by the development of new medications and the need for formal validated outcome measures for use in future clinical trials.

2 Peripheral Joint Disease

Several assessments of peripheral joint disease activity developed for RA have been utilized in PsA, including the American College of Rheumatology (ACR) joint count and the Ritchie Articular Index (RAI). *The ACR* (previously the American Rheumatism Association) *joint count* was developed for the evaluation of patients with RA in 1965 [1]. The ACR joint count records clinically involved joints, as painful or tender with pressure or passive movement, and swollen other than bony proliferation. Joints are examined bilaterally and include the temperomandibular, sternoclavicular, acromioclavicular (AC), shoulder, elbow, wrist, metacarpophalangeal (MCP) (*5*), proximal interphalangeal (PIP) (*4*), interphalangeal (IP) of the thumb (*1*), distal interphalangeal (DIP) (*4*), hip, knee, ankle, mid-tarsal (including subtalar), metatarsophalangeal (MTP) (*5*), IP joints of toes (*5* – proximal and distal IP joints of the toes counted as *1*). Separate values are usually recorded for numbers of tender joints (maximum 68) and swollen joints (maximum 66 – the hips are not included for assessment of swelling). The ACR joint count has been validated in RA for reproducibility and sensitivity to change [1].

The ACR joint count has also been evaluated in PsA. While it has been noted that patients with PsA are less tender than RA patients when active joints are evaluated [2], the ACR 66/68 joint count reliably recorded joint activity in patients with PsA with minimal interobserver variability despite significant differences in the severity of patients' disease [2, 3]. This validation study, however, was performed on only a small number of patients [3]. The 66 and 68 ACR joint counts have also been used in clinical trials of PsA patients treated with leflunomide [4], etanercept [5, 6], infliximab [7].

A simplified *28 joint count* that includes only shoulders, elbows, wrists, MCP and PIP joints of the hands, and knees has been used to follow clinical disease activity in practice and in clinical trials in RA [7]. This joint count has also been incorporated in a simplified version of the Disease Activity Scoring (DAS) system discussed further below. While attractive for its ease of use in trials and clinical practice, the 28 joint count has not been validated in PsA and may be inadequate for the assessment of PsA given the exclusion of the DIPs of the hands and feet, which are more commonly involved in PsA than RA [8]. In fact, DIP involvement in RA is uncommon.

The *Ritchie Articular Index* (RAI) was described in 1968 for the evaluation of RA [9]. Each joint is scored on a scale of 0–3 for severity of tenderness (0=none, 1=mild, 2=moderate, 3=severe). The original description included the assessment of 53 joints including the shoulders, cervical spine, elbows, wrists, hips, knees, ankles, subtalar joints, and midtarsals. For the following joints only one score is given for each group based on the highest score of any one joint in the group: the temporomandibular joints, sternoclavicular joints, acromioclavicular joints, the MCPs of each hand, the PIPs of each hand, and the MTPs of each foot. For example, all the MCPs of a single hand are counted together as a group and would have a maximum score of 3 on the RAI. The maximum score for the 26 units is 78. A modification of the RAI assesses tenderness of individual joints separately according to the ACR joint count with a 0–3 scale for tenderness, but does not include the IP joints of the feet. The original RAI has been used more frequently in Europe as it is one of the components of the original DAS measurement.

In a study evaluating four different articular indices in RA, the ACR joint count had less inter-observer variability compared to the RAI. The scaled grading of joint tenderness in the RAI was likely responsible for a greater variability seen in this measurement. A further modification by Hart of the Ritchie index, which excluded the scaled grading of severity, performed better than the original RAI and in fact had the least inter-observer variability of the 4 indices evaluated [10].

The different joint counts have also been evaluated for their sensitivity to change in a small study of 38 patients with PsA. The RAI, tender joint counts (*68* or *28*), and swollen joint counts (*66*, *44*, or *28*) were recorded before and after 1 year of different treatments for PsA and all were correlated with the assessor's global assessment (AGA) of disease activity after treatment. Only the RAI and swollen joint counts correlated with the AGA before treatment [11]. The best measure to assess swollen and tender joints in PsA, and the specific joints that should be recorded require further evaluation in larger groups of patients.

Spinal Measures

Measurements of spinal motion and tenderness have been developed for the evaluation of ankylosing spondylitis but have not been validated for PsA. Metrology developed for the spine in AS were established to evaluate symmetrical sacroiliitis and a continuous process of the spine. While these measurements may be applicable to AS-like patients with PsA, spondylitis is present in only a subset of patients with PsA. In addition, PsA spondyloarthropathy differs from AS in that it often involves the sacroiliac joints asymmetrically, may affect the spine in an asymmetric and discontinuous fashion, and result in less severe disease in regards to pain and restriction of motion [8].

The *Schober method* for measurement of lumbar flexion was defined by marking the lumbosacral junction (also defined as the spinal intersection of a line joining the dimples of Venus) with the patient erect and making another skin mark 10 cm above this [12]. When the patient bends forward, the distance between the two marks is measured, reflecting anterior lumbar flexion. The distance should increase by at least 5 cm (Fig. B1).

A *modification of the Schober test* was later developed by Macrae and Wright in which a second skin mark 5 cm below the lumbosacral junction was added, resulting in a 15-cm distance between the upper and lower marks [12].

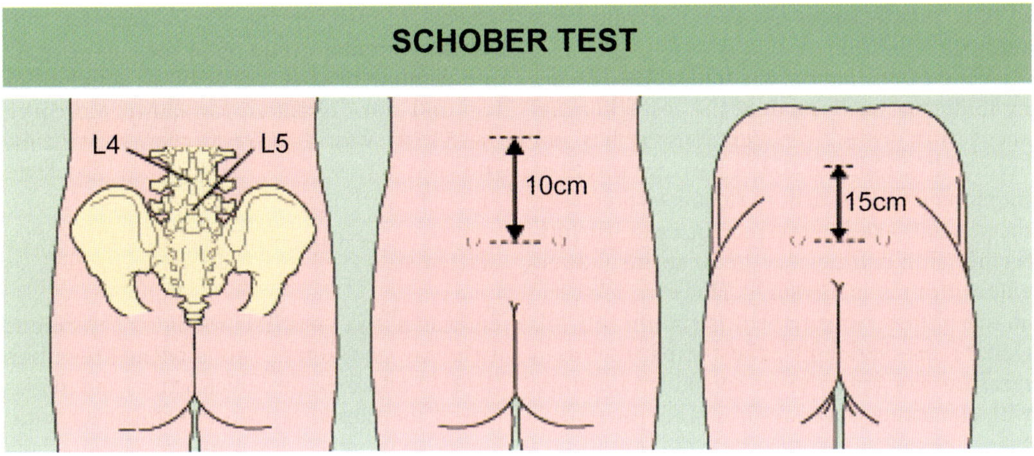

Fig. B1. Schober test (Hochberg, Electronic Image Collection for Rheumatology, CD, Fig. 103.12, with permission).

The increase in distance between the 2 marks was again measured with the patient bending forward. Macrae and Wright studied the Schober and modified Schober in ulcerative colitis subjects with and without spinal disease and their relatives and spouses. Both methods correlated well with radiographs of true forward flexion of the lumbar spine performed with lead skin markers, but the modified method had a higher correlation coefficient and a smaller standard error. The increased accuracy of the modified Schober is thought to be a function of the lower skin point being more closely tethered to the underlying structures which results in less upward movement of the mark with flexion. It was also noted in this study that the modified Schober score was affected by age and sex, with older age and female sex being associated with lower scores [12].

In contrast, Portek et al. found no correlation of the modified Schober method with biplanar radiographic data and poor inter-observer agreement in subjects without spinal disease [13]. Nonetheless, the Schober test has become a standard part of the assessment of patients in clinical practice and in clinical trials for AS, and discriminates between drug and placebo in clinical trials of medications [14]. It is not known if the Schober test is a reliable method for the assessment of spinal disease in PsA.

Measurement of the *fingertip-to-floor distance* has also been used in assessing thoraco-lumbar motion in patients with AS. With a patient bent forward in flexion at the hips and spine, the distance between the middle fingertip and floor is recorded. While this measure is reproducible, its validity as a measure of vertebral flexion is limited, as it is affected by other variables such as hip mobility and hamstring extensibility [15]. Assessments of *lateral spinal flexion* have also been evaluated in AS. The *fingertip to floor distance* is measured with the patient in full lateral flexion at the hip and lower spine, without flexing forward or bending the knees. This is also felt to reflect lumbar spinal movement, an early area of involvement in AS. This method was found to have good inter-observer correlation and low intra-observer variation [15]. Neither of these two measurements has have been evaluated in PsA.

The *occiput to wall distance* has been commonly used in the clinical assessment of patients with AS. This measurement of upper thoracic kyphosis and lower cervical flexion, is assessed with the patient standing with heels and buttocks touching the wall and knees straight. The back of the head is moved as close to the wall as possible and the distance between the occiput and the wall is measured. While this measurement is reliable and reproducible, it is only affected in very severe and later stage AS [15]. Nonetheless this measurement has been shown to be sensitive to change in response to therapy with etanercept [14]. The performance of this measurement in PsA has not been studied.

While *chest expansion* is frequently affected in AS due to involvement of the costochondral and posterior facet articulations, it has not been well studied in PsA. Chest expansion is measured at the level of the xiphisternum with the patient's hands placed on the head. The difference in circumference between inspiration and expiration is measured. However, the variability of this measurement is significant [15]. Despite this variability, chest expansion as a measure was found to be sensitive to change with etanercept treatment in a randomized placebo-controlled trial in AS patients [14].

The hips are commonly affected in spondyloarthropathies. Swelling cannot be accurately assessed in the hip joints. However, assessment of hip joint function is important to record in the spondyloarthropathies. The *intermalleolar distance*, a measure of hip function, is measured with the patient supine, knees straight and toes pointing upward. The patient maximally abducts the hips and the distance between the medial malleoli is measured [16]. In PsA patients, intermalleolar distance measurements of hip motion were reliable with good agreement among observers [17]. Another group has reported, however, that other measurements of hip flexion, abduction, adduction, internal and external rotation using a goniometer are unreliable, with high interobserver and intraobserver variability [15].

The *sacroiliac joints* are difficult to assess clinically due to their inaccessibility and immobility; they cannot be assessed for joint line tenderness accurately or pain with range of motion. Maneuvers to stress the SI are neither sensitive nor specific for AS and assessment of SI pain has not been used extensively in the evaluation of AS or PsA.

The *Bath Ankylosing Spondylitis Metrology Index* (BASMI) was developed by analyzing 20 different measures in 43 patients with AS. Five measurements were ultimately included that most accurately reflected axial disease. The five measurements included cervical rotation, occiput to wall distance, thoracolumbar lateral flexion, modified Schober, and intermalleolar distance. Each measure was scored from 0–2 for severity of involvement. The BASMI was validated in another group of 54 patients with AS and demonstrated reproducibility, with low inter- and intra-observer variability. Moreover, the BASMI was sensitive to change over time [16].

Enthesitis

Enthesitis is a characteristic feature of psoriatic arthritis and other spondyloarthropathies (SpA). Enthesopathy is defined as inflammation at the sites of tendon insertion into bone. Lower extremity enthesopathy is especially common in PsA. Investigators have demonstrated structural abnormalities at quadriceps tendon entheses in PsA that were not seen in RA, such as new bone deposition resulting in enthesophytes [18]. Similarly, subchondral bony lesions ("edema") adjacent to entheseal insertions was seen only in patients with SpA and not in RA knee effusions [19].

Enthesitis is difficult to assess clinically. Balint et al. showed that most entheseal abnormalities are not detected on clinical examination, consisting of examination for tenderness and swelling at each site [20]. In his study, clinical examination had a sensitivity of only 22.6% and a specificity of 79.7% for the detection of enthesitis compared to ultrasound in patients with SpA. The significance of asymptomatic enthesitis is not known.

Currently, there are two measures available for the clinical assessment of enthesitis in SpA. The *Mander Enthesis Index* (MEI) is comprehensive and includes 66 sites, each graded for intensity of tenderness to palpation from 0–3; no pain = 0, mild tenderness = 1, moderate tenderness = 2, wince or withdraw = 3. [21] (Fig. B2). The MEI was sensitive to change with treatment in one study, with decreased scores within 1 week of beginning treatment with nonsteroidal anti-inflammatory drugs (NSAIDs).

The *Maastricht Ankylosing Spondylitis Enthesis Score* (MASES) has also been validated in AS [22]. The MASES evaluates only the 13 most frequently involved of the 66 entheses and omits the grading of intensity, making it a simpler and more feasible tool for clinical assess-

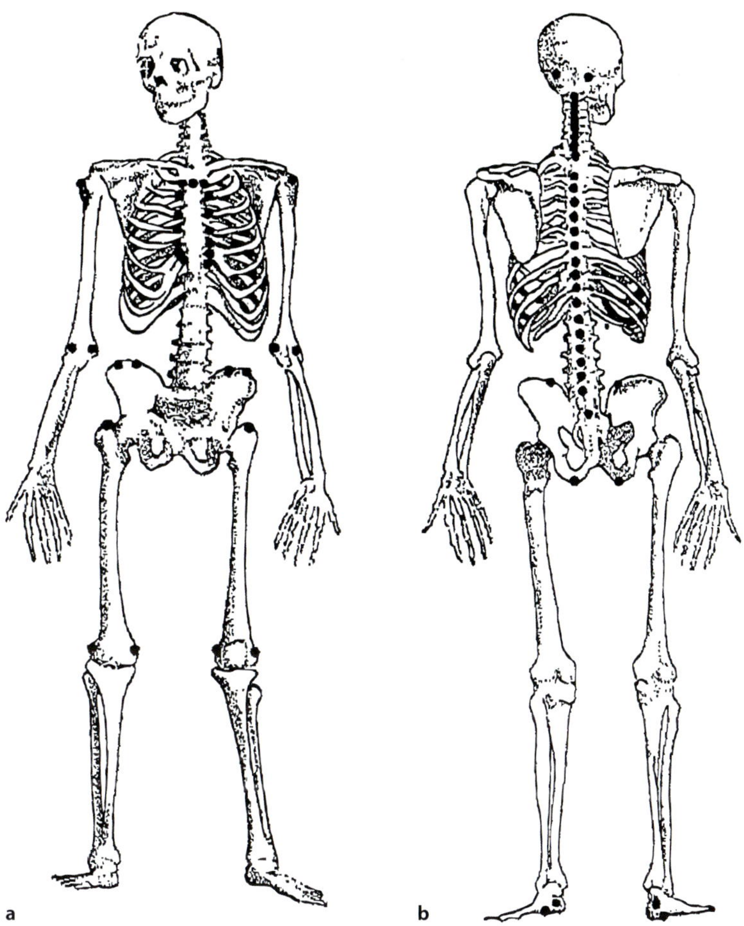

Fig. B2a, b. Mander Enthesis Index. From [21]

ments and clinical investigation. The MASES correlated well with the MEI, only showing discordance at low levels of activity measured by the MEI, the clinical significance of which is unknown. The MEI and MASES have both shown fair correlations with the Bath Ankylosing Spondylitis Disease Activity Index (BASDAI). The MASES has not been evaluated for its correlation with radiographic outcomes or its ability to detect treatment effects.

To date there have been no formal studies of the MEI or MASES entheses indices in PsA. The clinical assessment of enthesitis was included in a validation study of the Spondyloarthritis Research Consortium of Canada (SPARCC) using ten patients and ten rheumatologists. The observers had good agreement for the detection of plantar fasciitis but not for other entheses [17]. In a randomized, double blind trial of 102 active PsA patients treated with infliximab or placebo, Antoni et al. reported a decrease in the number of patients with enthesitis from 13 to 7 after treatment in the infliximab group compared to an increase from 13 to 15 in the placebo group after 16 weeks [23].

Dactylitis

Dactylitis, or sausage shaped swollen digit, is a classic finding in PsA resulting from a combination of flexor tenosynovitis and IP joint synovitis. In an ultrasound evaluation of 25 dactylitic digits in 17 PsA patients, flexor tenosynovitis was confirmed in 96% (24/25) and articular synovitis in 52% (13/25) of the dactylitic fingers [24]. Other investigators have reported a lower incidence of actual synovitis and a predominance of flexor tenosynovitis in dactylitic digits of patients with SpA [25]. The presence of dactylitis in PsA has been associated with increased radiographic damage compared to unaffected digits in some studies [24, 26]. Ultrasound (US) and Magnetic Resonance Imaging (MRI) both detect tendon structures that are not visualized on plain radiographs.

Currently, no measures have been validated for the clinical assessment of dactylitis. Dactylitis can be recorded as present (assigned a value of 1) or absent (assigned a value of 0) based on the presence of swelling, tenderness, and redness of an entire digit. Using this method to assess dactylitis in a clinical trial of infliximab for PsA, Antoni et al. reported that dactylitis scores decreased from a baseline of 2.33 to 0.24 with infliximab, compared to a change from 2.0 to 1.33 with placebo [23].

It is not clear if swelling of an entire digit in the absence of tenderness or erythema should be classified separately as chronic dactylitis. Clinical exam cannot distinguish dactylitis as a result of flexor tenosynovitis alone or in combination with synovitis. Based on ultrasound findings [24], synovitis is concurrently present in about half of dactylitic fingers; thus, some investigators recommend that all joints in a dactylitic finger should be counted in tender and swollen joint counts.

Biologic Markers of Inflammation

Both the erythrocyte sedimentation rate (ESR) and C-reactive protein (CRP) correlate with disease activity in RA and are responsive to treatment; however, these measurements have not performed as well in AS [27]. In PsA, only 40–60% of patients demonstrate an elevation in the ESR; this finding is seen particularly in patients with polyarticular involvement [28]. The mean ESR in one series of patients studied was 36 mm/h, and was found to correlate with assessor's global assessment and was sensitive to change after treatment [11]. One study of 36 PsA patients showed that the ESR was the best indicator of disease activity and severity [29]. In another study, a low ESR level was protective of progression of joint damage in PsA, and high ESR was associated with early mortality [30].

CRP is also elevated in some patients with PsA. Daunt et al. reported that 44% of PsA patients in their series had normal CRP levels [31]. In some studies, CRP correlated with radiographic scores and severity but not with disease activity [29], while in others it has been shown to correlate with disease activity [32].

In the recent Phase II randomized clinical trial of etanercept in PsA, the mean baseline ESR was 16 mm/h (placebo) and 22 mm/h (etanercept) and mean baseline CRP was 12 mg/l (placebo) and 14 mg/l (etanercept) [5]. Both parameters demonstrated significant decreases with treatment compared to placebo. In the Phase III study of etanercept in PsA, the baseline CRP was 1.7 mg/dl (placebo) and 2.2 mg/dl (etanercept) [6]. The CRP decreased with etanercept treatment but not in the placebo group. It should be noted that patients in both of these studies were required to have at least three tender and three swollen joints to be enrolled in the study. These clinical trial data suggest that in this subset of PsA patients with active disease, CRP is sensitive to change with treatment. However, in patients with minimal baseline elevations, the relevance of ESR and CRP is unknown.

In an open label pilot study of infliximab treatment which required elevated ESR levels for study entry, baseline ESR (44 mm/h) and CRP (1.79 mg/dl) significantly decreased by 57% and 68% respectively after 14 weeks of treatment [33]. Patients with CRP baseline values greater than 2.0 in this study had significantly more frequent improvement in several other outcome measures suggesting that patients with higher baseline CRP levels may have a better response to treatment with TNF antagonists.

ESR and CRP are inflammatory markers that may be useful in some patients in the assessment of PsA. These measurements change with treatment and correlate with clinical responses. Whether, as in RA, these will correlate with long term progression and disability will require further study. There is also a need to determine the level of elevations of CRP and ESR in larger non clinical trial populations of patients with PsA.

Anti-cyclic citrullinated peptides (anti-CCP) antibodies have recently received much attention in RA because of their high specificity and moderate sensitivity for the diagnosis of RA [34–36]. Anti-CCP antibodies have been correlated with the development of erosive disease in a few studies [34, 36–38]. Studies to date have not detected an increase in anti-CCP antibodies in PsA, but the number of patients studied has been small [38]. Lee et al. noted only 2 out of 21 PsA patients to have positive anti-CCP antibodies and no correlation with radiographic erosions was detected [34]. Another study of anti-CCP antibodies also did not detect an increase in 13 patients with PsA [39]. The currently available data does not suggest that anti-CCP antibodies are elevated in PsA, but the numbers of patients included so far have been small, and further studies are needed.

3 Imaging Methods

Radiography is an important tool in assessing the progression of disease in chronic inflammatory joint diseases. Increasingly, prevention of joint damage, measured by plain radiography, has become an important goal in the clinical care of patients as well as a major outcome measure in clinical drug trials. Numerous methods exist to interpret radiographic changes in rheumatoid arthritis (RA), and these have been subsequently applied to the assessment of psoriatic arthritis (PsA). Although the joint destruction in PsA has some similarities to RA, including erosions and joint space narrowing, the unique features of PsA, notably DIP involvement, periostitis, and ankylosis, are not captured using standard assessment tools for RA. Similarly, some tools to evaluate AS also may be appropriate for the evaluation of PsA spondylitis and sacroiliitis.

Peripheral Joint Radiographs

Several methods of radiographic assessment have been used to evaluate joint destruction in PsA. Each method was originally developed to assess RA. The Steinbrocker radiographic stage, modified Sharp score and Larsen method have all been demonstrated to correlate well with each other in RA [40].

The first scoring system to quantify radiographic evaluation in RA was developed by Steinbrocker et al. in 1949 [41]. The Steinbrocker method assigns one score to the entire joint based on all detected abnormalities. Normal joints are classified as Grade 0, evidence of soft-tissue swelling or juxta-articular osteopenia as Grade 1, evidence of erosions as Grade 2, evidence of erosions plus joint space narrowing as Grade 3, and total joint destruction as Grade 4. The patient's score is determined by the status of the worst joint. A modification of the Steinbrocker method includes a score for each joint.

The Larsen method assigns a score to each of ten hand joints and four wrist areas. This method assesses the amount of joint destruction with a single score of 0–4 for each joint based on comparison with standard radiographs [42]. Larsen's method was modified by Rau et al. in 1995, to include a semi-quantitative description of the loss of joint surface area [43].

In an attempt to validate existing radiographic scoring methods for RA in PsA, Rahman et al. compared the original Steinbrocker, which gives a single score based on the status of the worst joint; a modified Steinbrocker method, which was altered to include the DIP joints, MTPs and first IP of the feet; and the Larsen method, also modified to include the DIPs, MTPs, and IP of the feet for detecting change in PsA radiographs performed at least 2 years apart [44]. All three measures demonstrated good inter-observer and intra-observer reliability. As expected, the modified Steinbrocker and Larsen methods were superior to the original Steinbrocker to detect change over time in PsA.

The Sharp score is a detailed system that assigns separate scores for both erosions and joint space narrowing for each joint evaluated. The initial description included all joints in the hands and carpus but was eventually modified to include 17 areas for erosions and 18 areas for joint space narrowing. Erosions are scored from 0–5, with 0 being no erosion and 5 being more than 4 erosions in 1 joint. Joint space narrowing is scored from 0–4, with 0 being no loss of joint space and 4 being significant joint space narrowing. The erosion scores and joint space narrowing scores may be calculated separately and the sum of both scores equals the total Sharp score [45].

The modified Sharp score and its variations are the most widely used detailed scoring systems for RA. The van der Heijde modification includes scoring of the feet [46]. In this modification, 16 areas are evaluated for erosions and 15 areas for joint space narrowing in the hands. In the feet, the MTP joints and 1st IP joints are included. A further modification of the Sharp/van der Heijde method including the DIPs was evaluated in 120 patients with PsA and demonstrated significant correlation between radiographic scores and clinical damage scores. Other PsA specific radiographic features, such as juxta-articular new bone, osteolysis, and ankylosis, were also strongly correlated with the Sharp scores [47].

Recently, a randomized double-blind, placebo-controlled trial of etanercept in 205 PsA patients utilized a modified Sharp score that included assessment of the hands and wrists and was further modified to include the DIP joints. This modified Sharp score was able to distinguish change in radiographs over time in patients with PsA [48]. The modified Sharp score demonstrated, for the first time, the ability of a drug to reduce radiographic progression in PsA compared to placebo treated patients over 1 - year (total sharp score mean change from baseline at 1 year was −0.02 in the treatment arm vs. +1.03 in the placebo arm). The rate of Sharp score progression in the placebo group in this study is less than seen in most placebo groups in RA studies of 1 year duration. This likely relates both to disease differences and the decision not to score radiographs of the feet in the PsA trial. PsA-specific radiographic features, which are not accounted for in the Sharp score (pencil-in-cup, periostitis, osteolysis, etc.), were also evaluated in this trial, but no changes were detected at 1 year follow-up in either group [49].

As noted, PsA is characterized by many structural features that are unique to this disease and not present in RA. The radiographic scoring methods developed for the assessment of RA, do not take into account several of these features. The previously described scores only measure joint erosions or joint space narrowing, but PsA is characterized by both joint destruction and bony proliferation.

Wassenberg et al. in 2001 developed a new method to score radiographic change in PsA [50]. This method evaluated 40 joints of the hands and feet with separate destruction and proliferation scores. The destruction score ranged from 0–5, where 0 is normal, 1 is one or more erosions with an interruption of the cortical plate >1 mm with destruction of the total joint surface up to 10%, 2 is joint surface destruction of 11–25%, 3 is joint surface destruction of 26–50%, 4 is joint surface destruction of 51–75%, and 5 is >75% joint surface destruction. The proliferation scores range from 0–4 and includes any extra bone formation typical for PsA, where 0 is normal, 1 is 1–2 mm of bony proliferation or bone growth of <25% of the original size (diameter), 2 is 2–3 mm or 25–50% bone growth, 3 is >3 mm or >50% bone growth, and 4 is bony ankylosis. The maximum total score is 360, but destruction and proliferation scores can also be calculated separately. Their method was validated in 20 PsA patients treated with MTX who had baseline and 3-year radiographs, with good intra-observer and inter-observer agreement of the readings. The investigators also demonstrated the ability to detect change over time. This new method developed specifically for PsA has not yet been tested in randomized clinical drug trials and will need to be compared to other radiographic scoring methods.

Plain radiographs in PsA have demonstrated the ability to detect progression as early as 1 - year in the etanercept trial [48]. As new medications become available to slow radiographic progression in PsA, monitoring of such parameters will become increasingly important. Serial plain radiographs should be performed every 1–2 years in patients with PsA to assess progressive joint damage that may not be clinically evident. The overall rate of progression in patients with PsA (e.g., slow and fast progressors) is not well understood and may be slower than RA, based on the progression in the placebo group in the recent etanercept trial. An evaluation of data sets using probability plots may provide further insights into radiographic progression in PsA as in RA [51].

Radiographic Sacroiliitis

No radiographic methods have formally evaluated sacroiliac (SI) joints in PsA. SI involvement is less frequent in PsA than peripheral joint involvement. Asymmetric involvement of the SI joints is common in PsA compared to the typical bilateral involvement seen in AS. The anatomy of the sacroiliac joints makes them difficult to assess with x-rays. In AS, plain SI radiographs have demonstrated a sensitivity of 80–85% and a specificity of 71–75% for the diagnosis of sacroiliitis when compared to CT scans. Intra-observer agreement varies between 65–100% [52].

Radiographic Spinal Assessments

Spinal involvement in PsA is not as common as in AS. There are no methods for spinal radiographic assessment that have been validated or evaluated for use in PsA. In AS, the Bath Ankylosing Spondylitis Radiologic Index (BASRI) is a global grading system comparable to a Larsen score in RA. The BASRI evaluates the cervical spine, lumbar spine, SI joints, and hips with a score of 0–4 for each area for a maximum score of 16 [53, 54]. The BASRI has been employed in a randomized controlled trial of infliximab treatment in AS to assess changes after 2 years, but the results are not yet available [55]. The modified Stoke Ankylosing Spondylitis Spinal Score (mSASSS) is a detailed scoring system that evaluates lateral views of the cervical and lumbar spine with anterior sites scored for squaring, erosions, osteophytes, and syndesmophytes [56].

Serial changes in radiographs of the pelvis, SI joints, and spine have a low sensitivity to detect damage in AS and should be obtained no more frequently than every 1–2 years. The utility of serial radiographs of the pelvis, SI joints, and spine has not been formally evaluated in PsA. Given the discontinuous nature of spinal involvement in PsA, any formal assessment of the spine should be comprehensive and include the cervical, thoracic, and lumbar spine.

MRI and Ultrasound of Peripheral Joints

Magnetic resonance imaging (MRI) is an attractive imaging technique in the assessment of patients with inflammatory arthritis because of its greater sensitivity and its ability to detect inflammation. Plain radiographs are not sensitive to changes over short periods of time making MRI potentially more useful to assess short term responses to therapeutic agents. Gadolinium-DPTA uptake by joints directly correlated with severity of inflammatory arthritis in a study of eighteen patients with RA treated with infliximab [57].

The use of MRI has been studied in the evaluation of peripheral joints in PsA in an open label study of infliximab treatment. This study evaluated the joints of ten PsA patients before and after 10 weeks of infliximab treatment. There was a mean reduction of 82.5% in inflammation, as measured by gadolinium-DPTA uptake on MRI that correlated with improvement of other clinical parameters after infliximab treatment [58]. In RA, MRI is thought to have the ability to detect erosions with better resolution and at earlier stages, but the significance of these MRI findings is still unclear. MRI and ultrasound were both found to be better at detecting progression of erosions at 2 years in RA patients [59]. The definitive role of MRI and ultrasound in the evaluation of peripheral arthritis in RA has yet to be determined and has not been adequately addressed in PsA.

Entheses and Tendons

MRI and US are superior to plain x-rays in the detection of enthesopathy, an especially common feature of PsA. US is comparable to MRI for the detection of enthesitis and tendon pathology and has the advantage of being less expensive, and more convenient for repeated assessments. However, specialized training and experienced personnel may be required for US.

In AS, a sonographic entheseal index (SEI) has been used to evaluate entheseal abnormalities in the lower extremities [60]. Active injury signs include hypoechogenicity, increased tendon thickness, peritendinous edema, and bursitis. Chronic injury signs include insertional bone erosions, entheseal calcification, decreased tendon thickness, and tendon rupture. The SEI was evaluated in 35 patients with active AS and demonstrated good inter-observer correlation as well as correlation with disease severity parameters.

Balint et al. have also proposed a sonographic scoring system for enthesitis in SpA, the Glasgow Ultrasound Enthesitis Scoring System (GUESS) [20]. The GUESS evaluates various aspects of tendon thickness, bursitis, erosion, and enthesophytes at five sites in the lower extremity (quadriceps tendon, proximal patellar ligament, distal patellar ligament, Achilles tendon, plantar aponeurosis). GUESS scores did not correlate with ESR and CRP but were superior to clinical examination in the detection of enthesitis. Clinical examination had a sensitivity of only 22.6% compared to ultrasound for enthesitis.

MRI and US may be useful tools to assess response to therapy due to their sensitivity in detecting tendon and entheseal pathology and both require further study in AS and PsA [18, 19, 60, 61]. The clinical significance of asymptomatic detection of enthesopathy has not been studied in PsA.

MRI of Sacroiliac Joints and Spine

MRI has been demonstrated to be more sensitive than conventional radiographs for the detection of inflammation in the SI joints. Contrast enhanced US also has good sensitivity when compared to MRI for the detection of sacroiliitis [62]. In AS, MRI can predict development of sacroiliitis on radiography 3 years later [63]. The role of MRI in the evaluation of SI joints in PsA has not been studied. Similarly, MRI evaluation of the spine is thought to be superior to plain radiographs for detection of structural damage but has not been studied in PsA. In AS, some investigators have suggested a scoring system using MRI (ASspiMRI) to evaluate spinal inflammation with a separate activity and chronicity score [64].

The ASspiMRI was recently evaluated in a randomized double-blind, placebo-controlled trial of infliximab therapy in active AS. Twenty patients enrolled in the trial at one center had MRIs of the spine performed initially and after 3 months and all 40 images were read by two blinded assessors. Active inflammation, measured by gadolinium-DPTA scores, improved in the infliximab group by 40% compared to 6% in the placebo group, and the STIR image scores, measuring bone marrow edema, improved 60% in the infliximab group, versus a decrease of 21% in the placebo group. The T1 image score, representing chronic changes, improved only 7% in the infliximab group but deteriorated by 35% in the placebo group. These results suggest that this MRI scoring method is sensitive to change and able to detect treatment differences. The MRI changes and scores also correlated with clinical improvement as assessed by the BASDAI [65, 66]. This study is the first to show the ability of a medication, infliximab, to reduce spinal inflammation seen on MRI in active AS patients. The activity measures are sensitive to treatment changes but the chronicity measures require further validation. Further studies and comparison to plain radiographic changes are also required. This scoring system has not been tested in PsA.

4 Conclusion

Disease specific measures for PsA are lacking and are currently the focus of investigation. The majority of measures currently available, for both clinical and radiologic assessment, are borrowed from the assessment of RA and AS [67]. While this is a good starting point, given the similarities of some aspects of PsA to both RA and AS, many of these measures have not been adequately validated for use in PsA. The development of disease specific instruments may increase our understanding of this disease and allow us to follow disease activity over time in both clinical practice and clinical trials. These measures, along with skin specific measures, could ultimately be combined to reflect an aggregate index of the disease activity of psoriasis and psoriatic arthritis.

References

1. Deandrade JR, Casagrande PA (1965) A seven-day variability study of 499 patients with peripheral rheumatoid arthritis. Arthritis Rheum 19:302–334
2. Buskila D, Langevitz P, Gladman DD, Urowitz S, Smythe HA (1992) Patients with rheumatoid arthritis are more tender than those with psoriatic arthritis. J Rheumatol 19:1115–1119
3. Gladman DD, Farewell V, Buskila D, Goodman R, Hamilton L, Langevitz P, et al. (1990) Reliability of measurements of active and damaged joints in psoriatic arthritis. J Rheumatol 17:62–64
4. Kaltwasser J, Nash P, Gladman D, Rosen C, Behrens F, Mease P (2003) Leflunomide in the treatment of psoriatic arthritis and psoriasis: data from a double-blind, randomized, placebo-controlled clinical trial. Ann Rheum Dis 62(Suppl 1): abstract #OP0081
5. Mease PJ, Goffe BS, Metz J, VanderStoep A, Finck B, Burge DJ (2000) Etanercept in the treatment of psoriatic arthritis and psoriasis: a randomised trial. Lancet 356:385–390
6. Mease P, Kivitz A, Burch F, Siegel E, Cohen S, Burge D (2001) Improvement in disease activity in patients with psoriatic arthritis receiving etanercept (Enbrel): results of a phase 3 multicenter clinical trial [abstract]. Arthritis Rheum 44(Suppl 9):S90
7. Antoni C, Kavanaugh A, Kirkham B, Burmester G, Weisman M, Keystone E, et al. (2002) The Infliximab Multinational Psoriatic Arthritis Controlled Trial (IMPACT) [abstract]. Arthritis Rheum 46(Suppl 9): S381
8. Gladman DD (1998) Psoriatic arthritis. Rheum Dis Clin North Am 24:829–844
9. Ritchie DM, Boyle JA, McInnes JM, Jasani MK, Dalakos TG, Grieveson P, et al. (1968) Clinical studies with an articular index for the assessment of joint tenderness in patients with rheumatoid arthritis. Q J Med 37:393–406
10. Thompson PW, Hart LE, Goldsmith CH, Spector TD, Bell MJ, Ramsden MF (1991) Comparison of four articular indices for use in clinical trials in rheumatoid arthritis: patient, order and observer variation. J Rheumatol 18:661–665
11. Ujfalussy I, Koo E (2003) Measurement of disease activity in psoriatic arthritis. Extended report. Z Rheumatol 62:60–65
12. Macrae IF, Wright V (1969) Measurement of back movement. Ann Rheum Dis 28:584–589
13. Portek I, Pearcy MJ, Reader GP, Mowat AG (1983) Correlation between radiographic and clinical measurement of lumbar spine movement. Br J Rheumatol 22:197–205
14. Davis JC Jr, Van Der Heijde D, Braun J, Dougados M, Cush J, Clegg DO, et al. (2003) Recombinant human tumor necrosis factor receptor (etanercept) for treating ankylosing spondylitis: a randomized, controlled trial. Arthritis Rheum 48:3230–3236
15. Pile KD, Laurent MR, Salmond CE, Best MJ, Pyle EA, Moloney RO (1991) Clinical assessment of ankylosing spondylitis: a study of observer variation in spinal measurements. Br J Rheumatol 30:29–34
16. Jenkinson TR, Mallorie PA, Whitelock HC, Kennedy LG, Garrett SL, Calin A (1994) Defining spinal mobility in ankylosing spondylitis (AS). The Bath AS Metrology Index. J Rheumatol 21:1694–1698
17. Gladman DD, Cook RJ, Schentag C, Feletar M, Inman R, Hitchon C, et al. (2003) The Clinical Assessment of Patients with Psoriatic Arthritis (PsA): Results of a Validation Study of the Spondyloarthritis Research Consortium of Canada. Arthritis Rheum 48(Suppl 9):S168
18. Frediani B, Falsetti P, Storri L, Allegri A, Bisogno S, Baldi F, et al. (2002) Ultrasound and clinical evaluation of quadricipital tendon enthesitis in patients with psoriatic arthritis and rheumatoid arthritis. Clin Rheumatol 21:203–206
19. McGonagle D, Gibbon W, O'Connor P, Green M, Pease C, Emery P (1998) Characteristic magnetic resonance imaging entheseal changes of knee synovitis in spondylarthropathy. Arthritis Rheum 41: 694–700
20. Balint PV, Kane D, Wilson H, McInnes IB, Sturrock RD (2002) Ultrasonography of entheseal insertions in the lower limb in spondyloarthropathy. Ann Rheum Dis 61:905–910
21. Mander M, Simpson JM, McLellan A, Walker D, Goodacre JA, Dick WC (1987) Studies with an enthesis index as a method of clinical assessment in ankylosing spondylitis. Ann Rheum Dis 46: 197–202

22. Heuft-Dorenbosch L, Spoorenberg A, van Tubergen A, Landewe R, van der Tempel H, Mielants H, et al. (2003) Assessment of enthesitis in ankylosing spondylitis. Ann Rheum Dis 62 : 127–132
23. Antoni CE, Kavanaugh A, Kirkham B, Burmester G, Manger B, Tutuncu Z, et al. (2003) The Infliximab Multinational Psoriatic Arthritis Controlled Trial (IMPACT): Substantial Efficacy on Synovitis and Psoriatic Lesions With or Without DMARD Therapy. Ann Rheum Dis 62(Suppl 1) : abstract #OP0082
24. Kane D, Greaney T, Bresnihan B, Gibney R, FitzGerald O (1999) Ultrasonography in the diagnosis and management of psoriatic dactylitis. J Rheumatol 26 : 1746–1751
25. Olivieri I, Barozzi L, Favaro L, Pierro A, de Matteis M, Borghi C, et al. (1996) Dactylitis in patients with seronegative spondylarthropathy. Assessment by ultrasonography and magnetic resonance imaging. Arthritis Rheum 39 : 1524–1528
26. Brockbank J, Stein M, Schentag CT, Gladman DD (2000) Characteristics of dactylitis in psoriatic arthritis (abst.). Arthritis Rheum 43(Suppl 9) : S105
27. Spoorenberg A, van der Heijde D, de Klerk E, Dougados M, de Vlam K, Mielants H, et al. (1999) Relative value of erythrocyte sedimentation rate and C-reactive protein in assessment of disease activity in ankylosing spondylitis. J Rheumatol 26 : 980–984
28. Gladman DD, Rahman P (2001) Psoriatic arthritis, 6th edn, Chap 71. WB Saunders, Philadelphia
29. Helliwell PS, Marchesoni A, Peters M, Platt R, Wright V (1991) Cytidine deaminase activity, C reactive protein, histidine, and erythrocyte sedimentation rate as measures of disease activity in psoriatic arthritis. Ann Rheum Dis 50 : 362–365
30. Gladman DD, Farewell VT, Wong K, Husted J (1998) Mortality studies in psoriatic arthritis: results from a single outpatient center. II. Prognostic indicators for death. Arthritis Rheum 41 : 1103–1110
31. Daunt AO, Cox NL, Robertson JC, Cawley MI (1987) Indices of disease activity in psoriatic arthritis. J R Soc Med 80 : 556–558
32. Laurent MR, Panayi GS, Shepherd P (1981) Circulating immune complexes, serum immunoglobulins, and acute phase proteins in psoriasis and psoriatic arthritis. Ann Rheum Dis 40 : 66–69
33. Salvarani C, Cantini F, Olivieri I, Macchioni P, Padula A, Niccoli L, et al. (2003) Efficacy of infliximab in resistant psoriatic arthritis. Arthritis Rheum 49 : 541–545
34. Lee DM, Schur PH (2003) Clinical utility of the anti-CCP assay in patients with rheumatic diseases. Ann Rheum Dis 62 : 870–874
35. Jansen AL, van der Horst-Bruinsma I, van Schaardenburg D, van de Stadt RJ, de Koning MH, Dijkmans BA (2002) Rheumatoid factor and antibodies to cyclic citrullinated peptide differentiate rheumatoid arthritis from undifferentiated polyarthritis in patients with early arthritis. J Rheumatol 29 : 2074–2076
36. Terzoglou K, Papaventsis DC, Theodoropoulou G, Kremasmenou E, Cherouvim E, Boki K (2003) Anticitrullinated peptides detection and diagnosis of rheumatoid arthritis (abst.). Ann Rheum Dis 62 (Suppl 1) : THU0130
37. Kroot EJ, de Jong BA, van Leeuwen MA, Swinkels H, van den Hoogen FH, van't Hof M, et al. (2000) The prognostic value of anti-cyclic citrullinated peptide antibody in patients with recent-onset rheumatoid arthritis. Arthritis Rheum 43 : 1831–1835
38. Nell VPK, Machold KP, Eberl G, Hiesberger H, Hoefler E, Smolen JS, et al. (2003) The diagnostic and prognostic significance of autoantibodies in patients with very early arthritis (abst.). Ann Rheum Dis 62(Suppl 1) : abstract #OP0015
39. Mettler S, Roch A, Langer H (2003) Antibodies against cyclic citrullinated peptide (CCP; filaggrin) in daily rheumatology practice: highly specific in diagnosis of rheumatoid arthritis (abst.). EULAR 2003 Abstracts : AB0074
40. Pincus T, Callahan LF, Fuchs HA, Larsen A, Kaye J (1995) Quantitative analysis of hand radiographs in rheumatoid arthritis: time course of radiographic changes, relation to joint examination measures, and comparison of different scoring methods. J Rheumatol 22 : 1983–1989
41. Steinbrocker O, Traeger CH, Batterman RC (1949) Therapeutic criteria in rheumatoid arthritis. J Am Med Assoc 140 : 659–662
42. Larsen A, Dale K, Eek M (1977) Radiographic evaluation of rheumatoid arthritis and related conditions by standard reference films. Acta Radiol Diagn (Stockh) 18 : 481–491
43. Rau R, Herborn G (1995) A modified version of Larsen's scoring method to assess radiologic changes in rheumatoid arthritis. J Rheumatol 22 : 1976–1982
44. Rahman P, Gladman DD, Cook RJ, Zhou Y, Young G, Salonen D (1998) Radiological assessment in psoriatic arthritis. Br J Rheumatol 37 : 760–765
45. Sharp JT (2000) An overview of radiographic analysis of joint damage in rheumatoid arthritis and its use in metaanalysis. J Rheumatol 27 : 254–260
46. van der Heijde D (2000) How to read radiographs according to the Sharp/van der Heijde method. J Rheumatol 27 : 261–263
47. Arreghini M, Panni B, Arnoldi C, Battafarano N, Gibelli E, Tosi S, et al. (2003) Radiographic evaluation of long-standing peripheral psoriatic arthritis: usefulness of a modified version of the Sharp/Van der Heijde method (abst.). Ann Rheum Dis 62(Suppl 1) : abstract #FRI0155
48. Ory P, Sharp JT, Salonen D, Rubenstein J, Mease PJ, Kivitz AJ, et al. (2002) Etanercept inhibits radiographic progression in patients with psoriatic arthritis (abst.). Arthritis Rheum 46(Suppl 9) : S196
49. Ory P, Sharp JT, Salonen D, Rubenstein JD, Mease PJ, Ruderman EM, et al. (2003) Etanercept inhibits radiographic progression in patients with psoriatic arthritis. Ann Rheum Dis 62(Suppl 1) : abstract #OP0089

50. Wassenberg S, Fischer-Kahle V, Herborn G, Rau R (2001) A method to score radiographic change in psoriatic arthritis. Z Rheumatol 60:156–166
51. van der Heijde DM (2004) Assessment of radiographs in longitudinal observational studies. J Rheumatol Suppl 69:46–47
52. van Tubergen A, Heuft-Dorenbosch L, Schulpen G, Landewe R, Wijers R, van der Heijde D, et al. (2003) Radiographic assessment of sacroiliitis by radiologists and rheumatologists: does training improve quality? Ann Rheum Dis 62:519–525
53. MacKay K, Mack C, Brophy S, Calin A (1998) The Bath Ankylosing Spondylitis Radiology Index (BASRI): a new, validated approach to disease assessment. Arthritis Rheum 41:2263–2270
54. Calin A, Mackay K, Santos H, Brophy S (1999) A new dimension to outcome: application of the Bath Ankylosing Spondylitis Radiology Index. J Rheumatol 26:988–992
55. Braun J, Brandt J, Listing J, Zink A, Alten R, Golder W, et al. (2002) Treatment of active ankylosing spondylitis with infliximab: a randomised controlled multicentre trial. Lancet 359:1187–1193
56. Creemers M, Franssen M, Hof Mv M, Gribnau F, Van De Putte L, Van Riel P (2004) Assessment of outcome in ankylosing spondylitis: an extended radiographic scoring system. Ann Rheum Dis (in press)
57. Kalden-Nemeth D, Grebmeier J, Antoni C, Manger B, Wolf F, Kalden JR (1997) NMR monitoring of rheumatoid arthritis patients receiving anti-TNF-alpha monoclonal antibody therapy. Rheumatol Int 16:249–255
58. Antoni C, Dechant C, Hanns-Martin Lorenz PD, Wendler J, Ogilvie A, Lueftl M, et al. (2002) Open-label study of infliximab treatment for psoriatic arthritis: clinical and magnetic resonance imaging measurements of reduction of inflammation. Arthritis Rheum 47:506–512
59. Backhaus M, Burmester GR, Sandrock D, Loreck D, Hess D, Scholz A, et al. (2002) Prospective two year follow up study comparing novel and conventional imaging procedures in patients with arthritic finger joints. Ann Rheum Dis 61:895–904
60. Alcade M, Cruz M, Bordoy C, Gonzalez L, Acebes C, Sanchez-Pernaute O, et al. (2002) Assessment of entheseal injury in ankylosing spondylitis by ultrasound (abst.). Arthritis Rheum 46(Suppl 9):S427
61. Kamel M, Mansour R, Eid H, Ferandez I (2002) Ultrasound detection of patellar enthesitis: a comparison with MRI (abst.). Arthritis Rheum 46 (Suppl 9):S104
62. Klauser A, Springer P, Frauscher F, Schirmer M (2002) Comparison between magnetic resonance imaging, unenhanced and contrast enhanced ultrasound in the diagnosis of active sacroiliitis (abst.). Arthritis Rheum 46(Suppl 9):S426
63. Oostveen J, Prevo R, den Boer J, van de Laar M (1999) Early detection of sacroiliitis on magnetic resonance imaging and subsequent development of sacroiliitis on plain radiography. A prospective, longitudinal study. J Rheumatol 26:1953–1958
64. Braun J, Baraliakos X, Golder W, Brandt J, Rudwaleit M, Listing J, et al. (2003) Magnetic resonance imaging examinations of the spine in patients with ankylosing spondylitis, before and after successful therapy with infliximab: evaluation of a new scoring system. Arthritis Rheum 48:1126–1136
65. Braun J, Baraliakos X, Golden W, Listing J, Brandt J, Bollow M, et al. (2002) Ankylosing spondylitis (AS) – development and evaluation of a spinal scoring system (ASspiMRI) using magnetic resonance imaging (MRI) in patients with active disease (abst.). Arthritis Rheum 46(Suppl 9):S426
66. Braun J, Baraliakos X, Golden W, Listing J, Brandt J, Bollow M, et al. (2002) Improvement of spinal inflammation in ankylosing spondylitis (AS) by infliximab therapy as assessed by a magnetic resonance imaging (MRI) using a novel evaluated spinal scoring system – results of a double-blind placebo-controlled trial (abst.). Arthritis Rheum 46 (Suppl 9):S426–S427
67. Gladman DD, Helliwell P, Mease PJ, Nash P, Ritchlin C, Taylor W (2004) Assessment of patients with psoriatic arthritis: a review of currently available measures. Arthritis Rheum 50:24–35

Quality of Life

VII

A Psoriasis

Steven R. Feldman, Stephen R. Rapp

Contents

1 Introduction

Quality of life considerations for patients with psoriasis are central in any discussion of the impact of the disease. Improving quality of life is at least as important to successful treatment as is improvement in lesional scores. Moreover, addressing quality of life helps establish a collaborative relationship between the clinician and patients that should result in better control over all aspects of the disease. The most important considerations in understanding and improving quality of life are:

- 1. Understanding how the patient views the impact of their disease
- 2. Identifying relevant outcomes in addition to lesion properties
- 3. Helping convey to patients that their physician is someone who wants to understand them and their disease
- 4. Helping office staff recognize the magnitude of importance of what they do for patients
- 5. Confirming that treatments that improve psoriasis skin lesions in clinical trials are making meaningful improvements in the disease
- 6. Planning which treatments are appropriate for which patients

This chapter will provide an overview of quality of life in psoriasis, including both the qualitative concerns of patients and the quantitative assessment of quality of life. This chapter will strive to provide practical advice on the management of quality of life concerns of psoriasis patients.

2 Quality of Life: Background

Over the past several decades interest in how illnesses impact people's lives has steadily increased. This expansion of interest beyond disease symptoms to include patients' emotional, social, and physical functioning has been welcomed by an appreciative patient population. The challenge to health care providers is how to incorporate this broader focus into busy practices so that better patient outcomes can be achieved. Physicians and their patients may differ somewhat in what they consider important. Dermatologists have traditionally focused primarily on symptom management, while patients value symptom reduction but also the prevention or reduction of distress and disability imposed by the condition. The best care, therefore, incorporates both perspectives.

The construct of 'health-related quality of life' (HRQL) refers to patients' perceived distress and disability and therefore is central to our understanding of how diseases impact people. HRQL refers to a collection of primary functional capacities that each person values and that contribute significantly to satisfaction with life and self. While different models of HRQL can include different 'core' functional capacities, most emphasize physical functioning, emotional functioning, social functioning, occupational functioning, and leisure functioning. The study of HRQL has advanced rapidly offering clinicians and health researchers knowledge to guide them in assessing disease impact and excellent tools with which to do it.

3 HRQL: An Introduction

Health-related quality of life refers to people's subjective evaluations of the influence of their current health (and other factors) on their ability to achieve and maintain a level of overall functioning that allows them to pursue valued life goals and that is reflected in their general well-being. Perhaps the most fundamental feature of HRQL is that it represents the *patient's* perspective on major domains of their functioning. Health care providers and patients will differ in their estimates of impact [20]. Capturing patient perspective ensures that both the clinician's and patient's perspective are available and can be weighed in treatment decisions. Another key aspect of HRQL is its multidimensionality. By assessing several major functional domains, the impact of illness can be ascertained more completely. This permits comparisons within and between disease states and within and between individuals, a particularly valuable feature when trying to determine the efficacy of a particular treatment. The domains of function most commonly included in HRQL assessment are physical functioning (e.g., daily activities like walking, climbing stairs, lifting objects or getting dressed), social functioning (e.g., interacting with others, social support, intimacies), psychological-emotional functioning (e.g., positive and negative mood state, self-consciousness, self-esteem), occupational functioning (e.g., work or school activities), and leisure functioning (e.g., hobbies, recreational activities, pastimes). Some HRQL models also include domains of spiritual functioning, somatic functioning (e.g., pain, sleep, nausea, itching), and economic well being (e.g., adequacy of income). Note that specific disease symptoms are not included in HRQL concept. This is to avoid confounding disease with the impact of disease on functioning. Symptoms are measured separately and examined in relation to HRQL. Figure A1 depicts a schematic of a basic model of HRQL in which health is affected by a disease state leading to potential impacts on various domains of function. Anyone who has treated a patient is aware that a plethora of factors can influence the nature and extent of the impact a disease has on the individual. Some patients with very small, inconspicuous psoriatic plaques report significant psychological or social impact while other patients with extensive lesions report minimal HRQL impact. This is a reflection of the fact that there are modifying factors that can influence the HRQL impact of disease. Treatments, demographics (age, gender, and ethnicity), other disease states, stress, social support, personality, culture, and coping resources are examples of potential modifying factors.

4 HRQL: Significance and Assessment

Significance

The most compelling reason to consider patients' HRQL is that HRQL reflects what matters to patients. Patients evaluate treatment effectiveness by how much it reduces *suffering and disability*. Dissatisfaction with their doctors [19] may reflect that patient and provider are not focused on all the outcomes valued by the patient, that physicians often do not rate the

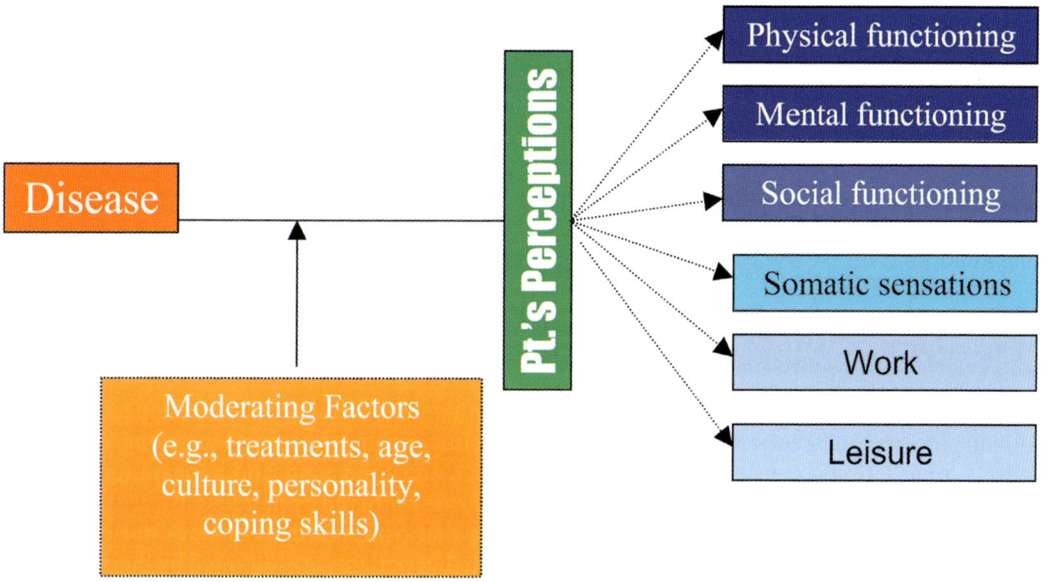

Fig. A1. Conceptual model of health related quality of life. The disability felt by patients with psoriasis is dependent on several factors. First is the severity of the skin lesions. These lesions are perceived differently by different people, depending on their personality, support structures and other variables. The disease results in effects on quality of life. Psoriasis affects all dimensions of health related quality of life

disease as severe as does the patient, and that the physician does not offer treatments sufficiently effective to control the disease. Dissatisfaction also may reflect that that the patient perceives the physician as not simply not caring enough about the disease. Another reason to treat based on HRQL is that many dermatological diseases including psoriasis are chronic and incurable, eroding patient's quality of life over many years. Symptomatic treatments do not confer improved life quality for some. Remembering to address HRQL issues with patients can improve their overall outcome. Third, skin disorders can impact many aspects of patients' lives. As noted above, physical functioning, psychological functioning, social functioning, vocational, and leisure activities are often adversely affected. Not paying sufficient attention to these domains of patients' lives can increase dissatisfaction with treatment and provider. In sum, a better understanding of how psoriasis impacts people's lives can help the specialist to become more effective in caring for them.

Assessment

Most dermatologists regularly assess patients' quality of life, both in their skin disease patients in general and in psoriasis patients in particular. When even psoriasis treatment "experts" are asked how they measure the impact of disease in their patients, most often they say they ask patients, "how are you doing?" and other questions that assess patients' quality of life as much or more than eliciting an objective assessment of skin lesion severity. In fact, many psoriasis treatment clinical trials incorporate a basic measure of global improvement (a patient global assessment) that simply represents a formalization of the "how are you doing?" concept.

Since HRQL is a multidimensional concept, assessments of it require multidimensional measurement models. In recent years we have developed multidimensional models for the assessment of HRQL for several skin diseases. In this section we will describe the development of such a model for psoriasis. First we describe the collection of qualitative information from patients. Next, we describe how we used that information to develop and test a quantitative measure of psoriasis-related quality of life impact. We also briefly review other published measures so the reader can gain a bird's eye view of available instruments. Additional information about individual instruments should be obtained from the primary references.

5 HRQL in Psoriasis

VII

Studies of the impact of psoriasis have corroborated clinicians' perceptions that psoriasis can have a quite serious impact on social and psychological functioning for some. Social embarrassment, feelings of stigmatization, and lowered self-esteem are common [8, 9] and severe psychological disturbance among some patients has been well documented [10–12, 16, 17, 19]. It has also become clearer that physical and occupational functioning can be affected [5, 7, 15, 17, 18, 21]. Studies have indicated that HRQL of psoriasis patients is comparable to that of patients with serious, even life threatening diseases like cancer, congestive heart failure, diabetes, chronic obstructive pulmonary disease, and clinical depression [18].

Research into the role of modifying factors has revealed that higher age is generally associated with better HRQL [17], that having a dispositional tendency to worry about the judgments of others is associated with poorer functioning, especially when severity increases [13], and that most of the social coping strategies patients use (e.g. concealing lesions, avoiding people) are not associated with improved HRQL [16]. We are just beginning to understand how modifying variables relate to HRQL. With greater attention to these variables, clinicians may be better able to identify sub-populations of their patients and offer them specific adjunctive interventions. For example, highly socially anxious and avoidant patients, if correctly identified, can be referred for specific counseling.

Qualitative Assessment

To begin to understand how psoriasis impacts patients' lives, open-ended focus groups were held with patients. In these sessions, psoriasis patients discussed how the disease impacted them and specifically what it was about the disease that bothered them most. This analysis identified many bothersome aspects of the disease that could be broadly grouped into three categories. First, there are the physical manifestations of the disease itself. The lesions are bothersome because of their appearance, the scaling, itching, burning sensations, skin soreness, and joint pain and appearance. Patients also are bothered by hair loss. We are not implying that psoriasis does or does not cause hair loss, but patients are bothered by their own perceptions of hair loss due to psoriasis. Finally, arthritis is a common symptom of psoriasis that adds considerably to the burden of the disease.

Second, several characteristics of treatment were identified as bothersome aspects of psoriasis. These include time spent caring for the disease, odors, stains on clothing and furniture, lost work time, the time of treatment, cost of treatment, messiness of treatments, medication side effects and the cost of medications. These are actually factors over which the physician probably exerts a great degree of control, perhaps more control than over the characteristics of the lesions that patients find bothersome.

The final group of bothersome aspects of the disease related to patients' psychosocial interactions. Patients are bothered by an inability to control the disease, people reacting negatively, being avoided by people and feeling self-conscious about their skin. The lack of support people with psoriasis perceive probably is a major contributor to the magnitude of impact experienced by patients with this chronic disease. Patients with other chronic diseases typically experience people rallying to support them, helping to mitigate the negative aspects of the disease. Typically, patients with psoriasis experience the opposite, other people do not understand the disease and shun the patient (certainly that is what the patient perceives, whether true or not); this magnifies the negative impact of the condition.

The sense of isolation and stigmatization in psoriasis extends to the physician-patient interaction. Patients commonly express that their doctor's attitude about psoriasis is one of the bothersome aspects of the disease. This is a striking finding. Patients often perceive a dismissive attitude on the part of the physician. They report their physicians are not sufficiently aggressive managing the disease. From the physician's perspective, it is easy to see how this may come about. A chronic disease like psoriasis is frustrating for the patient and the physician. These patients are psychologically needy, and physicians may not feel they have the time to invest in dealing with those needs. Moreover, traditional treatments have been of such limited efficacy that many physicians may (to an extent, rightly) feel that there is nothing more to be done for the disease.

Living in isolation with a severe chronic illness has an extraordinary impact on patients' lives. It is not surprising then that suicidal ideation is common in psoriasis patients. As many as one in four patients considers suicide because of psoriasis at some time in their lives. Eight percent were actively considering suicide in one cross sectional study. Over time, however, patients do tend to adapt to the disease. Psoriasis tends to have less impact on older patients than on younger patients. Palm and sole involvement is one risk factor that predicts greater impact, likely because of the pain and limitations on physical activity that such involvement entails [15].

Quantitative Assessment

Quantitative HRQL measurement can be at three levels of detail. The first level is *generic*. Generic HRQL refers to global HRQL, not related to skin disease. Generic measures permit comparisons across different disease states that can be useful for health policy decisions. For example, one might wish to determine whether psoriasis imparts a greater negative impact on patient function than heart disease. One disadvantage of generic HRQL assessment is the lack of specificity in relation to a particular disorder or group of disorders.

The Medical Outcomes Study Short-Form 36 Health Survey (SF-36) has become the most widely used global HRQL instrument in HRQL research. It was developed to permit comparisons across different disease states, ages or treatment groups. It consists of 36 items assessing eight domains of function including physical functioning, role functioning, pain, general health, vitality, social functioning, role-emotional functioning, and mental health. In addition to individual domain scores, two summary scores can also be generated, one for Mental Health and the other for Physical Health. The SF-36 has been exhaustively researched and has excellent reliability and validity. Very good norms are available for several disease states allowing easier interpretation of the scores.

The SF-36 has been applied to a population of patients with psoriasis in order to see how psoriasis compares to other serious medical diseases [14, 18]. In one study, the impact of psoriasis was as great as or greater than many other common medical conditions. Psoriasis was worse than hypertension, diabetes and myocardial infarction on both physical and mental dimensions of HRQL [18]. These data indicate that for some psoriasis are a significant medical condition and not simply a cosmetic disorder.

The next level of HRQL assessment is *population-specific*. Population-specific HRQL measures include items specific to a class of disease, like skin-diseases. They allow comparisons between diseases within that class. For example, if one were interested in comparing the efficacy of a particular treatment or skin care product used by psoriatics and by atopic dermatitis patients. Another practical use might be to collect data on HRQL within a dermatology practice. This is best accomplished by a measure that is relevant to all dermatological diseases. This level offers somewhat greater detail than the global level assessment, but may still lack adequate sensitivity to specific features of a particular disorder such as itching or scaliness. The Dermatology Life Quality Index (DLQI) [6], the Skindex [3], and the Dermatology-Specific Quality of Life (DSQL) [2] scale are three such instruments. The DLQI consists of ten questions covering six domains: symptoms and feelings, daily activities, leisure, work and school, personal relationships and bother with treatment. It has been widely used in research and has good reliability, validity, and sensitivity to change. The small number of items limits its sensitivity and the breadth of content. The Skindex exists in several versions of differing lengths [1, 4] making it convenient for the respondents. It assesses functioning, emotions, and skin symptoms. Its psychometric properties are excellent and it is easy to administer and score. The DSQL consists of 36 items organized a single global scale with 5 subscales: physical symptoms, daily activities, social activities and functioning, work/school, and self perception. Reliability and validity appear to be adequate.

The DLQI has been used in many clinical trials of pharmacological agents as a complement for measures of the severity of the skin lesions. Improvement in DLQI demonstrates that medical treatments can affect primary symptoms as well as the impact of these symptoms on patients' lives. Moreover, patients who have a 75% improvement in PASI score have improved DLQI scores demonstrating that 75% improvement in PASI is a good measure of treatment success, at least in so far as it correlates with an improvement in people's lives. Patients with 50% improvement in PASI also exhibit improved quality of life as measured with the DLQI

The last level is *disease-specific* HRQL assessment. At this level the detail is the greatest and measures are typically, therefore, most sensitive to changes in HRQL. Assessment at this level can yield very specific information regarding the impact of the disease. A disadvantage, however, is that one cannot compare outcomes across conditions within a class or between classes. Examples include the Psoriasis Disability Index [5] and the Psoriasis Disability Scale [19] both of which have good psychometric properties and are acceptable to patients.

The selection of a measure depends on the objective of assessment. To compare the impact of psoriasis on patients to the impact of acne would require a dermatology-specific measure, while contrasting psoriasis with heart disease would necessitate a global or generic measure. If one is evaluating a single disease state, a disease-specific measure is probably the best choice. One may have more than one objective in assessing HRQL. In that case a combined level of analysis may be suitable. For example, one may wish to compare the effect of a treatment for two dermatological diseases *and* to describe the impact of the treatment on specific features of these diseases. In this case, a small battery of measures that includes disease-specific HRQL tool and disease-specific scales is useful.

It is encouraging that in dermatology we have HRQL instruments at each level of analysis and that at least some have adequate psychometric properties to recommend their use in research if not clinical care as well.

6 Office Management of HRQL

While it is clear that psoriasis has a significant on patients' lives, it is of equal importance to discuss how to manage this impact. The simplest and most cost effective way to address many of patient's psychosocial concerns is to encourage patients to join a psoriasis support/advocacy group such as the National Psoriasis Foundation (www.psoriasis.org). These organizations are a very effective management tool for many patients. By joining, patients become part of a supportive group, reducing their sense of isolation. In the US, the Psoriasis Foundation has enumerable educational resources that increase patients' knowledge of the disease and treatments, and these are available worldwide through the website. Practical advice is offered for how to manage the day-to-day challenges that psoriasis presents. Useful information empowers patients to do something about the disease. Working together, psoriasis advocacy/support group members can also support research toward a cure or work for better access to treatment.

Physicians can incorporate other basic measures to address the psychosocial implications of psoriasis. Foremost among these is touching the lesions. Physicians should make a special effort to palpate the skin lesions. While it may appear to be done as a means to assess the induration and scaling of the lesions, the power of touch is in communicating caring and closeness. Patients need to hear that psoriasis is not cancer and that it is not contagious. Your touching the lesions reinforces this message in the best way possible. This is probably particularly important for younger patients with the disease who have stronger interpersonal concerns and sensitivities. It is important for physicians to communicate this to their office staff. Nurses and assistants in the clinic can support the physician's efforts by showing equal willingness to touch the affected areas. Staff can inadvertently sabotage physician's efforts if they appear to shun patients with the disease. On the other hand, staff can be energized by understanding how important their role is in improving the lives of patients who suffer as much as psoriasis patients do.

To help eliminate patients' perceptions that their physician dismisses the negative impact of the disease, it is helpful to proactively ask patients about the bothersome aspects of the disease described above. To help strengthen patients' sense of control, it is important to involve patients in treatment planning and to discuss how s/he is managing QOL issues like embarrassment or stigmatization. This also helps to avoid recommending treatment plans that patients find worse than the disease. One of the most important factors in determining the effectiveness of psoriasis treatments is patients' adherence to medication. Involving patients in the treatment plan is likely to help improve adherence and, therefore, clinical and HRQL outcomes.

Physicians should also set realistic expectations of treatment. Often patients with psoriasis are seeking the "holy grail" of cure. In order to reduce extreme disappointment, physicians should make clear that they will work with the patient to achieve "control" of the disease, as current treatments do not offer complete cures. Usually patients are satisfied with this approach, and if they are not, at least they know up front that cure is not to be expected. Setting realistic expectations is particularly important when patients come in having learned of new treatments that they think will be qualitatively different (i.e., cure) than previously available treatments. Finally, setting realistic expectations may help patients comply with treatments that are expected to work slowly.

Physicians caring for patients with psoriasis, or any chronic skin disease for that matter, should be alert to signs of depression and other serious emotional states. Spontaneous tearfulness, sad or irritable mood, flat affect, statements of hopelessness or helplessness may be visible signs of depression. Physicians can further assess this by asking non-confrontational questions about appetite and weight changes; sleep pattern changes (waking in the middle of the night and feeling unrested in the morning), low energy level, and a loss of interest in favorite activities that may confirm concerns about depression. Suicidal thought should also be queried if depression is present, and appropriate referral may be indicated.

Physicians caring for patients with psoriasis also should recognize their own feelings about the disease. Just as living with a chronic illness can be frustrating, caring for demanding patients with a chronic disease can be difficult. Recognizing this, and recognizing the profound positive impact physicians can make for their psoriasis patients, allows physicians to experience the pride and joy of improving patients' lives.

HRQL Treatment Algorithm

To help the busy dermatologist respond appropriately to patient distress and dysfunction we have developed guidelines captured in the acronym: I VOTE. *I*nquire about patients' functioning and possible distress. Explicitly validating patients' experience with an illness by acknowledging the distress and dysfunction without judgment of appropriateness communicates in a very strong way your respect for him/her and their experience. *V*alidation of distress is the foundation of the partnership of equals needed to manage the disease and its impact on life quality. *O*ffering assistance with the management of the impact of psoriasis as well as with the management of symptoms defines both as important. *T*alk with the patient about any

Table A1. Guidelines to help address patient distress and dysfunction: "IVOTE"

Distress/dysfunction level	Signs/symptoms	Possible action
Mild	Patient able to carry out all activities, but complains that psoriasis is mild to moderately disturbing or annoying	*I*nquire extent of impact *V*alidate patient's feelings *E*valuate distress/dysfunction at each visit
Moderate	Psoriasis is interfering with somewhat with physical or social functioning; or unpleasant moods (e.g., anxiety, depression, anger), or negative attitudes (lowered self-esteem, resentful toward others, hopeless/ helplessness) are evident	*I*nquire extent of impact *V*alidate patient's feelings *O*ffer to discuss these issues or to refer *E*valuate distress/dysfunction at each visit
Severe	Moderate to high distress or disability; or many complaints; or any self-injurious thoughts or actions	*I*nquire extent of impact *V*alidate patient's feelings *O*ffer to discuss these issues or to refer *T*alk with patient *E*valuate distress/dysfunction at each visit *R*efer to specialist after discussing it with patient

planned treatment. Patients can't be expected to be compliant with treatments they feel are worse than the disease. *E*valuating the efficacy of strategies to improve QOL problems is essential and guides subsequent intervention. Table A1 provides a guide for applying the I VOTE strategies.

7 Conclusion

Psoriasis has a profound impact on the lives of patients. No matter how much or little of the skin is involved, patients may experience physical, mental, and social effects of the disease. Arthritis is a major contributor to the impact of psoriasis and should be considered by all physicians caring for these patients.

There are several practical strategies physicians can use to help patients address the adverse impact of psoriasis on life quality. Sit close to the psoriasis patient. Casually palpate their lesions while talking to them. Proactively ask them about the bothersome aspects of psoriasis described in the qualitative section above. By doing so, patients will recognize you as someone who understands psoriasis and understands them. Encourage patients to join the National Psoriasis Foundation or other psoriasis advocacy/support groups. The patient will benefit greatly from the many educational resources these groups provide provides. Finally, involve patients in treatment planning. By presenting oneself as a physician who is empathetic and understanding of psoriasis and its impact, patients will be more likely to trust you and to adhere to the treatment regimen you propose.

References

1. Abeni D, Picardi A, Pasquini P, Melchi CF, Chren MM (2002) Further evidence of the validity and reliability of the Skindex-29: an Italian study on 2,242 dermatological outpatients. Dermatology 204:43–49
2. Anderson RT, Rajagopalan R (1997) Development and validation of a quality of life instrument for cutaneous diseases. J Am Acad Dermatol 37:41–50

3. Chren MM, Lasek RJ, Quinn LM, Mostow EN, Zyzanski SJ (1996) Skindex, a quality-of-life measure for patients with skin disease: reliability, validity, and responsiveness. J Invest Dermatol 107:707–713
4. Chren MM, Lasek RJ, Sahay AP, Sands LP (1989) Measurement properties of Skindex-16: a brief quality-of-life measure for patients with skin diseases. J Cutan Med Surg 5:105–110
5. Finlay AY, Kelly SE (1987) Psoriasis – an index of disability. Clin Exp Dermatol 12:8–11
6. Finlay AY, Khan GK (1994) Dermatology Life Quality Index (DLQI) – a simple practical measure for routine clinical use. Clin Exp Dermatol 19:210–216
7. Finlay AY, Khan GK, Luscombe DK, Salek MS (1990) Validation of Sickness Impact Profile and Psoriasis Disability Index in Psoriasis. Br J Dermatol 123: 751–756
8. Ginsburg IH, Link BG (1989) Feelings of stigmatization in patients with psoriasis. J Am Acad Dermatol 20:53–63
9. Ginsburg IH, Link BG (1993) Psychosocial consequences of rejection and stigma feelings in psoriasis patients. Int J Dermatol 32:587–591
10. Hughes JE, Barraclough BM, Hamblin LG, White JE (1983) Psychiatric symptoms in dermatology patients. Br J Psychiatry 143:51–54
11. Koblenzer CS (1993) Psychiatric syndromes of interest to dermatologists. Int J Dermatol 32:82–88
12. Koblenzer CS (1987) Psychocutaneous diseases. Grune and Stratton, New York
13. Leary MR, Rapp SR, Herbst KC, Exum ML, Feldman SR (1998) Interpersonal concerns and psychological difficulties of psoriasis patients: effects of disease severity and fear of negative evaluation. Health Psychol 17:530–536
14. Nichol MB, Margolies JE, Lippa E, Rowe M, Quell J (1996) The application of multiple quality-of-life instruments in individuals with mild-to-moderate psoriasis. Pharmacoeconomics 10:644–653
15. Pettey AA, Balkrishnan R, Rapp SR, Fleischer AB, Feldman SR (2003) Patients with palmoplantar psoriasis have more physical disability and discomfort than patients with other forms of psoriasis: implications for clinical practice. J Am Acad Dermatol 49:271–275
16. Rapp SR, Cottrell CA, Leary MR (2001) Social coping strategies associated with quality of life decrements among psoriasis patients. Br J Dermatol 145: 610–616
17. Rapp SR, Exum ML, Reboussin DM, Feldman SR, Fleischer A, Clark A (1997) The physical, psychological and social impact of psoriasis. J Health Psychol 2:525–537
18. Rapp SR, Feldman SR, Exum ML, Reboussin DM, Fleischer AB Jr (1999) Psoriasis causes as much disability as other major medical diseases. J Am Acad Dermatol 41:401–417
19. Rapp SR, Feldman SR, Fleischer AB Jr, Reboussin DM, Exum ML (1998) Health related quality of life in psoriasis: A biopsychosocial model and measures. In: Rajagopalan R, Sherertz E, Anderson R (eds) Care management of skin diseases: life quality and economic impact. Marcel Dekker, New York, pp 125–145
20. Sampogna F, Picardi A, Melchi CF, Pasquini P, Abeni D (2003) The impact of skin diseases on patients: comparing dermatologists' opinions with research data collected on their patients. Br J Dermatol 148: 989–995
21. Zachariae R, Zachariae C, Ibsen H, Mortensen JT, Wulf HC (2000) Dermatology life quality index: data from Danish inpatients and outpatients. Acta Derm Venereol 80:272–276

B Psoriatic Arthritis

Dafna D. Gladman

Contents

1 Introduction

Psoriatic arthritis (PsA) is an inflammatory arthritis that may affect some 30% of patients with psoriasis. While almost all patients suffer from arthritis in the peripheral joints, some 40–50% may also have a spondylitis, and about 4% have isolated inflammatory back disease. Until the mid 1980s PsA was considered less severe than rheumatoid arthritis (RA), the prototype of inflammatory arthritis. Wright's original description of PsA included a majority of patients who presented with an oligoarthritis (four or less peripheral joints affected) [1]. Compared to polyarticular RA this group appeared milder. However, a follow-up study from Wright's group in Leeds identified a larger proportion of patients with polyarticular disease (five or more peripheral joints involved), and demonstrated that there was disability and even mortality among these patients [2]. Although a study from Britain suggested that the majority of patients who had been admitted to an inpatient facility were doing well after 10 years of disease [3], more recent studies provide evidence for more severe disease among patients with PsA [4].

2 Assessment of Disability

The assessment of disability and quality of life in Rheumatology has included a number of tools, some that are completed by the physician, and others that are patient-derived questionnaires. A review of the use of these instruments in PsA as well as the level of disability in patients with PsA is provided in this chapter.

ACR Functional Class

The American College of Rheumatology (ACR, formerly American Rheumatism Association) developed a method to assess functional ability in the late 1940s. Similar to the functional classification for heart disease, patients are graded according to their ability to perform activities of daily living, based on limitations imposed by their disease (Table B1) [5]. While this classification is crude, as the levels of function as defined do not distinguish between patients who carry on despite marked disability and those who do not function well with mild disease, the ACR functional class does reflect the level of daily activity a patient reports at a given time. An analysis of 220 patients who were registered in the Psoriatic Arthritis Clinic revealed that about a fifth of the patients had severe disease, defined by the presence of 5 or more deformed joints, and that 11% of the patients had significant disability, as determined by the ACR functional class III and IV [6]. This study introduced the concept that PsA was more severe than previously thought. Over the past 20 years several studies have supported this view [7–9].

Table B1. ACR functional class

Class I	– able to carry on normally without pain or discomfort
Class II	– able to carry on with usual activities despite pain or discomfort
Class III	– activities of daily living limited to self care because of pain or disability
Class IV	– bedridden

The Health Assessment Questionnaire (HAQ)

Over the past 30 years a number of instruments have been developed to assess functional ability and quality of life in a more detailed way. Fries et al. described the Health Assessment Questionnaire (HAQ) [10], which was initially developed as a tool to assess patient function in rheumatoid arthritis, and has since been used generally in rheumatology. It is considered an instrument specific for arthritis. The HAQ evaluates patient's function in 8 different domains (Table B2). It is scored on a 0–3 scale where higher numbers represent more disability.

The HAQ was administered to 114 patients with PsA followed in a PsA Clinic [11]. Higher HAQ scores were associated with more actively inflamed joints as well as with measures of function (ACR functional class and grip strength) and with fibromyalgia tender points. The HAQ did not correlate with disease severity as measured by clinically and radiologically damaged joints.

One study reported that HAQ scores of 47 patients with PsA were not statistically different from those of 47 patients with RA matched on disease duration [12]. However, another study, which compared 107 patients with PsA and 43 patients with RA followed in an outpatient clinic, found that HAQ scores in PsA were lower than those reported in patients with RA [13]. The latter study did not control for disease duration, and the patients with PsA had a lower number of actively inflamed joints than the RA patients. Thus, it may be that patients with PsA with polyarticular disease have similar HAQ scores to patients with RA, confirming that PsA causes disability. Indeed, mean HAQ score of PsA patients included in the IMPACT trial of infliximab was 1.1, which is similar to that reported for RA patients [14]. Significant reductions in HAQ score were recently documented in randomized controlled trials of anti-TNF agents in PsA [15].

A modification of the HAQ for the spondyloarthropathies has been developed and validated [16]. This version includes two questions regarding disability due to back involvement. Since some 40–50% of patients with PsA have an associated spondyloarthritis, the modified HAQ was tested in PsA [11]. The summary scores of the modified HAQ (HAQ-S) were similar to the original HAQ (0.50 and 0.53 respectively). Like the original HAQ, the HAQ-S correlated with disease activity and function, but not with disease severity. There was no statistical difference between the HAQ and HAQ-S scores of patients with and without spondyloarthritis.

The HAQ was further modified by including questions related to psoriasis [17]. Patients with PsA were asked to identify the difficulties they encountered in activities of daily living related to their psoriasis. From the list generated by the patients several questions were identified and included in the HAQ to generate HAQ-SK. The HAQ-SK was then administered to 118 patients and provided almost identical scores to the original HAQ (0.56 and 0.55 respectively). While the HAQ-SK did not correlate with the Psoriasis Activity Severity Index (PASI) score, patient and physician rating of psoriasis did correlate. This study concluded that the HAQ-SK did not add important information to the original HAQ.

Table B2. HAQ tasks

- Dressing and grooming
- Arising
- Eating
- Walking
- Hygiene
- Reach
- Grip
- Activities

Other Measurements of Function

Meenan et al. described another instrument that was useful in patients with arthritis, called the Arthritis Impact Measurement Scales (AIMS) [18]. This instrument is longer than the HAQ and provides both functional assessment and a quality of life measurement. It was subsequently modified and described as AIMS2 [19].

The AIMS has been shown to be reliable and sensitive to change in patients with a variety of forms of arthritis.

Both the original AIMS and the AIMS2 were validated in PsA [20, 21]. The AIMS was administered to 145 patients with PsA. The physical function scales were correlated moderately to highly with measures of disease activity, function, and disease severity, and the pain scale was highly correlated with disease activity and function. The AIMS2 was administered to 124 patients with PsA and like the original AIMS was found to correlate with disease activity and function [21]. The finding that the AIMS was sensitive to articular changes that occurred in patients over a 4-year period provides further support for the utility of the AIMS as an outcome measure in clinical studies of PsA [22]. However, while the AIMS and AIMS2 appear to be valid instruments in the assessment of patients with PsA, it takes patients a relatively long time to complete these instruments Thus, AIMS and AIMS2 are less feasible to use in both clinical trials and clinic setting.

The Disabilities of Arm, Shoulder, and Hand (DASH) Questionnaire was developed as an outcome measure for patients with upper extremity musculoskeletal conditions [23]. It measures symptoms and functional status with a focus on physical functioning. The DASH was administered to 50 consecutive patients in the PsA clinic to assess its construct validity with respect to clinical measures of function, inflammatory joint disease activity, and joint deformity in the upper extremity [24]. The DASH correlated with clinical measures of upper extremity function such as grip strength and actively inflamed joint count in the upper extremity. However, there was no correlation between upper extremity damaged joints and the DASH in the group of patients tested.

The Bath Ankylosing Spondylitis Functional Index (BASFI) was developed for the assessment of patients with inflammatory back disease and functions well in patients with ankylosing spondylitis, the prototypical form of spondylitis [25]. It has not functioned very well in PsA in that it did not distinguish patients with spinal disease from those who had peripheral arthritis only [26].

3 Quality of Life Measures

The Medical Outcome Study short form 36 (SF-36) is a generic quality of life instrument which has been used extensively to describe quality of life and function in a number of medical conditions [27]. SF-36 has an advantage over disease specific instruments in that it allows for comparison between patients with different diseases. The SF-36 includes eight domains and can be evaluated in each individual domain or as a composite index. The SF-36 has been validated in PsA. It demonstrated that patients with PsA have lower function and quality of life than the general population [28]. Moreover, the SF-36 was at least as good as if not superior to the HAQ and the AIMS2 in reflecting changes in disease status over time [29]. Thus the SF-36 is a useful instrument in the assessment of quality of life in patients with PsA.

The European Quality of Life (EQ-5D) questionnaire is a generic measure of health status developed by the EuroQoL Group, an international research network established in 1987 by researchers from Finland, the Netherlands, Sweden, and the United Kingdom [30]. The EQ-5D questionnaire defines health in terms of five dimensions: mobility, self-care, usual activities (work, study, housework, family, or leisure), pain or discomfort, and anxiety or depression. Each dimension is subdivided into three categories, which indicate whether the respondent has no problem, a moderate problem, or an extreme problem. The EQ-D5 was administered to patients with PsA and found to be similar to scores of patients with RA matched for disease duration [12]. The EQ-D5 scores were similar even though patients with PsA had less severe joint disease than the patients with RA. The authors suggest that this may be due to the skin disease, as a gradient in scores for both HAQ and EuroQol-5D was found across the skin severity groupings.

Recently, the Psoriatic Arthritis Quality of Life questionnaire was developed as an instrument specifically for the assessment of quality of life in patients with PsA. Through interviews with 48 patients with PsA followed in hospital outpatient clinic, a questionnaire of 51 items was derived and tested. The questionnaire was administered by mail to 120 individuals, of whom 94 responded. Rash analysis allowed a reduction to 35 items. A subsequent mailing to 450 members of the Psoriatic Arthropathy alliance generated a response from 286, of whom 237 participated in a validation study. Further analysis reduced the items from 35 to 20. The final questionnaire was tested again with excellent reliability and internal consistency. It was further tested for external construct validity by correlating the scores with scores of generic instruments such as the EuroQoL and the National Health Survey. However, it was not compared to the currently used instruments such as the SF-36 and the HAQ [31].

The Dermatology Life Quality Index (DLQI) was developed to measure quality of life in patients with skin diseases. It has been used extensively in evaluating dermatological conditions, including the assessment of patients with psoriasis, and has been shown to have construct validity and sensitivity to change in clinical status [32]. Although it has not been tested specifically in PsA, it has been used in a number of studies to assess quality of life in patients. It is not clear whether the DLQI is different from the SF-36 in assessing quality of life in patients with psoriasis and PsA, as the two were not measured against each other. The DLQI correlated with a recently developed measure of quality of life in psoriasis, the PSORQoL instrument, but there was enough difference to prompt the authors to suggest that the latter may be measuring some additional aspects of the disease [33].

Patients with PsA suffer from fatigue more frequently than the general population. This was demonstrated by the administration of a modification of the Krupp Fatigue Severity Score (FSS) [34, 35]. This nine-item scale assesses the impact of fatigue on activities of daily living and is scored from 0 to 10, with higher scores indicating more severe fatigue. The FSS for 75 patients with PsA was higher than for the 100 healthy controls (5.2 ± 3.0 vs. 3.9 ± 2.1, $p=0.001$). Forty-five percent of the PsA patients reported the presence of fatigue on clinical assessment. The mean FSS score in this group was 6.9 compared to 3.8 in patients who did not report fatigue. Fatigue was associated with fibromyalgia tender point count, morning stiffness, clinically damaged joint count, active joint count, and hemoglobin [34]. Change in FSS over time analyzed for 90 patients with PsA was found to be related to changes in actively inflamed joints [36].

4 Conclusion

Following the recognition that PsA may be more severe than previously thought, a number of assessment instruments have been used to evaluate function and quality of life among patients who suffer from this disease. Although only one quality of life instrument was developed specifically for PsA, it has not been compared to more generic instruments. All instruments document a reduced function and quality of life compared with the general population. In at least one study, skin disease was found to contribute to the diminished quality of life associated with the joint disease. These aspects of the disease need to be included in the assessment of current and future drug therapies for PsA.

References

1. Wright V (1961) Psoriatic arthritis: a comparative radiographic study of rheumatoid arthritis and arthritis associated with psoriasis. Ann Rheum Dis 20:123–132
2. Roberts MET, Wright V, Hill AGS, Mehra AC (1976). Psoriatic arthritis: A follow-up study. Ann Rheum Dis 35:206–219
3. Coulton BL, Thomson K, Symmons DPM, Popert AJ (1989) Outcome in patients hospitalised for psoriatic arthritis. Clin Rheumatol 2:261–265
4. Gladman DD (1994) Natural history of psoriatic arthritis. Baillières Clin Rheumatol 8:379–394
5. Steinbrocker O, Traeger GH, Batterman RC (1949) Therapeutic criteria in rheumatoid arthritis. J Am Med Assoc 140:659–662
6. Gladman DD, Shuckett R, Russell ML, Thorne JC, Schachter RK (1987) Psoriatic arthritis (PSA) – an analysis of 220 patients. Q J Med 62:127–141

7. Torre-Alonso JC, Rodriguez-Perez A, Arribas-Castrillo JM, et al. (1991) Psoriatic arthritis (PA): a clinical, immunological and radiological study of 180 patients. Br J Rheumatol 30:245–250
8. McHugh NJ, Balachrishnan C, Jones SM (2003) Progression of peripheral joint disease in psoriatic arthritis: a 5-yr prospective study. Rheumatology (Oxford) 42:778–783
9. Queiro-Silva R, Torre-Alonso JC, Tinture-Eguren T, Lopez-Lagunas I (2003) A polyarticular onset predicts erosive and deforming disease in psoriatic arthritis. Ann Rheum Dis 62:68–70
10. Fries JF, Spitz PW, Young DY (1982) The dimensions of health outcomes: the health assessment questionnaire, disability and pain scales. J Rheumatol 9: 789–793
11. Blackmore M, Gladman DD, Husted J, Long J, Farewell VT (1995) Measuring Health Status in Psoriatic Arthritis: The Health Assessment Questionnaire and its modification. J Rheumatol 22:886–893
12. Sokoll KB, Helliwell PS (2001) Comparison of disability and quality of life in rheumatoid and psoriatic arthritis. J Rheumatol 28:1842–1846
13. Husted JA, Gladman DD, Farewell VT, Cook RJ (2001) Health-related quality of life of patients with psoriatic arthritis: a comparison with patients with rheumatoid arthritis. Arthritis Rheum 45:151–158
14. Antoni C, Kavanaugh A, Kikham B, Brumester G, et al. (2003) The one year results of the Infliximab Multinational Psoriatic Arthritis Clinical Trial (IMPACT). Arthritis Rheum 48(Suppl 9):S265 (Abstract)
15. Mease PJ, Gottlieb AB, Wanke LA, Burge DJ (2003) Sustained improvement in activities of daily living in patients with psoriatic arthritis treated with etanercept. Arthritis Rheum 48(Suppl 9): S167 (Abstract)
16. Daltroy LH, Larson MG, Roberts NW, Liang MH (1990) A modification of the Health Assessment Questionnaire for the spondyloarthropathies. J Rheumatol 17:946–950
17. Husted J, Gladman DD, Farewell V, Long J (1995) Modified HAQ in psoriatic arthritis. Clin Exp Rheumatol 13:439–444
18. Meenan RF, Gertman PM, Mason JH (1980) Measuring health status in arthritis. The arthritis impact measurement scales. Arthritis Rheum 23:146–152
19. Meenan RF, Mason JH, Anderson JJ, Guccione AA, Kazis LE (1992) AIMS2. The content and properties of a revised and expanded Arthritis Impact Measurement Scales Health Status Questionnaire. Arthritis Rheum 35:1–10
20. Duffy CM, Watanabe Duffy KN, Gladman DD, Brubacher BL, Buskila D, Langevitz P, Farewell V (1992) Utilization of the Arthritis Impact Measurement Scales (AIMS) for patients with psoriatic arthritis. J Rheumatol 19:1727–1732
21. Husted J, Gladman DD, Farewell VT, Long JA (1996) Validation of the revised and expanded version of the Arthritis Impact Measurement Scales for patients with psoriatic arthritis. J Rheumatol 23: 1015–1019
22. Husted J, Gladman DD, Long JA, Farewell VT (1996) Relationship of the Arthritis Impact Measurements Scales (AIMS) to changes in articular status and functional performance in patients with psoriatic arthritis (PsA). J Rheumatol 23:1932–1937
23. Hudak PL, Amadio PC, Bombardier C (1996) Development of an upper extremity outcome measure: the DASH (disabilities of the arm, shoulder, and hand). Am J Ind Med 29:602–608
24. Navsarikar A, Gladman DD, Husted JA, Cook RJ (1999) Validity assessment of the Disabilities of Arm, Shoulder, and Hand questionnaire (DASH) for patients with psoriatic arthritis (PsA). J Rheumatol 26:2191–2194
25. Calin A, Garrett S, Whitelock H, Kennedy LG, O'Hea J, Mallorie P, et al. (1994) A new approach to defining functional ability in ankylosing spondylitis: the development of the Bath Ankylosing Spondylitis Functional Index. J Rheumatol 21: 2281–2285
26. Brockbank JB, Schimmer K, Schentag C, Hyrich KL, Gladman DD (2001) Spinal disease assessment in psoriatic arthritis. J Rheumatol 28(Suppl 63):62 (Abstract)
27. McHorney CA, Ware JE Jr, Lu JF, Sherbourne CD (1994) The MOS 36-item Short-Form Health Survey (SF-36): III. Tests of data quality, scaling assumptions, and reliability across diverse patient groups. Med Care 32:40–66
28. Husted J Gladman DD, Long JA, Farewell VT, Cook R (1997) Validating the SF-36 health questionnaire in patients with psoriatic arthritis. J Rheumatol 24: 511–517
29. Husted JA, Gladman DD, Cook RJ, Farewell VJ (1998) Responsiveness of health status instruments to changes in articular status and perceived health in patients with psoriatic arthritis (PsA). J Rheumatol 25:2146–2155
30. Brooks RG (1996) EuroQoL – the current state of play. Health Policy 37:53–72
31. McKenna SP, Doward LC, Whalley D, Tennant A, Emery P, Veale DJ (2004) Development of the PsAQoL: a quality of life instrument specific to psoriatic arthritis. Ann Rheum 63:162–169
32. Shikiar R, Bresnahan BW, Stone SP, Thompson C, Koo J, Revicki DA. Validity and reliability of patient reported outcomes used in psoriasis: results from two randomized clinical trials. Health Qual Life Outcomes 1:53
33. McKenna SP, Cook SA, Whalley D, Doward LC, Richards HL, Griffiths CE, et al. (2003) Development of the PSORIQoL, a psoriasis-specific measure of quality of life designed for use in clinical practice and trials. Br J Dermatol 149:323–331
34. Schentag CT, Beaton M, Rahman P, Husted J, Gladman DD (2000) Prevalence and correlates of fatigue in psoriatic arthritis (PsA). Arthritis Rheum 43 (Suppl 9):S105 (Abstract)

VII

35. Schentag CT, Cichon J, MacKinnon A, Gladman DD, Urowitz MB (2000) Validation and normative data for the 0–10 point scale version of the fatigue severity scale (FSS). Arthritis Rheum 43(Suppl 9): S177 (Abstract)

36. Schentag C, Gladman DD (2002) Changes in fatigue in psoriatic arthritis: Disease activity or fibromyalgia. Arthritis Rheum 46(Suppl 9): S424 (Abstract)

Clinical Outcome Measurements VIII

A Psoriasis

Kenneth B. Gordon

Contents

1 Introduction

Measuring improvement in psoriasis, while seemingly straightforward, remains a perplexing problem. It is relatively easy to estimate the amount of the body covered with psoriatic plaques; however, this measurement does account for the severity of the lesions involved. Moreover, the severity of the disease can be distinct from the number or size of lesions. A recent consensus conference of the American Academy of Dermatology emphasized that any determination of the severity of psoriasis requires special attention to the impact of the disease on the patient's quality of life [1]. Since the impact of psoriasis may differ from one patient to the next, any physical measurement of psoriasis will necessarily be an incomplete assessment of the severity of the disease. In this chapter, the commonly used techniques for measuring the clinical severity of psoriasis will be discussed. The critically important measures of quality of life are reviewed in Chap. VIIA.

2 Psoriasis Area and Severity Index (PASI)

The most commonly used outcome measure for the extent and severity of psoriasis in clinical trials today is the PASI. The PASI is a complex formula (Table A1) that was introduced in studies of systemic retinoids in 1978 [7]. The PASI incorporates the elements in the clinical presentation of psoriasis that are readily visible on the skin: erythema, scaling, and desquamation. Each element is assessed separately on a 5 point (0–4) scale for each of the sections of the body: the head and neck, the trunk, the upper extremities, and the lower extremities. Scores for each of the three different factors are added, along with the score from a 6 point scale (1–6) representing the surface area involved on that body region. This number is multiplied by a correction factor that accounts for the area encompassed by that body region (0.1 for the head and neck, 0.2 for the upper extremities, 0.3 for the trunk, and 0.4 for the lower extremities). Finally, the scores for the 4 body regions are added to give the PASI score. The highest possible PASI is 72 though this number is generally considered impossible to attain. Scores in the 20's and 30's are considered to represent very severe disease.

Given the complexity of the PASI, it is not surprising that it is almost never used as a clinical measurement in dermatology offices. It is exclusively a tool for research purposes. The PASI can be manipulated in a number of ways as an outcome measurement. In clinical trials,

Table A1. Measurement of the Psoriasis Activity and Severity Index [7]

	Head and neck	Upper extremities	Trunk	Lower extremities
1 Erythema				
2 Induration				
3 Scale				
4 1+2+3				
5 Area				
6 4×5				
7 Body Segment Factor	0.1	0.2	0.3	0.4
8 6×7	A	B	C	D

Total PASI=A+B+C+D

Ratings for Erythema, Induration, and Scale:
0 – none
1 – mild
2 – moderate
3 – severe
4 – very severe

Ratings for Regional Surface Area:
1 – 1–<10%
2 – 10%–<30%
3 – 30%–<50%
4 – 50%–<70%
5 – 70%–<90%
6 – 90%–100%

the percentage change in PASI may be used as an endpoint. More commonly, however, the clinical endpoint of therapy is defined as the number of patients who reach a minimum percentage improvement in the PASI. The United States Food and Drug Administration (FDA) has used a 75% improvement in PASI as representing the clinically significant hurdle to define a patient response. Many researchers, however, believe that the PASI underestimates the clinical response to therapy and that a 50% improvement in PASI is a more reasonable endpoint [2]. Large changes in the quality of psoriasis lesions, without concomitant changes in surface area, is a common clinical scenario, and would result in a change in PASI that would be defined as non-responsive by the FDA criteria, but may be quite significant to the patient [2, 3].

Other difficulties with the PASI stem from the difficulty measuring it, as well as its lack of correlation with patient reported outcomes. Measurement of body surface area is inconsistent among researchers, leading to significant inter-observer variability [14]. More importantly, the PASI does not clearly predict the impact of the disease on patients. Studies examining the correlation of quality of life with PASI scores have demonstrated that there is little consistency [10]. On the positive side, PASI improvements do seem to correlate to improvements in quality of life in placebo controlled trials.

Several variations of the PASI have been proposed to improve upon these weaknesses, as well as to decrease the time and effort needed to perform this complex measurement. One particularly interesting variation is to have the patient perform a modified PASI on him-/herself. This measurement is called the Self Administered PASI (SAPASI) [4]. The SAPASI correlates well with PASI [6] and is responsive to therapy [5]. The SAPASI may be a particularly useful instrument in large, epidemiologic studies, where physician examination of all patients may be impractical [5].

3 Physician's Global Assessment (PGA)

Other measures of psoriasis severity have developed that are simpler to calculate than the PASI. One approach is to examine the overall quality of the lesions and assign a general severity score. This physician's global assessment (PGA) is most similar to the criteria used in a clinician's office to assess response. There are a number of different scales for the PGA and they are identified by many different names [8, 15]. The most important distinction is whether the PGA represents a static measure of disease severity at a single point in time, or as a dynamic measure of improvement following an intervention. Samples of each approach are shown in Table A2 [8, 13].

The primary endpoint used in static global assessments is the number of patients who reach the categories of "clear and almost clear." This is generally considered the point where almost all patients will be satisfied with their therapy. Interestingly, in studies where both a PASI 75 and static PGA have been measured, these numbers are generally very similar. Importantly, the PGA seems to have greater intra-rater and inter-rater reproducibility than the PASI, making it potentially a more effective research tool [14].

Table A2. Samples of the Physician's Global Assessment (PGA) [8]

Static Global Assessment	Dynamic Global Assessment
Very severe	Worse
Severe	Unchanged
Moderate	Slight improvement
Mild	Fair improvement
Minimal	Good improvement
Clear	Excellent improvement
	Cleared

A variation of the PGA that has been studied as a possible outcome measure is the Lattice System PGA (LS-PGA). This system relies on global ratings of scale, erythema, and lesion thickness to determine an overall rating for the patient. Particular emphasis is placed on lesional thickness with this instrument. In a small study, this measure had better intra-rater reproducibility than the PGA with similar inter-rater concordance [14].

4 Combination Outcome Measures

As noted above, measures of physical disease burden often do not represent the full impact of psoriasis on the patient. On the other hand, quality of life measures do not always indicate the full physiological effect of a medication. Combination outcome measures, incorporating both physical measures of disease burden and quality of life outcomes, have been proposed. This type of approach is commonly used in other areas of clinical research; the American College of Rheumatology (ACR) response criteria reviewed in Chap. VIIIB is a good example.

Two different combination criteria have been developed and validated in clinical trials, the National Psoriasis Foundation Psoriasis Score (NPF-PS) and the Salford Psoriasis Index (SPI). The NPF-PS incorporates elements of the PASI, and global assessments of both disease extent and symptoms. It has been compared to the PASI and the PGA in a small clinical trial and seems to correlate well [9]. Use of the NPF-PS has been limited by its complexity.

The SPI was developed to combine disease severity with the impact of psychosocial pressures faced by the patients. It is based on cancer staging methods, and incorporates separate scales for the amount of disease (PASI), a psychosocial instrument, and a record of disease treatment over time [11]. By combining these separate elements, it may be possible to better categorize the impact of disease on patients and to direct therapy based on this impact.

While this approach is still being developed, it seems a promising compromise for both research and clinical use [12].

5 Conclusion

Measuring the amount of psoriasis as well as its impact remains a significant challenge for clinical research in psoriasis. While the PASI and the physician's global assessment remain the standards, new criteria, including the NPF-PS and SPI are being developed that incorporate the impact of psoriasis on patients, not simply the physical amount of disease. Over time, evidence of the value of these types of outcome measures in other specialties, such the ACR criteria, will likely lead to greater acceptance of combination measures by dermatology researchers.

References

1. Callen JP, Krueger GG, Lebwohl M, McBurney EI, Mease P, Menter A, Paller AS, Pariser DM, Weinblatt M, Zimmerman G (2003) AAD consensus statement on psoriasis therapies. J Am Acad Dermatol 49: 897–899
2. Carlin CS, Feldman SR, Krueger JG, Menter A, Krueger GG (2004) A 50% reduction in the Psoriasis Area and Severity Index (PASI 50) is a clinically significant endpoint in the assessment of psoriasis. J Am Acad Dermatol 50:859–866
3. Feldman SR (2003) The design of clinical trials in psoriasis: lessons for clinical practice. J Am Acad Dermatol 49:S62–S65
4. Feldman SR, Fleischer AB Jr, Reboussin DM, Rapp SR, Exum ML, Clark AR, Nurre L (1996) The self-administered psoriasis area and severity index is valid and reliable. J Invest Dermatol 106:183–186
5. Fleischer AB Jr, Feldman SR, Dekle CL (1999) The SAPASI is valid and responsive to psoriasis disease severity changes in a multi-center clinical trial. J Dermatol 26:210–215
6. Fleischer AB Jr, Rapp SR, Reboussin DM, Vanarthos JC, Feldman SR (1994) Patient measurement of psoriasis disease severity with a structured instrument. J Invest Dermatol 102:967–969
7. Fredriksson T, Pettersson U (1978) Severe psoriasis – oral therapy with a new retinoid. Dermatologica 157:238–244
8. Gordon KB, Papp KA, Hamilton TK, Walicke PA, Dummer W, Li N, Bresnahan BW, Menter A (2003) Efalizumab for patients with moderate to severe plaque psoriasis: a randomized controlled trial. JAMA 290:3073–2080
9. Gottlieb AB, Chaudhari U, Baker DG, Perate M, Dooley LT (2003) The National Psoriasis Foundation Psoriasis Score (NPF-PS) system versus the Psoriasis Area Severity Index (PASI) and Physician's Global Assessment (PGA): a comparison. J. Drugs Dermatol 2:260–266
10. Heydendael VM, de Borgie CA, Spuls PI, Bossuyt PM, Bos JD, De Rie MA (2004) The burden of psoriasis is not determined by disease severity only. J Invest Dermatol Symp Proc 9:131–135
11. Kirby B, Fortune DG, Bhushan M, Chalmers RJ, Griffiths CE (2000) The Salford Psoriasis Index: an holistic measure of psoriasis severity. Br J Dermatol 142:728–732
12. Kirby B, Richards HL, Woo P, Hindle E, Main CJ, Griffiths CE (2001) Physical and psychologic measures are necessary to assess overall psoriasis severity. J Am Acad Dermatol 45:72–76
13. Krueger GG, Papp KA, Stough DB, Loven KH, Gulliver WP, Ellis CN (2002) A randomized, double-blind, placebo-controlled phase III study evaluating efficacy and tolerability of 2 courses of alefacept in patients with chronic plaque psoriasis. J Am Acad Dermatol 47:821–833
14. Langley RG, Ellis CN (2004) Evaluating psoriasis with psoriasis area and severity index (PASI), psoriasis global assessment (PGA), and lattice system physician's global assessment (LS-PGA). J Am Acad Dermatol (in press)
15. Weinstein GD, Koo JY, Krueger GG, Lebwohl MG, Lowe NJ, Menter MA, Lew-Kaya DA, Sefton J, Gibson JR, Walker PS (2003) Tazarotene cream in the treatment of psoriasis: Two multicenter, double-blind, randomized, vehicle-controlled studies of the safety and efficacy of tazarotene creams 0.05% and 0.1% applied once daily for 12 weeks. J Am Acad Dermatol 48:760–767

B Psoriatic Arthritis

Soumya M. Reddy,
Clifton O. Bingham III

Contents

1 Introduction

The development of criteria for therapeutic responses in arthritis was attempted as early as 1937, leading to the development of the Committee for Therapeutic Criteria of the New York Rheumatism Association in 1945 [1]. Since then, numerous different criteria have been suggested and employed for the evaluation of RA; however, only one response criterion has been specifically designed for PsA.

2 Psoriatic Arthritis Response Criteria

The Psoriatic Arthritis Response Criteria (PsARC) were developed by Clegg et al. in 1996 to assess responses to sulfasalazine in a clinical trial of 221 PsA patients [2]. The PsARC is defined as an improvement in at least four of four criteria, one of which must be the tender or swollen joint count, *and* no worsening in any criteria. The specific measures of improvement are: physician global assessment ≥1 unit on a 5-point scale, patient global assessment ≥1 unit, tender joint score ≥30%, and swollen joint score ≥30%.

In the study for which these criteria were developed, no significant differences were detected in the sulfasalazine vs. placebo group using the PsARC, perhaps reflecting limited efficacy of sulfasalazine, rather than the performance of the instrument. The PsARC has subsequently been used as an outcome measure in several clinical trials of psoriatic arthritis, including studies with leflunomide, etanercept, and infliximab [3–6]. In these studies, the PsARC detected differences with each treatment compared to placebo groups. For example, in a study of etanercept, 70% of patients receiving etanercept achieved a PsARC response compared to only 23% in the placebo arm after 24 weeks of treatment [4]. PsARC responses also correlated well in most instances with ACR 20% response criteria used in the same studies.

3 ACR Response Criteria

The ACR criteria for the definition of improvement in rheumatoid arthritis were developed in 1995 to standardize outcomes in clinical trials [7]. Prior to the development of the ACR criteria, numerous different measures and definitions were utilized. The most important clinical factors were selected by a group of rheumatologists evaluating standardized patients and then correlated with clinical trial data sets for their discrimination between treatment and placebo arms. The definition of response established was: a 20% improvement in the tender *and* swollen joint count plus 20% improvement in three out of five additional ACR core set measures (patient and physician global assessments, patient pain assessment, patient assessed disability, and an acute phase reactant-ESR or CRP).

The ACR 20% response criteria have been widely used as the primary outcome measure in RA clinical trials. Subsequently, ACR response criteria of 50% and 70% improvement were added with equivalent definitions. Some have questioned whether the ACR 20% improvement represents a clinically meaningful change in an individual patient. In addition, improvements based on these criteria are relative to baseline and do not give absolute information regarding the severity of disease. For example, a patient may have an ACR 50% response with a decrease in tender and swollen joint counts from 18 to 9 and still have significant disease activity.

The ACR response criteria incorporate several measures which may also be relevant in the assessment of PsA but have not been fully validated in this disease. These include the health assessment questionnaire (HAQ), and Patient and Physician global assessments of disease activity. Recent clinical trials of PsA have used a modification of the ACR response criteria with the DIPs of the hands and PIP and DIP joints of the feet (78 tender/76 swollen) used for joint counts [3, 4, 6]. The ACR 20/50/70 response criteria detected differences between the treatment and placebo groups and correlated well with other parameters. It is important to note, however, that these trials required an elevated joint count and/or ESR or CRP for study entry and it is not known if the ACR criteria would perform equally well in patients with less severe disease or without elevation of inflammatory markers.

VIII

4 European League Against Rheumatism and the Disease Activity Score

Investigators from the Netherlands created the *Disease Activity Score* (DAS) for the assessment of RA, incorporating tender and swollen joint counts, an acute phase reactant, and a patient assessment of disease activity. The DAS was developed to allow assessment of the aggregate amount of disease activity at any point in time, thus serving as a continuous variable. In addition, the DAS provides information about changes in disease activity over time, so that a response to a therapeutic intervention can be classified as good, moderate, or poor [8]. The DAS is defined as:

$$\begin{aligned} \text{DAS} = {} & 0.54\ (\text{square root of RAI}) \\ & + 0.065\ (\text{Swollen Joint Count}) \\ & + 0.33\ (\text{ESR mm/hr}) + 0.0072 \end{aligned}$$

Table B1 shows the European League Against Rheumatism (EULAR) response criteria for RA based on the DAS. Disease activity at a point in time can be defined as low if the DAS is ≤2.4, moderate if the DAS is >2.4 and ≤3.7, and high if the DAS is >3.7 [9].

The DAS has also been validated using a 28 joint swollen and tender joint count. For the DAS28, low disease activity is defined as a DAS ≤3.2, moderate if the DAS is >3.2 and ≤5.1, and high if the DAS is >5.1 [9, 10]. More recently, a DAS and DAS28 using a CRP rather than the ESR have been developed (http://www.das-score.nl/www.das-score.nl) [11, 12]. The DAS and DAS28 have been validated for ability to discriminate between treatment and placebo groups in RA and are associated with progression of radiographic joint damage and changes in functional capacity [8, 13].

The ACR and EULAR response criteria were compared at the OMERACT IV Conference in 1998 [13]. Seven large randomized RA trials were evaluated with ACR and EULAR criteria using the extended and 28 joint counts (ACR, ACR28, EULAR, EULAR28). The investigators found a high level of agreement between all four ACR and EULAR criteria and good corre-

Table B1. EULAR Response Criteria based on DAS [9]
EULAR criteria

DAS at endpoint	DAS28 at endpoint	Improvement in DAS or DAS28 from baseline		
		>1.2	>0.6 and ≤1.2	≤0.6
≤2.4	≤3.2	Good		
>2.4 and ≤3.7	>3.2 and ≤5.1		Moderate	
>3.7	>5.1			None

Table B2. Table comparing PsARC, ACR 20/50/70 and DAS responses

Drug (duration)	Patients	PsARC (%)		ACR 20/50/70	
	(*n*)	Drug	Placebo	Drug	Placebo
Leflunomide [3] (24 weeks)	190	59.0	29.7	26.3 (ACR 20)	20 (ACR 20)
Etanercept [4] (24 weeks)	205	70	23	50/37/9	13/4/1
Infliximab [15] (16 weeks)	102	76.5	18	69/49/29	8/0/0

lation with patient and investigator assessments of global disease activity and with radiographic progression.

The DAS has not yet been evaluated in published clinical trials of PsA. One group has recently evaluated correlations between ACR response criteria, EULAR DAS responses, and the PsARC criteria in thirty-eight patients with PsA [14]. The investigators showed a good correlation between the EULAR (DAS better than DAS28) and PsARC criteria, but 21% of patients had conflicting results between the ACR and DAS criteria and between ACR and PsARC [3, 4, 15] (Table B2).

5 Remission

Remission of PsA has been defined by Gladman et al. as a period of at least three consecutive visits with an actively inflamed joint count of 0 (no stress pain, joint line tenderness, or effusion) and was noted to occur in 17.6% of patients, lasting an average of 2.6 years; however, half of the patients had flares after a mean of 1.8 years [16]. The EULAR criteria for remission in RA, corresponding to the ARA definition of remission, are a DAS <1.6 and DAS28 <2.6 [17]. These cutoffs should not be used in PsA until they are validated against an accepted definition of remission.

6 Clinical Damage

The assessment of clinical damage has been defined by Gladman et al. as the number of deformed joints, which includes peripheral joints with limitation of >20% of range of motion that is not attributed to active inflammation, ankylosis, or loosening/subluxation [18]. This measurement has demonstrated reliability between observers. The relevance of clinical damage scores in the assessment of PsA is not known. This parameter is slow to change over time and is not likely to be useful for clinical trials or to monitor routine practice. Disability measures and radiographic changes will likely be more sensitive to change over shorter periods of time.

References

1. Steinbrocker O, Traeger CH, Batterman RC (1949) Therapeutic criteria in rheumatoid arthritis. J Am Med Assoc 140:659–662
2. Clegg DO, Reda DJ, Mejias E, Cannon GW, Weisman MH, Taylor T, et al. (1996) Comparison of sulfasalazine and placebo in the treatment of psoriatic arthritis. A Department of Veterans Affairs Cooperative Study. Arthritis Rheum 39:2013–2020
3. Kaltwasser J, Nash P, Gladman D, Rosen C, Behrens F, Mease P (2003) Leflunomide in the treatment of psoriatic arthritis and psoriasis: data from a double-blind, randomized, placebo-controlled clinical trial. Ann Rheum Dis 62(Suppl 1): abstract no. OP0081
4. Mease P, Kivitz A, Burch F, Siegel E, Cohen S, Burge D (2001) Improvement in disease activity in patients with psoriatic arthritis receiving etanercept (Enbrel): results of a phase 3 multicenter clinical trial [abstract]. Arthritis Rheum 44(Suppl 9): S90
5. Antoni C, Kavanaugh A, Kirkham B, Burmester G, Weisman M, Keystone E, et al. (2002) The Infliximab Multinational Psoriatic Arthritis Controlled Trial (IMPACT) [abstract]. Arthritis Rheum 46(Suppl 9): S381
6. Antoni CE, Kavanaugh A, Kirkham B, Burmester G, Manger B, Tutuncu Z, et al. (2003) The Infliximab Multinational Psoriatic Arthritis Controlled Trial (IMPACT): Substantial Efficacy on Synovitis and Psoriatic Lesions With or Without DMARD Therapy. Ann Rheum Dis 62 (Suppl 1): abstract no. OP0082

7. Felson DT, Anderson JJ, Boers M, Bombardier C, Furst D, Goldsmith C, et al. (1995) American College of Rheumatology. Preliminary definition of improvement in rheumatoid arthritis. Arthritis Rheum 38:727–735
8. van Gestel AM, Prevoo ML, van't Hof MA, van Rijswijk MH, van de Putte LB, van Riel PL (1996) Development and validation of the European League Against Rheumatism response criteria for rheumatoid arthritis. Comparison with the preliminary American College of Rheumatology and the World Health Organization/International League Against Rheumatism Criteria. Arthritis Rheum 39:34–40
9. Piet LCM, van Gestel AM, Scott DL (2000) EULAR Handbook of Clinical Assessments in Rheumatoid Arthritis. Van Zuiden Communications BV, Alphen aan den Rijn, The Netherlands
10. Prevoo ML, van't Hof MA, Kuper HH, van Leeuwen MA, van de Putte LB, van Riel PL (1995) Modified disease activity scores that include twenty-eight-joint counts. Development and validation in a prospective longitudinal study of patients with rheumatoid arthritis. Arthritis Rheum 38:44–48
11. Paulus HE, Ramos B, Wong WK, Ahmed A, Bulpitt K, Park G, et al. (1999) Equivalence of the acute phase reactants C-reactive protein, plasma viscosity, and Westergren erythrocyte sedimentation rate when used to calculate American College of Rheumatology 20% improvement criteria or the Disease Activity Score in patients with early rheumatoid arthritis. Western Consortium of Practicing Rheumatologists. J Rheumatol 26:2324–2331
12. Fransen J, Welsing PMJ, De Keijzer RMH, Van Riel PLCM (2003) Disease activity scores using C-reactive protein: CRP may replace ESR in the assessment of RA disease activity. Ann Rheum Dis 62(Suppl 1): abstract no. THU0138
13. van Gestel AM, Anderson JJ, van Riel PL, Boers M, Haagsma CJ, Rich B, et al. (1999) ACR and EULAR improvement criteria have comparable validity in rheumatoid arthritis trials. American College of Rheumatology European League of Associations for Rheumatology. J Rheumatol 26:705–711
14. Ujfalussy I, Koo E (2003) Measurement of disease activity in psoriatic arthritis. Extended report. Z Rheumatol 62:60–65
15. Gladman DD, Helliwell P, Mease PJ, Nash P, Ritchlin C, Taylor W (2004) Assessment of patients with psoriatic arthritis: a review of currently available measures. Arthritis Rheum 50:24–35
16. Gladman DD, Hing EN, Schentag CT, Cook RJ (2001) Remission in psoriatic arthritis. J Rheumatol 28: 1045–1048
17. Prevoo ML, van Gestel AM, van THMA, van Rijswijk MH, van de Putte LB, van Riel PL (1996) Remission in a prospective study of patients with rheumatoid arthritis. American Rheumatism Association preliminary remission criteria in relation to the disease activity score. Br J Rheumatol 35:1101–1105
18. Gladman DD, Farewell V, Buskila D, Goodman R, Hamilton L, Langevitz P, et al. (1990) Reliability of measurements of active and damaged joints in psoriatic arthritis. J Rheumatol 17:62–64

Conventional Therapy IX

A Psoriasis

Contents

1 Topical Therapy

Rachel Quinby

Introduction

Topical therapy has been, and remains, the primary therapeutic option for the treatment of limited psoriasis limited in the skin. It provides potential therapeutic efficacy and limits the effects of the treatment to the target tissue. It also can provide symptomatic improvement in the discomfort associated with psoriasis when used in conjunction with potentially more potent treatments like phototherapy and systemic medications. Unfortunately, topical treatments are limited by difficulty in application when the disease is wide-spread and are not always well accepted by patients do to potential tolerability issues, primarily skin irritation and cosmetic considerations. In this chapter, the common topical therapies in use for psoriasis are reviewed with a particular emphasis on the evidence for the use of these treatments and potential side-effects.

Topical Corticosteroids

Topical corticosteroids have long been the mainstay of therapy for mild-to-moderate psoriasis. They are available in varying strengths, ranging from the lowest potency, class 7 steroids to the superpotent class 1 steroids. They are formulated in a wide variety of vehicles including ointment, cream, foam, lotion, gel, solution, and tape. They can be used alone or in combination with other topical therapies. Although highly effective, their use is limited by potential side effects.

Corticosteroids are vasoconstrictive, antiproliferative, anti-inflammatory, and immunosuppressive. These effects are exerted through alterations in gene regulation. Corticosteroids form complexes with glucocorticoid receptors in the cytoplasm of cells after which this complex traverses the nuclear envelope and then binds to and modulates DNA transcription. The antiproliferative effects of topical corticosteroids are mediated by inhibition of DNA synthesis and mitosis that restricts the proliferation of keratinocytes and causes atrophy of the dermis through inhibition of fibroblasts. They exert their immunosuppressive and anti-inflammatory properties by inhibiting leukocytes, Langerhans cells, the formation of prostaglandins, and the production of cytokines such as IL-1, IL-2, and IFN-gamma. Vasoconstriction is caused by an augmented response to catecholamines [2, 9, 12, 40, 48, 57, 79].

The vasoconstrictive assay, initially described by McKenzie and Stoughton [103], has been widely used to measure the potency of topical corticosteroids and correlates well with clinical efficacy [23]. These assays, in combination with clinical trials, have been used to separate the topical corticosteroids into seven classes based on potency. Occlusive vehicles (such as ointments) and occlusive dressings enhance percutaneous absorption and thus tend to enhance potency [103, 142]. Absorption is also influenced by the condition of the skin and varies according to the skin site. Penetration correlates inversely with the thickness of the stratum corneum [142] and is greatly increased on areas such as the scrotum and the face [38]. Penetration is also increased on inflamed skin [147] and with increased hydration of the stratum corneum [142].

Randomized, controlled trials have established the clinical efficacy of class I corticosteroids in the treatment of plaque psoriasis [6, 11, 47, 60, 64, 65]. These superpotent steroids, such as halobetasol dipropionate and clobetasol propionate, have superior therapeutic efficacy compared to the less potent steroids [11, 102]. Treatment is generally twice a day for approximately 2 weeks followed by an intermittent dosing regimen to preserve remission. In a multicenter, double-blind study, patients who achieved remission of their psoriasis after 3–4 - weeks of twice-daily application of augmented betamethasone dipropionate ointment were treated with either the steroid or placebo for three consecutive applications (12 h apart) once a week. The psoriasis of 60% of the patients treated with the steroid was controlled for 6 - months while 80% of the placebo-treated patients experienced an exacerbation; there were no serious adverse events [66]. Another maintenance regimen of clobetasol propionate twice weekly achieved remission for an average of 4 - months in 75% of patients treated [131]. Gammon et al. described a form of intermittent maintenance treatment that consisted of 2-week bursts of continuous twice-daily application of clobetasol ointment with intervals of 1–2 weeks without treatment. However, only 15% of patients had remissions lasting more than 7 weeks [44].

Topical corticosteroids, in the form of lotions, solutions, and foams, are also effective in the treatment of scalp psoriasis [41, 67, 104, 114]. The newer foam formulations, clobetasol propionate and betamethasone valerate, have proven to be more effective and have higher patient acceptability than their solution and lotion counterparts [41, 105]. Both of these foams have also proven to be effective against non-scalp psoriasis [96, 129].

Topical corticosteroids can be used in combination with other topical therapies to increase efficacy and decrease side effects. When combined with the keratolytic agent, salicylic acid, there is a marked increase in the penetration and efficacy of topical corticosteroids [84, 93]. In two separate randomized, double-blind trials, mometasone furoate 0.1% plus salicylic acid 5% ointment twice daily was significantly more efficacious than twice daily mometasone ointment or fluocinonide 0.05% ointment alone in the treatment of plaque psoriasis [75, 104]. Topical corticosteroids can also be used in combination with calcipotriene and tazarotene (see below).

Studies of topical corticosteroids plus ultraviolet therapy have shown mixed results [107]. When used with psoralens and ultraviolet A (PUVA), topical corticosteroids increased the rate of clearing and decreased UVA exposure compared to PUVA alone [53]. However, one study demonstrated a higher relapse rate with corticosteroid use [111]. There does not appear to be any benefit from the use of UVB plus corticosteroids and is not recommended [31, 87, 107].

Used for short periods without occlusion, topical corticosteroids are usually free from adverse events [1]. However, cutaneous and systemic adverse effects do occur when corticosteroids are used with excessive duration, amount, occlusion, or on the face and intertriginous areas. Atrophy is one of the most common local side effects [130]. It is characterized by thinning of the epidermis and dermis, telangiectasias, skin fragility, easy bruising, and striae. While minor atrophy is usually reversible, striae generally are not [109]. Due to this risk, potent corticosteroids should not be used on the face or intertriginous sites. However, limited application over a period of 10 weeks of fluticasone propionate ointment 0.005%, a mid-potency corticosteroid, was found to be effective in facial and intertriginous psoriasis without causing atrophy or telangiectasias [95].

Other cutaneous side effects include acne, folliculitis, periorificial dermatitis, steroid-induced rosacea, and rebound flaring of rosacea after cessation of the topical corticosteroid [99, 116.125, 126]. Irritant and allergic contact dermatitis may occur to the steroid itself or to components of the vehicle [1, 29, 39]. Corticosteroids applied to periorbital skin can also cause cataracts and increase ocular pressure leading to glaucoma [25, 113]. With repeated use, tolerance (or tachyphylaxis) can develop and the steroid will lose efficacy [34].

Topical corticosteroids, particularly when used in high doses, can lead to a pustular flare of psoriasis when discontinued [19, 128]. They can also cause suppression of the hypothalamic-pituitary-adrenal (HPA) axis and iatrogenic Cushing's syndrome [98, 112]. Infants and small children may be more susceptible due to their increased skin surface-to-body mass ratio [137]. Osteonecrosis of the femoral head has also been reported with long-term application of corticosteroids [86]. In accordance with the Food and Drug Administration, superpotent corticosteroids applied twice-daily should generally be limited to a 2-week course and less than 50 g per week [140]. Special consideration may be necessary depending upon the clinical requirements of the patient and the location of the psoriatic involvement.

Calcipotriene

Calcipotriene, also known as calcipotriol, is a widely prescribed topical treatment for psoriasis. It is available in the United States as a 0.005% ointment, cream, and solution. Calcipotriene has similar efficacy to class II and III corticosteroids but has relatively few side effects. It can be combined with topical corticosteroids, systemic agents, and phototherapy to improve efficacy and decrease the dosage of the more toxic agents and adverse events.

Calcipotriene is a structural analog of 1, 25-dihydroxy vitamin D_3 (calcitriol). It binds to the vitamin D_3 receptor, a member of the nuclear transcription superfamily, which then binds to and regulates target genes. It exerts its clinical effects by inhibiting the proliferation and promoting the differentiation of keratinocytes [10, 78]. In addition, calcipotriene may act on cells involved in immunologic reactions such as Langerhans cells and T lymphocytes [108, 121]. Although calcipotriene is as potent as 1, 25-dihydroxy vitamin D_3 in the regulation of cell proliferation and differentiation, it is at least 100 times less potent in its effects on calcium metabolism [10].

IX

Placebo controlled, double-blind trials have demonstrated twice-daily calcipotriene to be a safe and effective treatment for plaque psoriasis [32, 58, 79], and these findings have been reinforced by long-term studies [118]. Twice-daily application of calcipotriene has been found superior to 15% coal tar [135] and more effective and acceptable than short-contact dithranol therapy [7]. When compared to topical corticosteroids in the treatment of psoriasis, trials have found calcipotriene equal or superior to betamethasone 17 valerate in like vehicles [24, 81, 110] and calcipotriene ointment was found to be more effective than fluocinonide ointment [18]. However, though some improvement is frequently seen after 2 weeks of therapy, the maximum response is usually not seen for 6–8 - weeks when calcipotriene is used as monotherapy [119].

Although as monotherapy calcipotriene is less effective than superpotent corticosteroids, combined use of the two agents has proven superior to either agent used alone. Lebwohl et al. demonstrated that application of calcipotriene ointment in the morning and halobetasol ointment in the evening was more efficacious than either agent applied twice daily [88]. Another trial demonstrated that 76% of patients who applied calcipotriene twice daily on weekdays and halobetasol twice daily on weekends were able to maintain remission for 6 - months compared to only 40% of patients who applied halobetasol on the weekends and the vehicle on the weekdays [92]. In yet another trial, augmented betamethasone cream applied daily on the 1st and 3rd weeks and calcipotriene ointment applied twice daily on the 2nd and 4th weeks proved more effective than augmented betamethasone applied once daily for 4 - weeks [124].

A new combination product of calcipotriene and betamethasone dipropionate has shown superior efficacy and more rapid onset of action than either constituent alone [30, 51, 68]. Additionally, one study found no statistical or clinically relevant difference in efficacy if the formulation was used once or twice daily [51]. This study also found a decreased frequency of adverse events with the combined formulation. Another combination product of calcipotriene and clobetasol propionate applied once daily was found to be superior to daily calcipotriene alone [63].

Care should be taken when using combination therapy as calcipotriene is a relatively unstable molecule that is inactivated by an acid pH [82]. Patel et al. [115] demonstrated that calcipotriene ointment is stable when mixed with 5% tar gel or with halobetasol ointment or cream. However, mixture with 6% salicylic acid, 12% ammonium lactate, or hydrocortisone-17-valerate ointment resulted in its degradation.

Calcipotriene, in solution, is also effective for the treatment of scalp psoriasis [49]. However, twice daily calcipotriene has been found less effective than twice daily betamethasone 17 valerate and is associated with increased scalp and facial irritation [35, 70]. An increased treatment response to calcipotriene has been achieved when it is used along with other treatment modalities such as corticosteroids or salicylic acid [134].

Topical calcipotriene can be used in combination with systemic agents for the treatment of psoriasis. Some trials have found this to enhance efficacy while decreasing the risk of side effects by limiting exposure to the systemic agent. A trial by van de Kerkhof et al. compared acitretin and calcipotriene with acitretin and placebo ointment, with clearance or marked improvement in 67% in the calcipotriene group vs. 41% in the placebo group; there was a significantly lower cumulative dose of acitretin in the calcipotriene group [141]. A study by Grossman et al. compared low-dose cyclosporine (2 mg/kg daily) with either calcipotriene or the vehicle applied twice daily. Complete clearing or 90% improvement occurred in 50% of the calcipotriene group vs. 12% of those in the vehicle group [50]. In a placebo-controlled trial by de Jong et al., the combination of calcipotriene and methotrexate resulted in a significantly lower cumulative dose of methotrexate needed to control psoriasis when compared to methotrexate and vehicle alone [27].

Calcipotriene can also be used in combination with UVB and PUVA therapies to produce a UV-sparing effect. In a double-blind study by Frappaz and Thivolet, patients treated with calcipotriene plus PUVA thrice weekly for 10 - weeks achieved a mean reduction of PASI from baseline of 91.4% and a cumulative UVA dose of 30 J/cm^2 compared to 75.7% and 57 J/cm^2 for the control group [42]. In a bilateral comparison study by Speight and Farr in which one side of the body was treated with calcipotriene and both sides received PUVA, the side treated with calcipotriene required fewer treatments and lower cumulative doses of UVA to clear [127]. The UV-sparing effects of calcipotriene also apply to UVB. A study by Ramsay et al. found that twice weekly broad-band UVB plus calcipotriene when compared to thrice weekly broad-band UVB plus vehicle required fewer exposures and less cumulative irradiance to achieve both an 80% reduction in PASI as well as total clearance [120]. A more recent study comparing thrice weekly narrow-band UVB combined with calcipotriene vs. placebo found a significantly lower mean cumulative UVB dose in the calcipotriene group [146].

When combining calcipotriene with phototherapy, Lebwohl et al. demonstrated that UVA can degrade calcipotriene [89]. Furthermore, other studies have suggested that calcipotriene can block the transmission of UV light [28, 100]. Therefore, it has been suggested that when combining calcipotriene with UV therapy, calcipotriene should be applied after the application of UVB or UVA and never immediately before [74].

Calcipotriene is a relatively safe medication with few side effects. The most common adverse reaction is skin irritation on or around the psoriatic plaques. This can occur as an irritant contact dermatitis or, less commonly, as an allergic contact dermatitis [83]. Dilution with petrolatum [73] or concomitant use with corticosteroids can help minimize the irritating effects. Although calcipotriene has been shown to be effective in treating psoriasis of the face and intertriginous sites [69], these areas are especially prone to irritation.

The primary potential adverse systemic reaction of calcipotriene is an alteration of calcium homeostasis. The risk is a function of the cumulative weekly dose, and calcipotriene is generally considered safe when the dose is limited to the recommended 100 g of 50 µm/g ointment per week [15, 52, 118]. However, hypercalcemia and hypercalciuria can occur with larger doses [13, 14, 45]. Additionally, there have been reports of hypercalcemia in two patients applying 80–90 g/week [54] and a small rise in urine calcium excretion when using 100 g/week [8]. The degree of toxicity is also related to body weight, and hypercalcemia has occurred when using more than 5.6 g/kg per week [16]. Caution, therefore, is required when prescribing calcipotriene for any patient with known hypercalciuria or a history of renal stone formation.

Tazarotene

Tazarotene, a vitamin A derivative, is the first synthetically developed retinoid indicated for the topical treatment of psoriasis. It was approved for use in the United States in 1997 and is available as a 0.1% and 0.05% gel and cream. Although effective as monotherapy, irritation can be a limiting side effect. However, irritation can be reduced and efficacy increased when used in combination with corticosteroids. Tazarotene has an added benefit of sustained therapeutic efficacy after therapy has been stopped.

Tazarotene is metabolized in the skin to its active metabolite tazarotenic acid, which is a selective retinoic acid receptor (RAR) agonist that primarily binds to RAR β and γ [20, 21]. By binding these receptors, tazarotenic acid modulates the expression of certain genes. It has its clinical effect on psoriasis through normalization of keratinocyte differentiation and proliferation and through a decrease of inflammation [33, 37].

In a double-blind, randomized, vehicle-controlled trial, once-daily tazarotene 0.1% and 0.05% gel were superior to vehicle in efficacy (≥50% improvement) and time to initial success in the treatment of stable plaque psoriasis. The effectiveness of the tazarotene was seen as early one week, and the tazarotene treated patients had a sustained therapeutic effect that was observed 12 weeks after treatment was stopped [144]. In another double-blind trial, treatment success (>75% improvement) with once or twice-daily 0.05% or 0.1% tazarotene gel was superior to vehicle and also displayed a maintenance of therapeutic effect during the 8-week follow-up [85]. In a recent study, tazarotene 0.1% and 0.05% cream applied daily for 12 weeks was found to be more effective than vehicle in plaque psoriasis, and like the gel formulation, exhibited good maintenance of therapeutic effect [145]. When once-daily tazarotene 0.1% or 0.05% gel was compared to twice-daily fluocinonide 0.05% cream in a 12-week trial involving 348 patients, fluocinonide had an overall higher rate of treatment success (≥50% improvement) and significantly greater reduction in erythema during the treatment period. However, tazarotene demonstrated a prolonged therapeutic effect and significantly lower probability of relapse after 12 weeks off treatment [90].

In order to increase efficacy and decrease adverse effects, tazarotene has been used in combination with corticosteroids. In a trial involving 300 patients by Lebwohl et al. [91], tazarotene 0.1% gel plus placebo cream was compared to tazarotene plus a low-potency steroid (fluocinolone acetonide 0.01% cream), a mid-potency steroid (mometasone furoate 0.1% cream), or a high-potency steroid (fluocinonide 0.05% cream). The tazarotene was applied once in the evenings and the placebo or corticosteroid was applied once in the morning. The tazarotene plus the mid or high-potency steroid demonstrated significantly more rapid improvement, efficacy, and decreased irritation compared to tazarotene plus placebo. In a different study, a randomized, investigator-masked trial compared tazarotene 0.1% gel applied in the evenings plus mometasone furoate 0.1% cream (a mid-potency corticosteroid) applied in the mornings to mometasone applied twice-daily for 12 weeks. Tazarotene plus mometasone not only demonstrated greater efficacy and more rapid improvement than corticosteroid monotherapy but also had sustained improvement in the 12 weeks following treatment compared to a lessening of improvement in the mometasone only group [77]. Additionally, in an open-label, right-left comparison in 15 patients, once-daily tazarotene 0.1% gel plus twice-daily calcipotriene ointment was comparable in efficacy to twice-daily clobetasol 0.05% ointment over a 2-week treatment period [17].

While the addition of a topical corticosteroid can enhance the efficacy of tazarotene and diminish its irritation, topical retinoids have been shown to prevent corticosteroid induced skin atrophy in mice [97]. Unpublished data, reported in an article by Lebwohl, demonstrated tazarotene's ability to increase epidermal thickness and decrease the epidermal thinning effects of topical corticosteroids [94]. Furthermore, in a study by Hecker et al., tazarotene gel proved to be stable when combined with a number of commonly used topical psoriasis treatments and did not impact the stability of the other products [56]. The products tested included 6 different corticosteroids in a variety of vehicles as well as calcipotriene.

Tazarotene can also be combined with phototherapy in the treatment of psoriasis. In an investigator-masked trial by Koo et al. [76], 54 patients were treated with tazarotene 0.1% gel, vehicle gel, or no treatment for 14 days. These same treatments were then applied after UVB phototherapy thrice weekly for an additional 67 days. The tazarotene group achieved significantly greater efficacy and increased speed of improvement along with significantly lower median cumulative UVB exposure than the vehicle group plus UVB or UVB alone. There was no instance of photosensitivity. In a study investigating narrow-band UVB, tazarotene 0.05% gel or an emollient was applied nightly to one-half of the body and the whole body was treated with UVB 311 nm 5 times/week. The tazarotene plus narrow-band UVB resulted in more effective and faster clearing of psoriasis than narrow-band monotherapy [5]. There was no phototoxicity or significant tazarotene irritation, and the decreased irritation was hypothesized to be secondary to an enhanced skin barrier from phototherapy.

Tazarotene can also be used in conjunction with PUVA photochemotherapy. In a study of 12 patients, tazarotene 0.05% gel was applied once daily to psoriatic plaques on one side of the body and vehicle on the other side, and both sides of the body were treated with PUVA bath therapy four times per week. The tazarotene treated side was clinically and statistically superior to the control side and the treatments were well tolerated [4]. In another study, tazarotene applied in the evening combined with PUVA four times per week was comparably effective as PUVA monotherapy but with significantly fewer treatment requirements and less cumulative UVA exposure [138].

Tazarotene appears to be chemically stable when used in conjunction with UVB or UVA, and the use of tazarotene can reduce the minimal erythema dose (MED) for UVB and the amount of UVA required to induce immediate pigment darkening. Therefore, to prevent burning, it has been suggested to initiate UVB at 50–75% of the MED and PUVA at slightly lower doses than usual when used in conjunction with tazarotene [55].

The most common side effect of tazarotene is localized irritation characterized by pruritus, burning, and erythema [144]. Topically applied tazarotene has low systemic absorption and therefore has little potential for systemic adverse effects [133]. Hematologic, blood chemistry, and urinalysis studies have shown no consistent, clinically significant, drug-related effects, and women who became pregnant during clinical trials delivered healthy children with no incidence of teratogenicity [144]. However, tazarotene is rated as a pregnancy category X, and patients should be advised to use reliable contraception while using the medication and to discontinue use should pregnancy occur [106].

Tars and Anthralin

Coal tar is a chemically heterogeneous mixture of compounds including aromatic hydrocarbons such as benzenes and phenols [22]. Tars have a long history in the treatment of psoriasis, but their mechanism of action is not well defined and evidence-based research is limited. Their undesirable side effect profile also makes them an unpopular treatment option.

Although tars are photosensitizing [61], and are often used in combination with ultraviolet light (UVL), the therapeutic response seen in patients treated with tar and UVL may not be from tar photoxicity [132]. In the Goeckerman regimen, hospitalized patients were treated with an ointment of coal tar, zinc oxide, and petrolatum for 24 h followed by UVB phototherapy [46]. However, studies have shown that UVB plus crude coal tar ointment is no more effective than UVB plus the ointment vehicle [36].

In a randomized, double-blind, bilaterally controlled study of 18 patients by Kanzler and Gorsulowsky [62], 5% liquor carbonis detergens, a tar extract, resulted in significantly more improvement in psoriasis than its vehicle emollient base. In a randomized, observer-blinded intrapatient trial, a new 1% coal tar formulation was compared to calcipotriene in forty patients. The products showed comparable efficacy, but calcipotriene had more tolerability and cosmetic acceptability [139]. Other comparative studies have found calcipotriene superior to coal tar therapy [135]. Side effects of tar include folliculitis, phototoxicity, irritation, and staining [123].

Anthralin, also known as dithranol, is the synthetic version of chrysarobin, a product derived from the *Vouacopoua araroba* tree. Its mode of action in psoriasis is unknown, although it may affect DNA synthesis and cell proliferation [71]. Anthralin was used by Ingram as a substitution for crude coal tar in Goeckerman's regimen [59], and others have reported successful treatment with various concentrations and formulations [3]. Salicylic acid is frequently added to improve the stability of anthralin and to increase its penetration and efficacy [72].

Short-contact anthralin therapy (SCAT) was developed to optimize effectiveness and minimize staining and irritation. Runne and Kunze [122] compared "3-hour" therapy using 0.1–2% anthralin and "minutes" therapy using 1–3% anthralin to the traditional 24-hour method using lower concentrations. A high concentration of anthralin (1–3%) applied for 10–20 min was significantly better than standard therapy and the 3-hour therapy was equally effective as standard therapy. They concluded that a 10-min application of 2% anthralin was optimal. However, twice-daily calcipotriene has been found to be superior to SCAT and with better patient acceptability [7]. Micanol is a 1% anthralin formulation in a temperature-sensitive vehicle that releases active medication at skin surface temperatures. Staining of the skin can still occur, but not fabrics or other household items. It is removed by washing with cold water, which leads to recrystallization. It has been found effective in short and long-contact regimens [136].

Side effects of anthralin include inflammation and erythema, allergic contact dermatitis [26], and staining of skin, hair, fabrics, and porcelain sinks and bathtubs. Triethanolamine, applied after the removal of anthralin, prevents staining and irritation [117]. Chlorine bleach can be used to remove stains from household items [143].

Tacrolimus

Tacrolimus is a topical formulation of the immunomodulatory agent FK 506 and is available as a 0.03% and 0.1% ointment in the United States. Originally used for atopic dermatitis, tacrolimus modulates immune-cell function by inhibiting calcineurin-dependent dephosphorylation-activation of specific nuclear factors and therefore preventing transcription of proinflammatory cytokines [101]. Early studies suggest that it is of limited efficacy in the treatment of plaque psoriasis of the body. This may be due to its inability to penetrate thick hyperkeratotic lesions [148], but this difficulty may be overcome with the addition of salicylic acid or a gel vehicle (Feldman, unpublished data). However, studies have found it useful for psoriasis of the face and intertriginous areas. In an open-label trial of 21 patients, patients applied 0.1% tacrolimus twice-daily to psoriasis on the face or intertriginous areas for 8 weeks. There was statistically significant improvement in the physician's assessment and 81% experienced complete clearing. Furthermore, no atrophy, telangiectasia, or striae developed during the study and only two patients reported itching or warmth at the application site [43]. Side effects of tacrolimus include a localized burning sensation and pruritus.

Conclusion

Despite advances in the systemic treatment of psoriasis, topical therapy is used in almost all patients treated for psoriasis. As reviewed here, these agents can be greatly efficacious with limited side effects when used properly. Many of these agents have been used for many years and have a proven track record that is comforting for physicians and patients alike.

References

1. Akers WA (1980) Risks of unoccluded topical steroids in clinical trials. Arch Dermatol 116:786–788
2. Barnes PJ, Adcock I (1993) Anti-inflammatory actions of steroids: molecular mechanisms. Trends Pharmacol Sci 14:436–441
3. Beerman H, Kulchar GV, Pillbury DM, et al. (1935) Dioxyanthranol 1-8 as a substitute for chrysarobin. JAMA 104:26–29
4. Behrens S, Grundmann-Kollmann M, Peter RU, Kerscher M (1999) Combination treatment of psoriasis with photochemotherapy and tazarotene gel, a receptor-selective topical retinoid. Br J Dermatol 141:177
5. Behrens S, Grundmann-Kollmann M, Schiener R, Peter RU, Kerscher M (2000) Combination phototherapy of psoriasis with narrow-band UVB irradiation and topical tazarotene gel. J Am Acad Dermatol 42:493–495
6. Bernhard J, Whitmore C, Guzzo C, Kantor I, Kalb RE, Ellis C, Urbach F, Schwartzel EH, Gibson JR (1991) Evaluation of halobetasol propionate ointment in the treatment of plaque psoriasis: report on two double-blind, vehicle-controlled studies. J Am Acad Dermatol 25:1170–1174
7. Berth-Jones J, Chu AC, Dodd WA, et al. (1992) A multicentre, parallel-group comparison of calcipotriol ointment and short-contact dithranol therapy in chronic plaque psoriasis. Br J Dermatol 127: 266–271
8. Berth-Jones J, Bourke JF, Iqbal SJ, Hutchinson PE (1993) Urine calcium excretion during treatment of psoriasis with topical calcipotriol. Br J Dermatol 129:411–414
9. Besse JC, Bass AD (1966) Potentiation by hydrocortisone of responses to catecholamines in vascular smooth muscle. J Pharmacol Exp Ther 154: 224–238
10. Binderup L, Bramm E (1988) Effects of a novel vitamin D analogue MC903 on cell proliferation and differentiation *in vitro* and on calcium metabolism *in vivo*. Biochem Pharmacol 37:889–895
11. Blum G, Yawalkar S (1991) A comparative, multicenter, double-blind trial of 0.05% halobetasol propionate ointment and 0.1% betamethasone valerate ointment in the treatment of patients with chronic, localized, plaque psoriasis. J Am Acad Dermatol 25:1153–1156
12. Boumpas DT, Chrousos GP, Wilder RL, Cupps TR, Balow JE (1993) Glucocorticoid therapy for immune-mediated diseases: basic and clinical correlates. Ann Intern Med 119:1198–1208
13. Bourke JF, Berth-Jones J, Hutchinson PE (1993) Hypercalcaemia with topical calcipotriol. BMJ 306: 1344–1345
14. Bourke JF, Berth-Jones J, Iqbal SJ, Hutchinson PE (1993) High-dose topical calcipotriol in the treatment of extensive psoriasis vulgaris. Br J Dermatol 129:74–76
15. Bourke JF, Iqbal SJ, Hutchinson PE (1996) Vitamin D analogues in psoriasis: effects on systemic calcium homeostasis. Br J Dermatol 135:347–354
16. Bourke JF, Mumford R, Whittaker P, Iqbal SJ, Le Van LW, Trevellyan A, Hutchinson PE (1997) The effects of topical calcipotriol on systemic calcium homeostasis in patients with chronic plaque psoriasis. J Am Acad Dermatol 37:929–934
17. Bowman PH, Maloney JE, Koo JY (2002) Combination of calcipotriene (Dovonex) ointment and tazarotene (Tazorac) gel versus clobetasol ointment in the treatment of plaque psoriasis: a pilot study. J Am Acad Dermatol 46:907–913
18. Bruce S, Epinette WW, Funicella T, et al. (1994) Comparative study of calcipotriene (MC 903) ointment and fluocinonide ointment in the treatment of psoriasis. J Am Acad Dermatol 31:755–759
19. Carruthers JA, August PJ, Staughton RCD (1975) Observations on the systemic effect of topical clobetasol propionate (Dermovate). Br Med J 4:203
20. Chandraratna RA (1996) Tazarotene – first of a new generation of receptor-selective retinoids. Br J Dermatol 135 Suppl 49:18–25
21. Chandraratna RA (1997) Tazarotene: the first receptor-selective topical retinoid for the treatment of psoriasis. J Am Acad Dermatol 37:S12–17
22. Comaish JS (1981) Tar and related compounds in the therapy of psoriasis. Arch Dermatol 92:56–58
23. Cornell RC, Stoughton RB (1985) Correlation of the vasoconstrictive assay and clinical activity in psoriasis. Arch Dermatol 121:63–67
24. Cunliffe WJ, Berth-Jones J, Claudy A, et al. (1992) Comparative study of calcipotriol (MC 903) ointment and betamethasone 17-valerate ointment in patients with psoriasis vulgaris. J Am Acad Dermatol 26:736–743
25. Dahl MGC (1985) Hazards of topical steroid therapy. Adverse Drug Reaction Bull 115:428–431
26. DeGroot AC, Nater JP (1981) Contact allergy to dithranol. Contact Dermatitis 7:5–8
27. de Jong EM, Mork NJ, Seijger MM, et al. (1993) The combination of calcipotriol and methotrexate compared with methotrexate and vehicle in psoriasis: results of a multicentre placebo-controlled randomized trial. Br J Dermatol 148:318–325
28. De Rie MA, Di Nuzzo S, Brands S, Hansen AB, Bos JD (2000) Calcipotriol ointment and cream or their vehicles applied immediately before irradiation inhibit ultraviolet B-induced erythema. Br J Dermatol 142:1160–1165
29. Dooms-Goossens AE, Degreef HJ, Marien KJ, Coopman SA (1989) Contact allergy to corticosteroids: a frequently missed diagnosis? J Am Acad Dermatol 21:538–543
30. Douglas WS, Poulin Y, Decroix J, et al. (2002) A new calcipotriol/betamethasone formulation with rapid onset of action was superior to monotherapy with betamethasone dipropionate or calcipotriol in psoriasis vulgaris. Acta Derm Venereol 82: 131–135

31. Dover JS, McEvoy MT, Rosen CF, Arndt KA, Stern RS (1989) Are topical corticosteroids useful in phototherapy for psoriasis? J Am Acad Dermatol 20:748–754
32. Dubertret L, Wallach D, Souteyrand P, et al. (1992) Efficacy and safety of calcipotriol (MC 903) ointment in psoriasis vulgaris. A randomized, double-blind, right/left comparative, vehicle-controlled study. J Am Acad Dermatol 27:983–988
33. Duvic M, Asano AT, Hager C, Mays S (1998) The pathogenesis of psoriasis and the mechanism of action of tazarotene. J Am Acad Dermatol 39: S129–133
34. du Vivier A, Stoughton RB (1975) Tachyphylaxis to the action of topically applied corticosteroids. Arch Dermatol 111:581–583
35. Duweb GA, Abuzariba O, Rahim M, al-Taweel M, Abdulla SA (2000) Scalp psoriasis: topical calcipotriol 50 micrograms/g/ml solution vs. betamethasone valerate 1% lotion. Int J Clin Pharmacol Res 20:65–68
36. Eells LD, Wolff JM, Garloff J, et al. (1984) Comparison of suberythromogenic and maximally aggressive ultraviolet B therapy for psoriasis. J Am Acad Dermatol 11:105–110
37. Esgleyes-Ribot T, Chandraratna RA, Lew-Kaya DA, Sefton J, Duvic M (1994) Response of psoriasis to a new topical retinoid, AGN 190168. J Am Acad Dermatol 30:581–590
38. Feldman RJ, Maibach HI (1967) Regional variation in percutaneous penetration of 14 C cortisol in man. J Invest Dermatol 48:181–183
39. Fisher AA, Pascher F, Kanoff NB (1971) Allergic contact dermatitis due to ingredients of vehicles. A "vehicle tray" for patch testing. Arch Dermatol 104:286–290
40. Fisher LB, Maibach HI (1971) The effect of corticosteroids on human epidermal mitotic activity. Arch Dermatol 103:39–44
41. Franz TJ, Parsell DA, Halualani RM, Hannigan JF, Kalbach JP, Harkonen WS (1999) Betamethasone valerate foam 0.12%: a novel vehicle with enhanced delivery and efficacy. Int J Dermatol 38: 628–632
42. Frappaz A, Thivolet J (1993) Calcipotriol in combination with PUVA: a randomized double-blind placebo study in severe psoriasis. Eur J Dermatol 3 :351–354
43. Freeman AK, Linowski GJ, Brady C, et al. (2003) Tacrolimus ointment for the treatment of psoriasis on the face and intertriginous areas. J Am Acad Dermatol 48:564–568
44. Gammon WR, Krueger GG, Van Scott EJ, et al. (1987) Intermittent short courses of clobetasol propionate ointment 0.05% in the treatment of psoriasis. Curr Ther Res 42:419–427
45. Georgiou S, Tsambaos D (1999) Hypercalcaemia and hypercalciuria after topical treatment of psoriasis with excessive amounts of calcipotriol. Acta Derm Venereol 79:86
46. Goeckerman WH (1925) Treatment of psoriasis. Northwest Med 24:229–231
47. Goldberg B, Hartdegen R, Presbury D, Smith EH, Yawalkar S (1991) A double-blind, multicenter comparison of 0.05% halobetasol propionate ointment and 0.05% clobetasol propionate ointment in patients with chronic, localized plaque psoriasis. J Am Acad Dermatol 25:1145–1148
48. Gower WR (1993) Mechanism of glucocorticoid action. J Fla Med Assoc 80:697–700
49. Green C, Ganpule M, Harris D, Kavanagh G, Kennedy C, Mallett R, Rustin M, Downes N (1994) Comparative effects of calcipotriol (MC903) solution and placebo (vehicle of MC903) in the treatment of psoriasis of the scalp. Br J Dermatol 130: 483–487
50. Grossman RM, Thivolet J, Claudy A, et al. (1994) A novel therapeutic approach to psoriasis with combination calcipotriol ointment and very low-dose cyclosporine: results of a multicenter placebo-controlled study. J Am Acad Dermatol 31:68–74
51. Guenther L, Van de Kerkhof PC, Snellman E, et al. (2002) Efficacy and safety of a new combination of calcipotriol and betamethasone dipropionate (once or twice daily) compared to calcipotriol (twice daily) in the treatment of psoriasis vulgaris: a randomized, double-blind, vehicle-controlled clinical trial. Br J Dermatol 147:316–323
52. Guzzo C, Lazarus G, Goffe BS, Katz HI, Lowe NJ, Pincus SH (1996) Topical calcipotriene has no short-term effect on calcium and bone metabolism of patients with psoriasis. J Am Acad Dermatol 34:429–433
53. Hanke CW, Steck WD, Roegnick HH Jr (1979) Combination therapy for psoriasis. Psoralens plus long-wave ultraviolet radiation with betamethasone valerate. Arch Dermatol 115:1074–1077
54. Hardman KA, Heath DA, Nelson HM (1993) Hypercalcaemia associated with calcipotriol (Dovonex) treatment. BMJ 306:896
55. Hecker D, Worsley J, Yueh G, Kuroda K, Lebwohl M (1999) Interactions between tazarotene and ultraviolet light. J Am Acad Dermatol 41:927–930
56. Hecker D, Worsley J, Yueh G, Lebwohl M (2000) In vitro compatibility of tazarotene with other topical treatments of psoriasis. J Am Acad Dermatol 42:1008–1011
57. Hein R, Krieg T (1988) Effects of corticosteroids on human fibroblasts in vitro. In: Christophers E, Schopf E, Kligman AM, et al. (eds) Topical corticosteroid therapy: a novel approach to safer drugs. Raven Press, New York, pp 57–65
58. Highton A, Quell J (1995) Calcipotriene ointment 0.005% for psoriasis: a safety and efficacy study. Calcipotriene Study Group. J Am Acad Dermatol 32:67–72
59. Ingram JT (1953) The approach to psoriasis. Br Med J 2:591
60. Jorizzo JL, Magee K, Stewart DM, et al. (1997) Clobetasol propionate emollient 0.05%: hypothalam-

ic-pituitary-adrenal-axis safety and four-week clinical efficacy results in plaque-type psoriasis. Cutis 60:55–60

61. Kaidbey KH, Kligman AM (1977) Clinical and histological study of coal tar phototoxicity in humans. Arch Dermatol 113:592–595
62. Kanzler MH, Gorsulowsky DC (1993) Efficacy of topical 5% liquor carbonis detergens vs. its emollient base in the treatment of psoriasis. Br J Dermatol 129:310–314
63. Katoh N, Kishimoto S (2003) Combination of calcipotriol and clobetasol propionate as a premixed ointment for the treatment of psoriasis. Eur J Dermatol 13:382–384
64. Katz HI, Hien NT, Pauer SE, et al. (1987) Superpotent topical steroid treatment of psoriasis vulgaris – clinical efficacy and adrenal function. J Am Acad Dermatol 16:804–811
65. Katz HI, Gross E, Buxman M, Prawer SE, Schwartzel EH, Gibson JR (1991) A double-blind, vehicle-controlled paired comparison of halobetasol propionate cream on patients with plaque psoriasis. J Am Acad Dermatol 25:1175–1188
66. Katz HI, Prawer SE, Medansky RS, Kreuger GG, Mooney JJ, Jones ML, Samson CR (1991) Intermittent corticosteroid maintenance treatment of psoriasis: a double-blind, multi-center trial of augmented betamethasone dipropionate ointment in a pulse dose regimen. Dermatologica 183:269–274
67. Katz HI, Lindholm JS, Weiss JS, Shavin JS, Morman M, Bressinck R, Cornell R, Pariser DM, Pariser RJ, Weng W, et al. (1995) Efficacy and safety of twice-daily augmented betamethasone lotion versus clobetasol propionate solution in patients with moderate-to-severe scalp psoriasis. Clin Ther 17: 390–401
68. Kaufmann R, Bibby AJ, Bissonnette R, et al. (2002) A new calcipotriol/betamethasone dipropionate formulation (Daivobet) is an effective once-daily treatment for psoriasis vulgaris. Dermatology 205: 389–393
69. Kienbaum S, Lehmann P, Ruzicka T (1996) Topical calcipotriol in the treatment of intertriginous psoriasis. Br J Dermatol 135:647–650
70. Klaber MR, Hutchinson PE, Pedvis-Leftick A, et al. (1994) Comparative effects of calcipotriol solution (50 micrograms/ml) and betamethasone 17-valerate solution (1 mg/ml) in the treatment of scalp psoriasis. Br J Dermatol 131:678–683
71. Klem EB (1978) Effects of antipsoriasis drugs and metabolic inhibitors on the growth of epidermal cells in culture. J Invest Dermatol 70:27–32
72. Kneczke M, Rahm C, Landersjo L (1990) The influence of salicylic acid on the in vitro release of anthralin from an o/w cream. Acta Pharm Nordica 2: 313–318
73. Koo J (1995) Diluting Dovonex. Psoriasis Forum 1:6
74. Koo J (1997) Calcipotriol/calcipotriene (Dovonex/Daivonex) in combination with phototherapy: a review. J Am Acad Dermatol 37:S59–61
75. Koo J, Cuffie CA, Tanner DJ, et al. (1998) Mometasone furoate 0.1%-salicylic acid 5% ointment versus mometasone furoate 0.1% ointment in the treatment of moderate-to-severe psoriasis: a multicenter study. Clin Ther 20:283–291
76. Koo JY, Lowe NJ, Lew-Kaya DA, Vasilopoulos AI, Lue JC, Sefton J, Gibson JR (2000) Tazarotene plus UVB phototherapy in the treatment of psoriasis. J Am Acad Dermatol 43:821–828
77. Koo JY, Martin D (2001) Investigator-masked comparison of tazarotene gel q.d. plus mometasone furoate cream q.d. vs. mometasone furoate cream b.i.d. in the treatment of plaque psoriasis. Int J Dermatol 40:210–212
78. Kragbelle K (1988) MC903, a non-calciotropic vitamin D_3 analogue stimulates differentiation and inhibits proliferation of cultured human keratinocytes. J Invest Dermatol 91:383
79. Kragbelle K (1989) Topical corticosteroids: mechanisms of action. Acta Derm Venereol Suppl (Stockh) 151:7–10; 47–52
80. Kragballe K (1989) Treatment of psoriasis by the topical application of the novel cholecalciferol analogue calcipotriol (MC 903). Arch Dermatol 125: 1647–1652
81. Kragballe K, Gjertsen BT, De Hoop D, et al. (1991) Double-blind, right/left comparison of calcipotriol and betamethasone valerate in treatment of psoriasis vulgaris. Lancet 26; 337(8735):193–196
82. Kragbelle K (1996) Vitamin D_3 analogues. Dermatol Clin 13:835–838
83. Krayenbuhl BH, Elsner P (1999) Allergic and irritant contact dermatitis to calcipotriol. Am J Contact Dermat 10:78–80
84. Krochmal L, Wang JC, Patel B, Rodgers J (1989) Topical corticosteroid compounding: effects on physiochemical stability and skin penetration rate. J Am Acad Dermatol 21:979–984
85. Krueger GG, Drake LA, Elias PM, et al. (1998) The safety and efficacy of tazarotene gel, a topical acetylenic retinoid, in the treatment of psoriasis. Arch Dermatol 134:57–60
86. Kubo T, Kojima A, Yamazoe S, Ueshima K, Yamamoto T, Hirasawa Y (2001) Osteonecrosis of the femoral head that developed after long-term topical steroid application. J Orthop Sci 6:92–94
87. Larko O, Swanbeck G, Svartholm H (1984) The effect on psoriasis of clobetasol propionate used alone or in combination with UVB. Acta Derm Venereol 64:151–154
88. Lebwohl M, Siskin SB, Epinette W, Breneman D, Funicella T, Kalb R, Moore J (1996) A multicenter trial of calcipotriene ointment and halobetasol ointment compared with either agent alone for the treatment of psoriasis. J Am Acad Dermatol 35: 268–269
89. Lebwohl M, Hecker D, Martinez J, Sapadin A, Patel B (1997) Interactions between calcipotriene and ultraviolet light. J Am Acad Dermatol 37:93–95
90. Lebwohl M, Ast E, Callen JP, et al. (1998) Once-daily tazarotene gel versus twice-daily fluocinonide

cream in the treatment of plaque psoriasis. J Am Acad Dermatol 38:705–711
91. Lebwohl MG, Breneman DL, Goffe BS, et al. (1998) Tazarotene 0.1% gel plus corticosteroid cream in the treatment of plaque psoriasis. J Am Acad Dermatol 39:590–596
92. Lebwohl M, Yoles A, Lombardi K, Lou W (1998) Calcipotriene ointment and halobetasol ointment in the long-term treatment of psoriasis: effects on the duration of improvement. J Am Acad Dermatol 39:447–450
93. Lebwohl M (1999) The role of salicylic acid in the treatment of psoriasis. Int J Dermatol 38:16–24
94. Lebwohl M (2000) Strategies to optimize efficacy, duration of remission, and safety in the treatment of plaque psoriasis by using tazarotene in combination with a corticosteroid. J Am Acad Dermatol 43:S43–46
95. Lebwohl MG, Tan MH, Meador SL, Singer G (2001) Limited application of fluticasone propionate ointment 0.005% in patients with psoriasis of the face and intertriginous areas. J Am Acad Dermatol 44:77–82
96. Lebwohl M, Sherer D, Washenik K, Krueger GG, Menter A, Koo J, Feldman SR (2002) A randomized, double-blind, placebo-controlled study of clobetasol propionate 0.05% foam in the treatment of nonscalp psoriasis. Int J Dermatol 41:269–274
97. Lesnik RH, Mezick JA, Capetola R, Kligman LH (1989) Topical all-trans-retinoic acid prevents corticosteroid-induced skin atrophy without abrogating the anti-inflammatory effect. J Am Acad Dermatol 21:186–190
98. Levin C, Maibach HI (2002) Topical corticosteroid-induced adrenocortical insufficiency: clinical implications. Am J Clin Dermatol 3:141–147
99. Leyden JJ, Thew M, Kligman AM (1974) Steroid rosacea. Arch Dermatol 110:619–622
100. Marsico RE, Dijkstra JW (1996) UVB blocking effect of calcipotriene ointment 0.005%. J Am Acad Dermatol 34:539–540
101. Marsland AM, Griffiths CE (2002) The macrolide immunosuppressants in dermatology: mechanisms of action. Eur J Dermatol 12:618–622
102. Mason J, Mason AR, Cork MJ (2002) Topical preparations for the treatment of psoriasis: a systematic review. Br J Dermatol 146:351–364
103. McKenzie AW, Stoughton RB (1962) Methods for comparing percutaneous absorption of steroids. Arch Dermatol 86:608–610
104. Medansky RS, Cuffie CA, Tanner DJ (1997) Mometasone furoate 0.1%-salicylic acid 5% ointment twice daily versus fluocinonide 0.05% ointment twice daily in the management of patients with psoriasis. Clin Ther 19:701–709
105. Melian EB, Spencer CM, Jarvis B (2001) Clobetasol propionate foam, 0.05%. Am J Dermatol 2:89–92
106. Menter A (2000) Pharmacokinetics and safety of tazarotene. J Am Acad Dermatol 43:S31–35
107. Meola T Jr, Soter NA, Lim HW (1991) Are topical corticosteroids useful adjunctive therapy for the treatment of psoriasis with ultraviolet radiation? A review of the literature. Arch Dermatol 127:1708–1713
108. Milde P, Hauser U, Simon T, Mall G, Ernst V, Haussler MR, Frosch P, Rauterberg EW (1991) Expression of 1,25-dihydroxyvitamin D_3 receptors in normal and psoriatic skin. J Invest Dermatol 97:230–239
109. Miller JA, Munro DD (1980) Topical corticosteroids: clinical pharmacology and therapeutic use. Drugs 19:119–134
110. Molin L, Cutler TP, Helander I, Nyfors B, Downes N (1997) Comparative efficacy of calcipotriol (MC903) cream and betamethasone 17-valerate cream in the treatment of chronic plaque psoriasis. A randomized, double-blind, parallel group multicentre study. Calcipotriol Study Group. Br J Dermatol 136:89–93
111. Morison WL, Parrish JA, Fitzpatrick TB (1978) Controlled study of PUVA and adjunctive topical therapy in the management of psoriasis. Br J Dermatol 98:125–132
112. Nathan AW, Rose GL (1979) Fatal iatrogenic Cushing's syndrome. Lancet 1:207
113. Nielson NV, Sorensen PN (1978) Glaucoma induced by application of corticosteroids to the periorbital region. Arch Dermatol 114:953–954
114. Olsen EA, Cram DL, Ellis CN, Hickman JG, Jacobson C, Jenkins EE, Lasser AE, Lebwohl M, Leibsohn E, Medansky RS, et al. (1991) A double-blind, vehicle-controlled study of clobetasol propionate 0.05% (Temovate) scalp application in the treatment of moderate to severe scalp psoriasis. J Am Acad Dermatol 24:443–447
115. Patel B, Siskin S, Krazmien R, Lebwohl M (1998) Compatibility of calcipotriene with other topical medications. J Am Acad Dermatol 38:1010–1011
116. Plewig G, Kligman AM (1973) Induction of acne by topical steroids. Arch Dermatol Forsch 247:29–52
117. Ramsay B, Lawrence CM, Bruce JM, Shuster S (1990) The effect of triethanolamine on anthralin-induced inflammation and therapeutic effect in psoriasis. J Am Acad Dermatol 23:73–76
118. Ramsay CA, Berth-Jones J, Brundin G, et al. (1994) Long-term use of topical calcipotriol in chronic plaque psoriasis. Dermatology 189:260–264
119. Ramsay C (1997) Management of psoriasis with calcipotriol used as monotherapy. J Am Acad Dermatol 37:S53–S54
120. Ramsay CA, Schwartz BE, Lowson D, Papp K, Bolduc A, Gilbert M (2000) Calcipotriol cream combined with twice weekly broad-band UVB phototherapy: a safe, effective and UVB-sparing antipsoriatic combination treatment. The Canadian Calcipotriol and UVB Study Group. Dermatology 200:17–24
121. Rigby WFC (1988) The immunobiology of vitamin D. Immunol Today 9:54–58

122. Runne U, Kunze J (1982) Short duration ("minutes") therapy with dithranol for psoriasis: A new outpatient regimen. Br J Dermatol 106:135–139
123. Silverman A, Menter A (1995) Tars and anthralins. Dermatol Clin 13:817–833
124. Singh S, Reddy DC, Pandey SS (2000) Topical therapy for psoriasis with the use of augmented betamethasone and calcipotriene on alternate weeks. J Am Acad Dermatol 43:61–65
125. Sneddon I (1969) Adverse effect of topical fluorinated corticosteroids in rosacea. Br Med J 1: 671–673
126. Sneddon IB (1980) Perioral dermatitis. Br J Dermatol 102:239–240
127. Speight EL, Farr PM (1994) Calcipotriol improves the response of psoriasis to PUVA. Br J Dermatol 130:79–82
128. Stegman SJ (1974) Pustular dermatosis on withdrawal of topically applied steroid. Arch Dermatol 109:100
129. Stein LF, Sherr A, Solodkina G, Gottlieb AB, Chaudhari U (2001) Betamethasone valerate foam for treatment of nonscalp psoriasis. J Cutan Med Surg 5:303–307
130. Stevanovic DV (1972) Corticosteroid-induced atrophy of the skin with telangiectasia. A clinical and experimental study. Br J Dermatol 87:548–556
131. Svartholm H, Larsson L, Fredereiksen B (1982) Intermittent topical treatment of psoriasis with clobetasol propionate (Dermovate). Curr Med Res Opin 8:154–157
132. Tanenbaum L, Parrish JA, Pathak MA, Anderson RR, Fitzpatrick TB (1975) Tar phototoxicity and phototherapy for psoriasis. Arch Dermatol 111: 467–470
133. Tang-Liu DD, Matsumoto RM, Usansky JI (1999) Clinical pharmacokinetics and drug metabolism of tazarotene: a novel topical treatment for acne and psoriasis. Clin Pharmacokinet 37:273–287
134. Thaci D, Daiber W, Boehncke WH, Kaufmann R (2001) Calcipotriol solution for the treatment of scalp psoriasis: evaluation of efficacy, safety and acceptance in 3,396 patients. Dermatology 203: 153–156
135. Tham SN, Lun KC, Cheong WK (1994) A comparative study of calcipotriol ointment and tar in chronic plaque psoriasis. Br J Dermatol 131: 673–677
136. Thune P, Brolund L (1992) Short- and long-contact therapy using a new dithranol formulation in individually adjusted doses in the management of psoriasis. Acta Derm Venereol Suppl (Stockh) 172: 28–29
137. Turpeinen M, Salo OP, Leisti S (1986) Effect of percutaneous absorption of hydrocortisone on adrenocortical responsiveness in infants with severe skin disease. Br J Dermatol 115:475–484
138. Tzaneva S, Honigsmann H, Tanew A, Seeber A (2002) A comparison of psoralen plus ultraviolet A (PUVA) monotherapy, tacalcitol plus PUVA and tazarotene plus PUVA in patients with chronic plaque-type psoriasis. Br J Dermatol 147:748–753
139. Tzaneva S, Honigsmann H, Tanew A (2003) Observer-blind, randomized, intrapatient comparison of a novel 1% coal tar preparation (Exorex) and calcipotriol cream in the treatment of plaque type psoriasis. Br J Dermatol 149:350–353
140. Ultravate [package insert] (2000) Bristol-Myers-Squibb Dermatology, Princeton, NJ
141. van de Kerkhof PC, Cambazard F, Hutchinson PE, et al. (1998) The effect of addition of calcipotriol ointment (50 micrograms/g) to acitretin therapy in psoriasis. Br J Dermatol 138:84–89
142. Vicker CFH (1963) Existence of a reservoir in the stratum corneum. Arch Dermatol 88:20–23
143. Wang JC, Krazmien RJ, Dahlheim CE, et al. (1986) Anthralin stain removal. J Am Acad Dermatol 15: 951–955
144. Weinstein GD, Krueger GG, Lowe NJ, et al. (1997) Tazarotene gel, a new retinoid, for topical therapy of psoriasis: vehicle-controlled study of safety, efficacy, and duration of therapeutic effect. J Am Acad Dermatol 37:85–92
145. Weinstein GD, Koo JY, Krueger GG, et al. (2003) Tazarotene cream in the treatment of psoriasis: Two multicenter, double-blind, randomized, vehicle-controlled studies of the safety and efficacy of tazarotene creams 0.05% and 0.1% applied once daily for 12 weeks. J Am Acad Dermatol 48:760–767
146. Woo WK, McKenna KE (2003) Combination TL01 ultraviolet B phototherapy and topical calcipotriol for psoriasis: a prospective randomized placebo-controlled clinical trial. Br J Dermatol 149:146–150
147. Yohn JJ, Weston WL (1990) Topical glucocorticosteroids. Curr Probl Dermatol 2:38–63
148. Zonneveld IM, Rubins A, Jablonska S, et al. (1998) Topical tacrolimus is not effective in chronic plaque psoriasis. A pilot study. Arch Dermatol 134: 1101–1102

2 Phototherapy

Jennifer Dempsey, Michael Zanolli[1]

Introduction

It has long been recognized that natural sunlight ameliorates psoriasis in many patients. With the advent of artificial fluorescent light,

[1] Neither Dr. Dempsey nor Dr. Zanolli received any compensation for the production of this manuscript. There are no conflicts of interest in regard to any phototherapy device manufacturer or medication mentioned in this chapter.

office based phototherapy became available as a routine treatment for psoriasis. Over the last half century, numerous advances have led to safer, more effective forms of ultraviolet therapy. Phototherapy may be used as a monotherapy or in combination with other agents to effectively treat mild, moderate or severe psoriasis. Despite the introduction of numerous effective systemic medications and biologic agents into the psoriasis treatment armamentarium, phototherapy remains a reliable, and often preferred, option for many psoriasis patients.

Historical Aspects of Ultraviolet Therapy

Most of the insight into the therapeutic benefit of phototherapy gained in previous centuries was related to the observed effects of natural sunlight. Therapeutic intervention with artificial sources of light was introduced in the late nineteenth century. In 1893, Neils Finsen used carbon arc lamps to treat cutaneous mycobacterial infection on the face (lupus vulgaris). He was later awarded the Nobel Prize in 1903 for his pioneering application of UV light as a medical treatment. Hot quartz lamps were employed as one of the mainstays of treatment throughout the middle of the twentieth century when used as a part of the Goeckerman treatment, in which UV light was combined with tar, and for the Ingram method of treatment, which combined UV light and anthralin. However, traditional delivery of the Goeckerman or Ingram methods required weeks of hospitalization in specialized facilities. The delivery of UVB therapy in the office, despite poor dosimetry in the early years of use, provided effective treatment for psoriasis. However, it was not until after 1945 that modern fluorescent UVB lamps were readily available for routine medical purposes.

The development of photochemotherapy combining psoralens and ultraviolet A light (PUVA) was a major advance. It was remarkably effective with a rapid onset of action as compared with traditional treatments. The outpatient delivery of PUVA treatment allowed patients to maintain a relatively normal lifestyle even though they were required to wear protective UV glasses during therapy and sometimes endured common short-term side effects, such as nausea.

Further application and modification of fluorescent lamps and high output metal halide lamps in the 1980s provided the foundation for therapeutic delivery of UVA and UVB light for treatment of psoriasis and other skin diseases. Applying specific wavelengths of UV light based on the action spectrum for treatment of psoriasis has been the most important development in phototherapy of the last decade. The development of narrowband (NB) fluorescent tubes allowed delivery of the most effective UVB wavelength for treatment for psoriasis. The use of NBUVB is almost as effective as PUVA without the problems associated with the concomitant use of a psoralen molecule, thereby making office use of phototherapy much easier to perform with fewer side effects. A further refinement of delivery of UV light therapy has been the application of localized delivery of UV light with either a narrow spectrum of UVB or 308 nm laser generated light. This localized delivery allows for higher fluence of UV energy at or near the wavelength of UVB most effective for psoriasis, while leaving unaffected skin spared from UV effects. The practical application of such units will depend on the continued demonstration of improved delivery, efficacy, decreased side effects, and cost effectiveness [38].

Photoimmunology of the Skin

Experience has demonstrated that ultraviolet light has both specific and broad modulatory effects on the immune system [9]. The immunomodulatory effects of UVB radiation primarily affect the epidermis and superficial dermis, while UVA radiation penetrates further into the dermis prior to absorption or scattering. T lymphocytes and antigen-presenting cells appear to be more susceptible to the effects of ultraviolet B therapy than do keratinocytes [28]. UV radiation-induced immunomodulation results from absorption of light by a chromophore in the skin, which initiates a cascade of events. Through the production of soluble mediators, such as reactive oxygen species and modification of cell surface receptors, UV radiation may modulate the actions of keratinocytes, leukocytes, and antigen presenting cells [5, 19].

One of the major mechanisms for identifying effects of ultraviolet light therapy on cells was to identify "sunburn" cells, keratinocytes undergoing apoptosis when seen through light microscopy. However, as lower doses of ultraviolet light may also be effective in treating psoriasis, it is clear that one does not have to use erythemogenic doses, which induces the formation of sunburn cells, of narrowband UVB therapy to produce the same clearing of psoriasis [13]. High doses of UV light may cause severe damage and destruction of cells in the skin, resulting in apoptosis of immune competent cells, while low dose UV light may merely affect the cutaneous immune system through modification of the process of antigen presentation and the production of cytokines.

UV light can cause two main categories of observable changes. The first consists of rapid changes, which include membrane damage, induction of cytoplasmic transcription factors, DNA damage, and isomerization of urocanic acid (UCA). The second category of subacute changes includes alteration of antigen-presenting cell populations and the modification of intracellular and intercellular signaling mechanisms. This overall effect creates a change in the environment of the cytokines in the dermis and epidermis, one that favors the development of a type 2 helper T cell response as a result of UV effects on the skin [5].

UCA is one of the major chromophores of UV light in the skin and is a known immune modifier. UVB light causes UCA to be isomerized from *trans*-UCA to *cis*-UCA. This effect is maximized between 290–310 nm of the UVB spectrum. The transformation from *trans*- to *cis*-UCA is dose dependent until equal parts of both are present in the skin [10, 16]. The presence of *cis*-UCA contributes to the overall effects of UV induced subacute changes in the cutaneous immune system shifting cytokine production from a Th-1 to a Th-2 environment in the skin [5].

Therapeutic Action Spectrum for Psoriasis

The spectrum of therapeutic ultraviolet light therapy for psoriasis includes broadband UVB, selected portions of the UVB spectrum, narrowband UVB at 311–313 nm, laser light at 308 nm, and UVA plus psoralen (PUVA). The determination of a therapeutic action spectrum for psoriasis provides the basis for selecting the best wavelengths of UV light for treating this condition when used as a monotherapy and offers insight into disease pathogenesis.

In 1976, Turkel Fisher reported on the action spectrum of psoriasis [7]. Although somewhat limited by the number of wavelengths tested, his work demonstrated beneficial effects for plaque-type psoriasis and indicated the wavelength of 313 nm was the most effective for treatment of psoriasis. In 1981, Parrish and Jaenicke [29] expanded this line of investigation, adding to it appreciably by including a more extensive number of wavelengths [29]. This pivotal work, in conjunction with Fisher's data, helped initiate the development of current phototherapy devices, resulting in more efficient and effective treatment for psoriasis.

Parrish found between 310 and 315 nm to be most effective for treatment of plaque-type psoriasis. An important observation made during these experiments was that erythemogenic doses below 300 nm produced significant clearing; however, these wavelengths also produce the greatest amount of erythema and burning. The wavelengths within the action spectrum for psoriasis, providing the best therapeutic response at suberythemogenic doses of UV light therapy, are between 310–315 nm.

Ultraviolet B Therapy

Background

The use of UVB continues to be an important therapeutic intervention for mild to moderate psoriasis. Because of the long duration of remission and the high rate of clearing associated with Goeckerman therapy, this combination method is still one of the standards by which other therapies are measured. UVB monotherapy therapy works best in treatment of primarily eruptive guttate and thin plaque forms of psoriasis and is less effective in chronic thick plaque-type psoriasis and other morphologies of psoriasis [14].

Clinical Application

Although effective, the use of broadband UVB (290–320 nm) is limited by its erythemogenic potential at relatively low doses because patients do not generally tolerate the uncomfortable sensation associated with repeated sunburn like reactions. This is primarily because it contains wavelengths below 300 nm, which are known to have the highest erythemogenic potential within the UVB spectrum [29]. The protocols devised for broadband UVB take this observation into account. The most effective approach to treatment with broadband UVB is with mildly erythemogenic doses of UVB so the patient gets slightly pink from the treatment within 8 h but this diminished at 24 h or the usual time for the next treatment. The most accurate method to determine the starting dose for the more aggressive effective treatment protocol with broadband UVB is to obtain the MED for the patient.

The dose range to produce erythema with narrow band UVB is from 400 to above 1800 mJ/cm², which is a much higher and broader range than that associated with broadband UVB. However, the range of the dose to produce erythema, relative to Fitzpatrick's skin type assignment, varies greatly from one skin type to another and is not as predictable as with BBUVB [38]. Therefore it is more difficult to accurately predict the most effective starting point for NBUVB therapy by assigning skin type to a patient.

Despite evidence that the most effective wavelengths for treatment of psoriasis are between 310 and 315 nm, it was not until the late 1980s that commercially manufactured lamps with the proper phosphor to emit a narrow band of UVB became available. The Philips TL01 lamp (Philips Medical Systems, Bothell, WA) has a peak emission between 310 and 313 nm. The clinical use of such lamps was initially implemented in Europe and the precedent setting clinical trials that followed demonstrated efficacy for treatment of plaque-type psoriasis [11, 20]. The shift to use of narrowband UVB occurred in Europe earlier than in the United States. Use of narrowband UVB has been shown to be superior to conventional broadband with respect to both clearing and remission times [11, 35, 37]. Some studies suggest that NBUVB is nearly as effective in PUVA in clearing psoriasis but does not produce a similar long duration of remission [33, 36].

Treatment Protocol

Although determination of an initial dose of phototherapy by assignment of a Fitzpatrick skin type (Table A1) is an accepted practice, determining a minimal erythema dose (MED) prior to the initiation of therapy provides a more accurate indication of the proper initial dose for an individual patient. The MED is determined by a single procedure which takes 10–15 min to complete. This can be done at the initial visit and is determined by irradiating a sun-protected area with incremental doses of UVB light. A positive reading is considered as identifiable erythema within the margins of phototesting (Table A2).

There are a number of requirements for all patients receiving UVB. Patients must wear eye protection and male patients should wear ap-

Table A1. Skin types

Skin type	History	Examination
I	Always burns, never tans	
II	Always burns, sometimes tans	
III	Sometimes burns, always tans	
IV	Never burns, always tans	
V		Brown[a]
VI		Black

[a]Asian, Hispanic, American Indian

Table A2. Determination of MED

- Test on sun-protected area (hip, lower back)
- Six or more ports should be used for phototesting (specific garments are available for testing)
- Ports to be irradiated should be uniform in size and at least 2 cm^2
- Patient should return for evaluation in 24 h
- A positive reading is considered as identifiable erythema within the margins of the phototesting ports

BBUVB		NBVUB	
Skin types I–III	Skin types IV–VI	Skin types I–III	Skin types IV–VI
20 mJ/cm^2	60 mJ/cm^2	400 mJ/cm^2	800 mJ/cm^2
30 mJ/cm^2	70 mJ/cm^2	600 mJ/cm^2	1000 mJ/cm^2
40 mJ/cm^2	80 mJ/cm^2	800 mJ/cm^2	1200 mJ/cm^2
50 mJ/cm^2	90 mJ/cm^2	1000 mJ/cm^2	1400 mJ/cm^2
60 mJ/cm^2	100 mJ/cm^2	1200 mJ/cm^2	1600 mJ/cm^2
80 mJ/cm^2	120 mJ/cm^2	1400 mJ/cm^2	1800 mJ/cm^2

propriate garments to shield the genitals with every treatment. It is beneficial to apply a non-UVB absorbing lubricant, such as mineral oil, to the plaques immediately prior to therapy as this decreases reflectance from the scale on the plaques, thus increasing transmittance of UV into the epidermis and improving efficacy. Agents containing salicylic acid and crude coal tar should be avoided immediately prior to therapy since these agents act as UVB absorbers. They should only be used after light treatments or at least 8 h prior to UV.

■ **Broad-band UVB.** The usual starting dose of BB-UVB is 50–70% of the MED and this can be initiated as early as 24 h after MED testing. Treatment frequency can range from three to five times weekly. On subsequent visits the patients should be asked about redness or tenderness of the skin related to the previous treatment. The dose should be held constant if the skin is pink and should be delayed 24 h if the skin is red. If no erythema is noted the doses should be increased by 25% of the MED for treatments 1–10, 10% of the MED for treatments 11–20, and held constant for subsequent treatments based on the treating physician's judgment. In general if only a partial response has been realized, the dose continues to be increased by 10% on subsequent treatments over 20. If the interval between treatments extends beyond 3 days, treatment protocol should be adjusted according to the time interval (Fig. A1). A treatment protocol for using BBUVB based on skin type outlines the starting dose and incremental increases during a treatment course following the same principles (Fig. A2).

■ **Narrow-band UVB.** The usual starting dose of NBUVB is 50–70% of the MED. More aggressive use of NBUVB therapy using 70–90% of the MED was not statistically superior to 50% of the MED when near versus far erythemogenic doses of NBUVB were used [13]. The frequency of treatments is generally three times weekly, although treatment frequency can range from two to four times per week. Comparison trials to determine the most effective methods for the delivery of NBUVB showed no statistical difference with increased frequency of visits to five times per week [4]. The dose should be held constant if the skin is pink and should be delayed 24 h if the skin is red. If no erythema is noted, the doses should be increased by 10–20% of the MED based on the treating physician's judgment. If the interval between treatments extends beyond 3 days, treatment protocol should be adjusted according to the length of the time interval (Fig. A3).

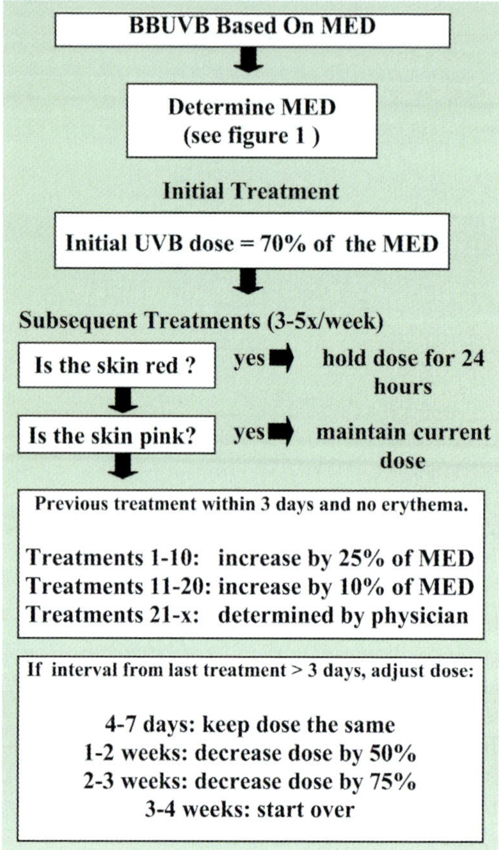

Fig. A1. BBUVB based on MED

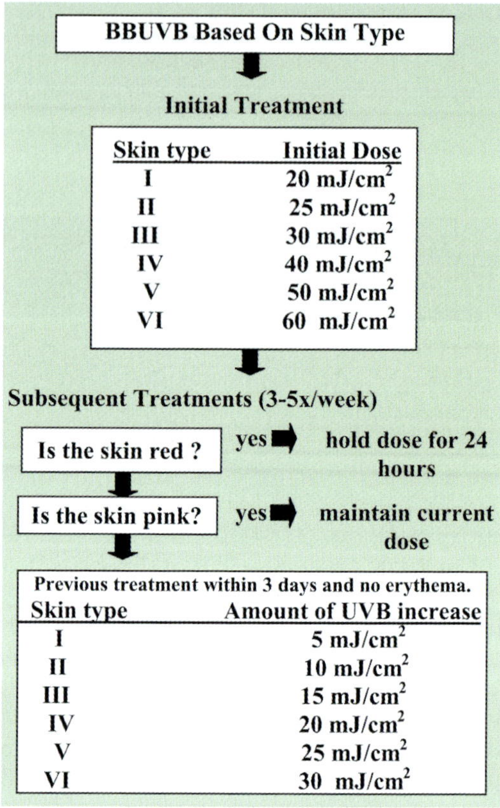

Fig. A2. BBUVB based on skin type

A treatment protocol using NBUVB based on skin type is outlined in Fig. A4.

■ **Maintenance Therapy.** Maintenance therapy can be initiated once the patient has experienced acceptable improvement in the severity of the psoriasis. An appropriate treatment options includes tapering phototherapy to once a week for several months with or without the concomitant use of adjuvant therapies, such as retinoids. Some patients may only require NBUVB treatments every 10–14 days. It should be noted that seasonal variation also occurs with the majority of psoriasis patients, which makes the use of maintenance therapy more likely needed during the winter months. The use of maintenance therapy will not necessarily prevent recurrence or flare of the disease process, however.

Side Effects

Short term side effects include erythema, swelling, dry skin, pruritus, occasional blistering, skin desquamation, and increased frequency of recurrent herpes simplex infection [14]. Photoaging is the major long-term side effect associated with UVB phototherapy. Although carcinogenesis may be a potential long-term consequence of UVB phototherapy, all published literature to date has failed to demonstrate any increased risk of skin cancer associated with therapeutic doses of UVB therapy when compared to adequate control populations of psoriasis patients [21, 32].

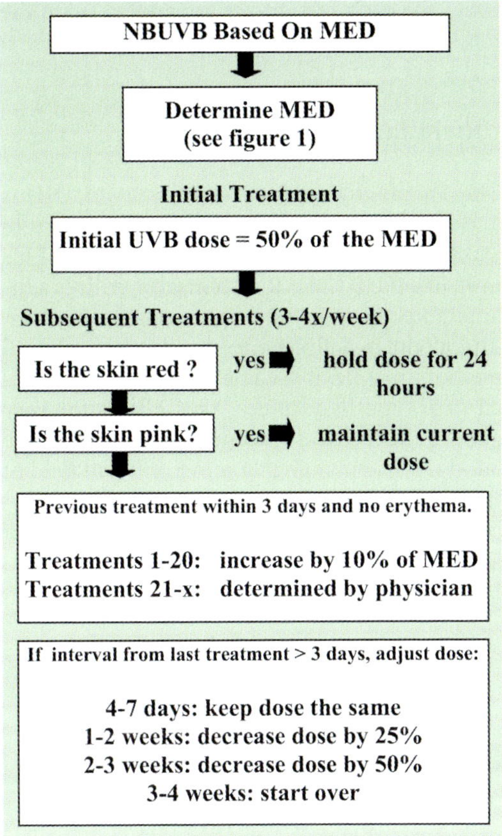

Fig. A3. NBUVB based on MED

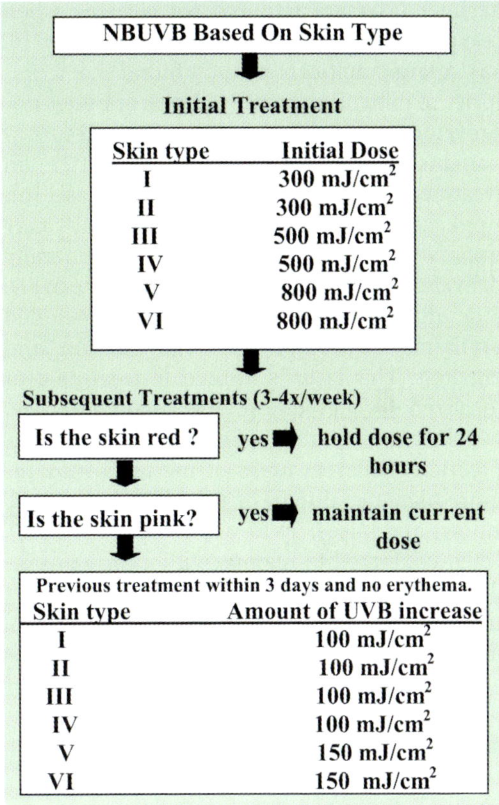

Fig. A4. NBUVB based on skin type

Localized Delivery of UVB

Specialized, high energy use of UVB light relies mainly on the types of effects that erythemogenic or super erythemogenic doses have on the skin. The histologic changes associated with delivery of multiples of an erythemogenic amount of UVB light are injury to the epidermis and superficial dermis with apoptosis of keratinocytes and immunocytes. The production of these changes is very rapid and more readily apparent by light microscopy than with low energy suberythemogenic doses. Consequently, local use of multiples of erythemogenic doses results in more inherent cell death than doses of UV light within the action spectrum that may also be delivered to uninvolved skin. The basic principle, then, for treatment with any of the delivery systems utilizing the localized delivery of UVB, is to determine the MED and then exceed it therapeutically, leaving normal skin unaltered. The therapeutic effect of a low number of treatments with 5 times the MED followed by a significant duration of remission after healing cannot be accomplished with low doses of UVB, which takes many more treatment sessions to produce clinical effectiveness.

Excimer Laser

The recent advent of the EXTRAC XeCl excimer laser (PhotoMedex, Radnor, PA) has made phototherapy a viable option for patients with localized disease. This laser emits monochromatic light at 308 nm and has a spot size of 3.2 cm^2. Studies have shown fewer treatments with the excimer laser are required for clearing when compared to standard UVB phototherapy [6, 34]. A large multicenter study found that a majority of patients experienced 75% or better improvement after only ten treatments and 50% of patients showed 90% improvement after ten treatments to targeted plaques of psoriasis [6]. Application of mineral oil prior to therapy may improve results [1, 34]. This laser is generally delivered twice weekly at multiples of the MED. Side effects were well tolerated and included erythema, blistering, hyperpigmentation, and erosions. This laser is limited to treatment of localized plaques due to the small spot size, which makes treating large surface areas impractical. Different areas of the body may require higher multiples of the MED such as the elbows and knees, up to 5 or 6 times the MED, when compared to regions with a thinner epidermis. The average for the body is a dose of 3 times the MED. Patients undergoing such treatments need to expect the bright red tender areas at the sites of treatment and that it would not be uncommon for blistering and crusting to occur at treatment sites.

B CLEAR

Another phototherapy delivery system which is useful for the localized treatment of psoriasis is the B CLEAR system (Lumenins, Santa Clara, CA). The light source for this device is a filamentous element that produces an incoherent source of UV light delivered through fiber optics to a hand held mechanism for final delivery to the skin surface at a peak emission between 300 and 320 nm. Prior to treatment, a MED must be determined, and subsequently multiples of the MED are delivered for treatment as determined by the clinician. Treatment with this device is based on the same principles as with treatment with the excimer laser, i.e. deliver multiples of the MED to localized areas to produce more rapid clearing while sparing non-involved skin the high doses of UVB light. The dosing for the treatments is facilitated by the electronics of the unit, which provides a clear display of the dose and a very easy-to-use handpiece for delivery of the UVB. Treatment times for each session are dependent upon the total area to be treated.

Theralight

The Theralight system (Daavlin, Bryan, OH) is another option in which localized delivery of UVB is used in the treatment of psoriasis. This unit, like the B CLEAR system, also utilizes a filamentous element as a light source. However, Theralight is delivered to the skin via a liquid medium in a flexible cable to a cylindrical pencil grip type hand piece. This allows for very good uniformity of the energy delivered at the handpiece, which gives a more uniform field of treatment for each delivery of light. The Theralight system has the utility to also switch to a low fluence UVA if localized PUVA is a consideration for therapy.

Photochemotherapy

Background

UVA is most commonly utilized in combination with a psoralen molecule in treatment of psoriasis (PUVA). Although it is remarkably effective, providing rapid results with long-term remissions, it requires ingestion of a systemic psoralen, use of specialized glasses and has a higher risk of long-term side effects compared to UVB. It is most useful in patients who have been treatment resistant to previous therapies, including those with thick chronic plaque-type psoriasis and dark-skinned individuals who are less responsive to UVB.

Practical Application

Over the last several decades, photochemotherapy has been a demonstrably effective treatment in psoriasis, with more than 80% of individuals expected to obtain good to excellent results. A psoralen molecule is an integral part of the treatment and must be ingested at a precise interval prior to therapy. In North America the psoralen molecule used is 8-methoxypsoralen

(8-MOP), while in Europe the use of 5-MOP is increasing due to decreased gastrointestinal side effects while maintaining efficacy. Up to 30% of patients experience nausea with 8-MOP sometimes resulting in discontinuation of PUVA therapy. In addition to nausea, another parameter making the use of photochemotherapy more complicated is the variable serum level of the psoralen molecule which can occur in an individual. This can be minimized by encouraging patients to have a consistent approach to ingestion of the psoralen molecule, including the same foods or liquids, if any, taken with the medication and consistent timing of the dose prior to delivery of UVA. Psoralen may be applied topically in certain circumstances, bypassing the gastrointestinal side effects.

PUVA effects can produce both oxygen dependent and oxygen independent photochemical reactions. Oxygen independent (type I) reactions may result in DNA crosslinks and development of cyclobutane rings. The construct of the covalent bonds in the cyclobutane rings gives a theoretical link to the observation of an increased risk of basal and squamous cell carcinoma associated with long-term use. Other factors must also be taken into consideration in this regard, however. The oxygen dependent (type II) reactions known to occur as a result of PUVA therapy produce reactive oxygen species such as superoxide dismutase and singlet oxygen. These molecules produce membrane damage in mitochondria and cell walls. T lymphocytes and antigen presenting cells appear to be more susceptible to this type of injury than keratinocytes. Depletion of CD3 lymphocytes in the epidermis of psoriasis skin correlates with the clinical response [3].

In North America there has been a prospective analysis of a large cohort of patients treated with PUVA starting in the early seventies. Some of these patients have had long-term PUVA in combination with other treatment approaches for psoriasis either in combination with or prior to PUVA. There is a statistical increase in the development of both basal cell carcinoma and squamous cell carcinoma in this group. It is a significant increase in the light skinned individuals who have skin types I–III. The incidence appears to be dose dependent and increases with a higher number of treatments after reaching the threshold of at least 250 treatments. This is especially true for males and the development of squamous cell carcinoma on the genitals if left unprotected [31]. Thus, early in the general use of PUVA as a treatment for psoriasis, recognition of this possible complication made male protection a standard part of the protocol.

Effects of psoralen molecules in combination with UVA light are known to cause ocular changes such as cataract formation in mice. Even prior to acceptance of PUVA as an approved treatment modality, the use of eye protection following treatment until there was clearance of the psoralen from circulation was standard. This has been a great success in preventive medicine for the patients treated with PUVA. Eye protection shielding UVB and UVA wavelengths should be utilized for 18 h post-treatment on the day of PUVA treatments. A more complicated consideration regarding PUVA therapy is, and has been, the observation of an increased risk of melanoma reported in the same North American cohort of patients discussed above. Though there are confounding factors which may have influence on this patient population, there is statistical evidence that long-term PUVA patients with light skin (types I–III) and a high number of treatments (>250) appear to develop atypical pigmented lentigines and produce melanomas at a rate higher than expected over the general population. Many of these patients have also had other topical and systemic agents which may have influenced this observation. The same increase in melanoma production has not been seen in other large series of PUVA patients in Europe however. Nevertheless, the diligence of the continued observation of the North American cohort of patients has modified the practical use of PUVA to generally limit the number of treatments to <200 in light skinned individuals. A change to another form of therapy or a combination of ultraviolet light therapy with systemic retinoids is usually done at that point. Fortunately, in the 21st century new advances have been realized in the treatment of psoriasis that broaden the options available for the clinician.

Treatment Protocol

The standard method of PUVA delivery in North America uses an initial dose of UVA determined by Fitzpatrick's skin types. The psoralen molecule, usually 8-MOP, is ingested 1.5 h prior to treatment. PUVA is delivered two to three times weekly. Patients should be asked about redness or tenderness related to the antecedent therapy and the time of psoralen ingestion prior to each treatment.

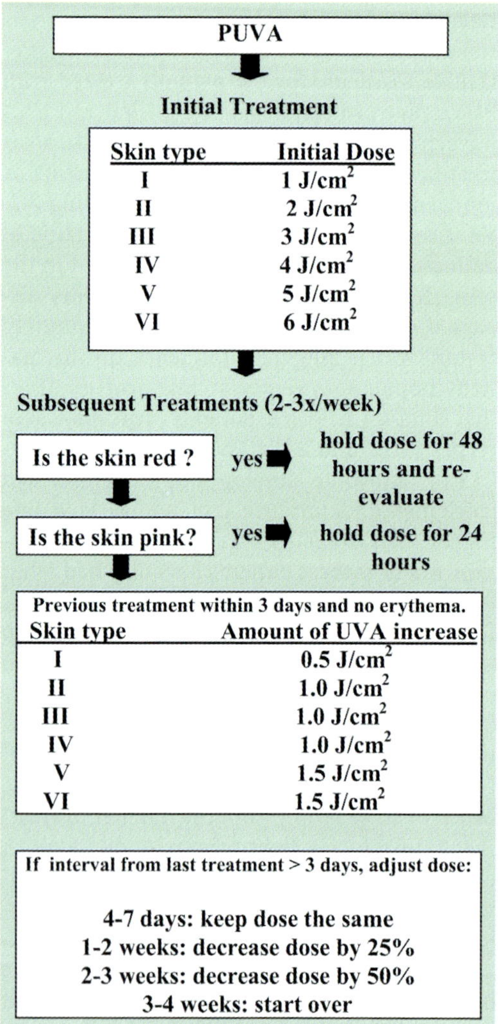

Fig. A5. PUVA

The dose should be withheld if the skin is pink and should be delayed for 48 h if the skin is red. If no erythema is noted the doses should be increased by 0.5–1.5 J/cm^2 based on skin type. If the interval between treatments extends beyond 3 days, then treatment protocol should be adjusted according to the time interval (Fig. A5). Once the patient has experienced acceptable improvement in the psoriasis, the frequency and dose may be tapered and long-term maintenance with or without combination therapy may be considered. Laboratory evaluation for any preexisting hepatic or renal disease should be done at baseline and then every 6 - months. An ophthalmologic exam should be obtained prior to initiation of treatment for patients with existing ocular disease and scheduled for patients without known risk factors for lens or retinal abnormalities. Follow-up ocular exams should be done every 6–12 months during therapy.

Side Effects

All patients should be warned of potential side effects including sunburn reaction, corneal burn or cataract formation (if eyes are unprotected), photoallergic dermatitis, reactivation of herpes simplex, freckling of the skin, aging of the skin, and the potential increased risk of both melanoma and non-melanoma skin cancers.

Combination Therapy

Topical Agents

Topical agents are used on a daily basis in combination with phototherapy. In fact, it is rare for phototherapy to be used alone without the combination of a topical agent. Mineral oil applied prior to the delivery of phototherapy enhances the overall transmittance of UV light into the epidermis and produces better results. Topical application of corticosteroids, retinoids, and vitamin D analogs have all been shown to be useful adjuncts to phototherapy. These agents may result in more rapid clearing of skin lesions or have an ultraviolet light sparing effect by requiring fewer treatments [17, 18, 26]. Calcipotriol must be applied after delivery of phototherapy as it is inactivated by ultraviolet light and the vehicle may impair transmission of ultraviolet wavelengths [22]. Caution should be used when advancing the dose of UVB or PUVA in the circumstance of combining topical retinoids with UV light because the retinoid effect on the plaques of psoriasis will produce thinning of the epidermis and stratum corneum [12]. Patients with moderate to severe psoriasis who are unresponsive to UV monotherapy or combination therapy with topical agents, are an appropriate population for consideration of use of systemic agents with or without phototherapy.

Retinoids Plus Ultraviolet Light

The overall goal of combination therapy is to maximize efficacy and decrease the potential side effects associated with a medication or treatment. The most effective class of medication commonly used in combination with ultraviolet light is systemic retinoids. There have been several reports of clinical trials concerning the use of systemic retinoids (acitretin) plus UVB therapy or PUVA treatments dating back to late 1980s [15]. The overall findings of the combination of UV therapy with systemic retinoids demonstrate that lower numbers of treatments are required to produce the same amount of clearing. Consequently, this therapy provides a lower total dose of UV radiation during a treatment course. Even low dose acitretin can enhance the overall effect of UV therapy, thereby making the systemic retinoid easier to tolerate because of decreased retinoid side effects [21, 23].

A consensus conference regarding adjunctive therapy with retinoids and ultraviolet light indicated this combination is underutilized. Retinoids if used 2 weeks prior to the initiation of ultraviolet light therapy produce effects in the skin and plaques of psoriasis which allow for a more efficient penetration of UV light into the skin. The retinoid effects of decreasing the thickness of the keratin layer and starting to decrease the overall thickness of the epidermis in plaques of psoriasis facilitate the transmittance and decrease the reflectance of UV throughout the outer layer of skin into the lower epidermis and superficial dermis. The MED of normal skin is affected by the retinoid effect and will allow less tolerance to UVB demonstrated by a lowering of the MED post-retinoid use. The most reliable and efficient use of retinoids would be to initiate retinoid therapy 10–14 days prior to either UVB, NBUVB, or PUVA followed by determination of an MED for UVB treatments or lowering the estimated skin type determination for a PUVA protocol. Treatments may then proceed in a standard manner.

If retinoids are to added to an ongoing treatment with ultraviolet light, caution must be taken to adjust for the retinoid effect by decreasing the dose of the UV light by 50% for 10–14 days, then one can proceed with advancement of the treatment dose. The usual frequency of the treatment protocol does not have to change and should be continued during this adjustment period. If this precaution is not taken, a phototoxic reaction will likely occur even though the patient had previously been tolerating the same dose of UV without difficulty.

Although acitretin is the systemic retinoid used most commonly in the treatment of psoriasis, 13-*cis*-retinoic acid (Accutane) can also be used in combination with phototherapy. Clinicians and patients must be cognizant of the general precautions needed for use of retinoids, including strict avoidance of pregnancy. There may be times when 13-*cis*-retinoic acid is preferred over acitretin because of the long-term bioavailability of acitretin metabolites when combined with alcohol. This causes a potential for long-term storage in fat, thus requiring prolonged years of strict adherence to contraception.

Ultraviolet therapy should be administered under physician supervision. Due in part to both the efficacy of physician-directed ultraviolet therapy and unavailability of this treatment in certain geographic areas, investigators have considered the use of non-prescription light treatment via commercial tanning beds in treatment of psoriasis. A small prospective trial found that combination treatment with systemic retinoids and commercial tanning bed light therapy had beneficial effects for psoriasis patients [2]. Extreme caution must be used with these non-prescription ultraviolet therapies as there is marked variability in tanning bed light output, dosimety, and quality. Tanning bed lamps were not designed or studied as efficient UV sources for the treatment of psoriasis; they were designed to maximize tanning. It should be noted that prescribing psoralens for use with a non-medical tanning device should never occur as this has the potential for disastrous outcomes.

Methotrexate Plus UV

Methotrexate (MTX) has frequently been used in combination with UV light for treatment of psoriasis [27, 30]. It is particularly helpful when used to control episodes of mild exacerbation of disease activity during the long-term course of MTX treatment. As an alternative to raising the dose of MTX, a 2- to 3-week course of UVB therapy might be added to MTX to bring this back under control. Another instance when MTX may be effectively used in combination with UVB is as pretreatment for very thick, hard to control areas of psoriasis. The effects of MTX initially would help thin the plaque and decrease scale, thereby facilitating the delivery and penetration of UVB to the epidermis and upper dermis, which are the sites for effective therapy. Care must be taken to use only suberythemogenic doses when MTX is combined with UV therapy to avoid the potential for a MTX sunburn recall reaction. Even though this is a very uncommon side effect, the development of generalized erythema would cause marked discomfort for the patient and require days to subside. MTX has also been used in combination with PUVA, although less commonly than UVB [27]. The long-term combination of these two relative immunosuppressive agents would theoretically have a more profound effect on the potential for cutaneous squamous cell carcinoma. Unfortunately, no long-term study specifically addresses this question.

Cyclosporin and Ultraviolet Light Therapy

This combination is mentioned because of the potential for complications, especially in patients who have previously undergone long-term PUVA therapy. There is a known increased risk of squamous cell carcinoma in psoriasis patients who have undergone more than 250 PUVA therapies over time. The addition of cyclosporine may increase this risk over and above the inherent risk of PUVA alone [25]. Accordingly, it is important to obtain a proper treatment history before the initiation of long-term therapy with cyclosporin.

Combination Therapy with Biologics

The most recent advance in the treatment of psoriasis is the use of genetically engineered protein molecules that target the cutaneous immune system. These biologic medications will undoubtedly be used in combination with ultraviolet light therapy. The relatively recent completion of phase II and III clinical trials to identify the effectiveness and dose for each agent did not include the necessary prospective comparison trials to produce reliable data concerning combination therapy. Early small series of patients having combination NBUVB and alefacept have been promising but further more controlled studies are necessary. There are currently phase IV investigations underway to better identify the most efficient manner to incorporate ultraviolet light into a treatment plan with biologic agents.

The need for combination therapy will arise in those patients who have had a partial response to treatment. In this instance a short course of UV light, most likely NBUVB, may be the most efficient and least immunosuppressive choice for many patients. The question regarding the timing of the addition of UV will be dependent upon each individual agent. Whether or not the addition of UV provides a reduction in the total dose of UV and is more effective than monotherapy alone must be addressed. Will there be an increase in the development of cutaneous malignancy such as basal cell or squamous cell carcinoma? Is there a safe treatment threshold which does not predispose to an increased incidence for these common tumors? Although biologic agents, in combination with phototherapy, may result in improvement of psoriasis, cumulative risk of cutaneous malignancy must be considered with their use. Further studies are needed to ascertain this potential risk. These questions require long-term studies and judicious, limited use of combination therapy only in those patients which need additional treatment. Even with this thoughtful concern in mind, the theoretical benefit of utilizing a treatment which primarily affects the immunologic mechanisms of antigen presentation and T-cell activation in the skin with a systemic agent which may modify the trafficking or potentiation of existing activated immune cells in the dermis or circulation is appealing for control of psoriasis. A combination of low dose UV light may in fact decrease the need for more profound systemic immunosuppression, thus following the basic premise for use of combination therapy of increasing efficacy while decreasing overall side effects of each combination agent.

References

1. Asawanonda P, Anderson RR, Chang Y, Taylor CR (2000) 308 nm excimer laser for the treatment of psoriasis: a dose-response study. Arch Dermatol 136:619–624
2. Carlin CS, Callis KP, Krueger GG (2003) Efficacy of acitretin and commercial tanning bed therapy for psoriasis. Arch Dermatol 139:436–442
3. Coven TR, Walters IB, Cardinale I, Kruger JP (1999) PUVA-induced lymphocyte apoptosis: mechanism of action in psoriasis. Photodermatol Photoimmunol Photomed 15(1):22–27
4. Dawes RS, Wainright NJ, Cameron H, Ferguson J (1998) Narrowband ultraviolet B phototherapy for chronic plaque psoriasis: three times or five times weekly treatment? Br J Dermatol 138:833–839
5. Duthie MS, Kimber I, Norval M (1999) The effects of ultraviolet radiation on the human immune system. Br J Dermatol 140:995–1009
6. Feldman SR, et al. (2002) Efficacy of the 308 nm excimer laser for treatment of psoriasis: results of a multicenter study. J Am Acad Dermatol 46:732–737
7. Fisher T (1976) UV-light treatment of psoriasis. Acta Derm Venereol 56:473–479
8. Fleischer AB Jr, Clark AR, Rapp SR, Reboussin DM, Feldman SR (1997) Commercial tanning bed treatment is an effective psoriasis treatment: results from an uncontrolled clinical trial. J Invest Dermatol 109:170–174
9. Garssen J, van Loveren H (2001) Effects of ultraviolet exposure on the immune system. Crit Rev Immunol 21:359–397
10. Gibbs ND, McCloone RP, Simics E (1997) An action spectrum for urocanic acid in human skin in vivo. Photochem Photobiol 65:103S-104S
11. Green C, Ferguson J, Lakshmipathi T, Johnson BE (1988) 311 nm UVB phototherapy – an effective treatment for psoriasis. Br J Dermatol 119:691–696
12. Guenther LC (2003) Optimizing treatment with topical tazarotene. Am J Clin Dermatol 4:197–202
13. Hofer A, Fink-Puches R, Kerl H, Wolf P (1998) Comparison of phototherapy with near vs. far erythemogenic doses of narrow band ultraviolet B in patients with psoriasis. Br J Dermatol 138:96–100
14. Honigsmann H (2001) Phototherapy for psoriasis. Clin Exp Dermatol 26:343–350
15. Iest J, Boer J (1989) Combined treatment of psoriasis with acitretin and UVB phototherapy compared with acitretin alone and UVB alone. Br J Dermatol 120:665–670
16. Kammeyer A, Teunissen MB, Pavel S, de Rie MA, Bos JD (1995) Photoisomerization spectrum of urocanic acid in human skin and in vitro: effects of simulated solar and artificial ultraviolet radiation. Br J Dermatol 132:884–891
17. Koo J, Behnam SE, Behnam SM (2003) The efficacy of topical tazarotene monotherapy and combination therapies in psoriasis. Expert Opin Pharmacother 4:2347–2354
18. Kragballe K (2002) Vitamin D and UVB radiation therapy. Cutis 70:9–12
19. Krutmann J (1998) Therapeutic photoimmunology: photoimmunological mechanisms in photo(chemo)-therapy. J Photochem Photobiol B 44:159–164
20. Larko O (1989) Treatment of psoriasis with a new UVB-lamp. Acta Derm Venereol 69:357–359
21. Lebwohl M, Drake L, Menter A, Koo J, Gottlieb AB, Zanolli M, et al. (2001) Consensus conference: Acitretin in combination with UVB or PUVA in the treatment of psoriasis. J Am Acad Dermatol 45:544–553
22. Lebwohl M, Quijije J, Gilliard J, Rollin T, Watts O (2003) Topical calcitriol is degraded by ultraviolet light. J Invest Dermatol 121:594–595
23. Lowe N, Prystowsky JH, Gourget T, Edelstein J, Nychay S, Armstrong R (1991) Acitretin plus UVB therapy for psoriasis. Comparisons with placebo plus UVB and acitretin alone. J Am Acad Dermatol 24:591–594
24. Lowe, Iest, Tanew, Lebwohl (1999)
25. Marcil I, Stern RS (2001) Squamous-cell cancer of the skin in patients given PUVA and cyclosporine: nested cohort crossover study. Lancet 358:1042–1045

26. Mascaro JM (2002) Vitamin D and psoralens plus UVA radiation. Cutis 70:13–15
27. Morison WL, Momtax K, Parrish JA, Fitzpatrick TB (1982) Combined methotrexate-PUVA therapy in the treatment of psoriasis. J Am Acad Dermatol 6: 46–51
28. Ozawa M, Ferenczi K, Kikuchi T, et al. (1999) 312 nm UV induces apoptosis of T cells. J Exp Med 189: 711–718
29. Parrish JA, Jaenicke KF (1981) Action spectrum for phototherapy of psoriasis. J Invest Dermatol 76: 359–362
30. Paul BS, Momtax K, Stern RS, Arndt KA, Parrish JA (1982) Combined methotrexate-ultraviolet B therapy in the treatment of psoriasis. J Am Acad Dermatol 7:758–762
31. Stern RS, Laird N, Melski J, Parrish JA, Fitzpatrick TB, Bleich HL (1982) Cutaneous squamous cell carcinoma in patients treated with PUVA. N Engl J Med 310:1156–1161
32. Stern RS, Laird N (1994) The carcinogenic risk of treatments for severe psoriasis. Photochemotherapy follow-up study. Cancer 77:2759–2764
33. Tanew A, Guggenbilcher A, Honigsmann H, Geiger JM, Fritsch P (1999) Photochemotherapy for severe psoriasis without or in combination with acitretin: a randomized, double blind comparison study. J Am Acad Dermatol 41:S25–28
34. Trehan M, Taylor CR (2002) High dose 308 nm laser for the treatment of psoriasis. J Am Acad Dermatol 46:732–737
35. Van Weelden H, De La Faille HB, Young E, Van der Leun IC (1988) A new development in UVB phototherapy of psoriasis. Br J Dermatol 119:11–19
36. Van Weelden H, Baart de la Faille H, Young E, Van der Leun JC (1990) Comparison of narrow-band UVB phototherapy and PUVA photochemotherapy in the treatment of psoriasis. Acta Derm Venereol 70:212–215
37. Walters IB, Burack LH, Coven TR, Gilleaudeu P, Krueger JG (1999) Suberythemogenic narrowband UVB is markedly more effective than conventional UVB treatment of psoriasis vulgaris. J Am Acad Dermatol 40:893–900
38. Zanolli M (2003) The modern paradigm of phototherapy. Clin Dermatol 21:398–406

IX

3 Systemic Retinoids

Milan J. Anadkat, Michael P. Heffernan

Introduction

The term *retinoids* refers to a group of natural and synthetic compounds with biologic activity similar to vitamin A. This includes the naturally occurring forms of vitamin A along with three generations of synthetic retinoids. Retinoids have had a role in dermatology since the early 1900s when vitamin A deficiency was associated with epidermal hyperkeratosis, keratinization disorders, squamous metaplasia of mucous membranes, and various precancerous conditions [74]. Therapy with high dose vitamin A was first used for the ichthyoses, Darier's disease, psoriasis, and other disorders of cornification [53].

Natural Retinoids

Vitamin A cannot be synthesized in vivo and must be acquired through diet. The natural analogs of vitamin A are retinol, retinal, and retinoic acid. Retinol (alcohol form) is the most potent natural analog and is the primary dietary, transport, and storage form. Retinyl esters derived from meat and animal products, including eggs and milk, are hydrolyzed to retinol in the intestines. Retinol is essential to reproductive function.

Retinal (aldehyde form) is derived from the ingestion of carotenoids. Carotenoids are synthesized in plants where they serve an important role as ultraviolet filters. Green leafy plants along with yellow and orange vegetables are a primary source of beta-carotene. Beta-carotene can be absorbed directly or converted to retinal in the gut. Two retinal molecules are formed for every one molecule of beta-carotene ingested in the intestines prior to absorption [75]. Retinal isomers are critical to biochemical reactions for visual function.

Retinol and retinal are inter-converted freely by retinol dehydrogenase. Retinal is irreversibly metabolized to all-*trans*-retinoic acid by retinal dehydrogenase [60]. Retinoic acid (acid form) is the most oxidized and water-soluble form of vitamin A. It is less toxic than other naturally occurring forms of vitamin A as it does not accumulate within the liver or other tissues. Both retinal and retinoic acid have roles in the promotion of epithelial growth and differentiation.

Synthetic Retinoids

Synthetic retinoids were formed to emulate the clinical utility of vitamin A while minimizing its associated toxicity. The US Food and Drug Administration (FDA) have approved four synthetic retinoids: isotretinoin, etretinate, acitretin, and bexarotene. Another agent, tazarotene, was submitted to the FDA for approval in December 2003. The retinoids are classified according to their chemical structure as either first, second, or third generation. Figure A6 displays the chemical structures of these agents. The three generations of systemic retinoids differ in pharmacokinetic, therapeutic, and toxicity profiles.

First generation retinoids are comprised of nonaromatic compounds formed through manipulation of the polyene side chain of vitamin A. Well known members of this class include the naturally occurring compounds tretinoin

Retinol (Vitamin A)
$C_{20}H_{28}O$

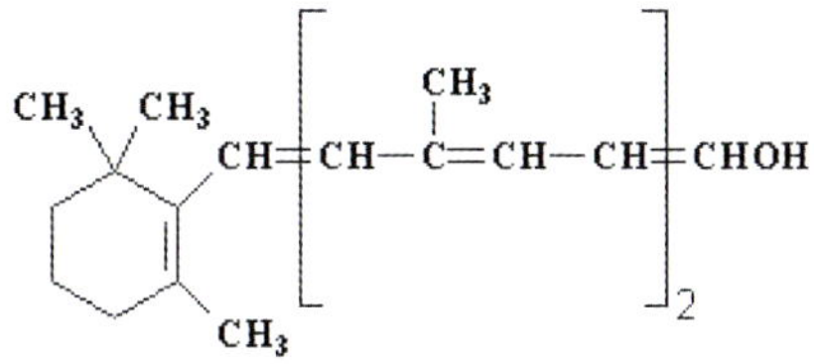

Isotretinoin
$C_{20}H_{28}O_2$

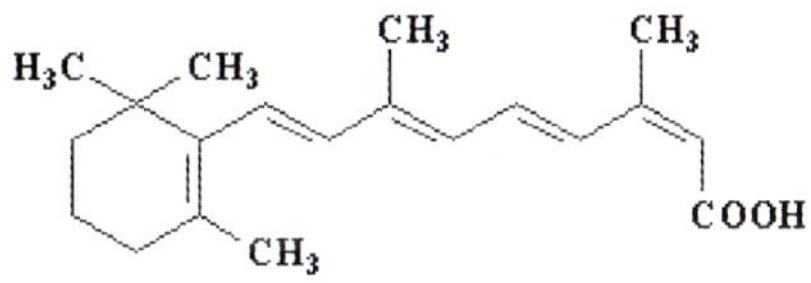

Acitretin
$C_{21}H_{27}O_3$

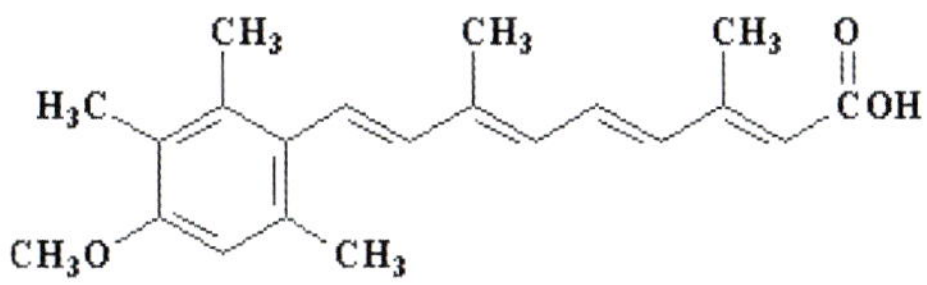

Etretinate
$C_{23}H_{30}O_3$

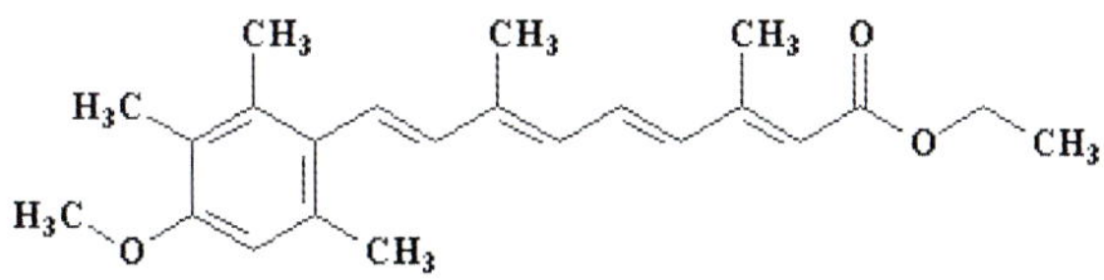

Bexarotene
$C_{24}H_{28}O_2$

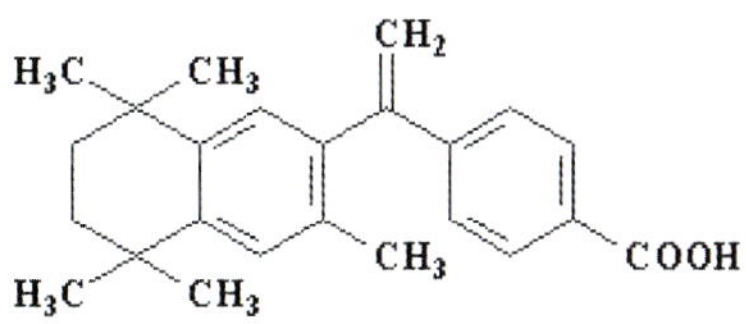

Tazarotene
$C_{21}H_{21}NO_2S$

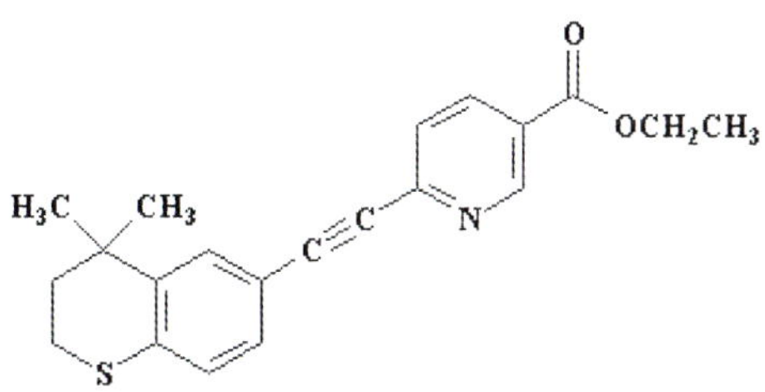

Fig. A6.
Chemical structures of systemic retinoids

(all-*trans*-retinoic acid) and alitretinoin (9-*cis*-retinoic acid). Tretinoin (Retin-A) is currently approved for the topical treatment of acne vulgaris. Isotretinoin (13-*cis*-retinoic acid; Accutane), a synthetic compound, is the only first generation retinoid approved for systemic use. Isotretinoin was first synthesized in 1955, but did not gain FDA approval until 1982 when it was released for the treatment of severe nodulocystic acne.

Monoaromatic compounds comprise the second generation of retinoids, the class first shown to have promise in the treatment of psoriasis. These agents are formed through substitution of the cyclic end of vitamin A with substituted and nonsubstituted ring systems. Etretinate (Tegison) and its metabolite, acitretin (Soriatane), constitute the clinically significant members of this class. Both were approved for the treatment of psoriasis and are also beneficial in the treatment of keratinizing disorders. Etretinate was FDA approved in 1986, but was later removed by its manufacturer (Roche) from US markets in March 1998 due to an unfavorable pharmacokinetic profile. A similar recall had occurred in Europe approximately one decade earlier. Acitretin was FDA approved in 1997 and has since largely replaced the use of etretinate. Etretinate is currently only available in Japan.

Third generation retinoids are polyaromatic compounds formed through cyclization of the polyene side chain of vitamin A. These agents have a more rigid structure with less variability in shape. Third generation retinoids are more potent and bind target receptors more selectively than first or second generation retinoids [12]. Adapalene (Differin) and tazarotene (Tazorac) are members of this class approved for topical use. An oral form of tazarotene is under clinical development for the treatment of moderate to severe plaque psoriasis and chemotherapy for multiple solid organ tumors (lung, breast, etc.) [27]. Bexarotene (Targretin) is currently approved in both topical and systemic forms for the treatment of cutaneous T-cell lymphoma (CTCL).

Our section will focus on acitretin, as it is the only systemic retinoid currently approved for the treatment of psoriasis. We will also briefly discuss older agents such as etretinate along with future agents such as tazarotene. In addition, the toxicities associated with systemic retinoids along with monitoring guidelines for prescribing physicians will be reviewed.

Mechanism of Action

Retinoids act as steroid hormones, passing freely through cell membranes en route to the nucleus. Cytosolic binding proteins transport retinoids to nuclear receptors resulting in alteration of gene transcription. There exist two main families of retinoid receptors, the retinoic acid receptor (RAR) and the retinoid X receptor (RXR), each with three subtypes (α, β, γ). These receptors belong to the superfamily of DNA-binding receptors, which include glucocorticosteroid, vitamin-D3, peroxisome proliferator, and thyroid hormone receptors.

Retinoids exert both direct and indirect effects on gene transcription. Short DNA sequences within the promoter region of target genes contain retinoic acid response elements. These response elements are bound *directly* by activated retinoid nuclear receptors, resulting in downstream stimulation or suppression of target gene transcription. Many genes do not contain retinoic acid response elements, however. In these instances, an *indirect* negative effect on gene transcription results [12].

All-*trans*-retinoic acid (tretinoin) is the naturally occurring RAR ligand. 9-*cis*-retinoic acid (alitretinoin) is a naturally occurring ligand for both RAR and RXR subtypes. Both RARs and RXRs can form homodimers or RAR-RXR heterodimers upon ligand binding. They may also form heterodimers with other DNA-binding steroid hormone receptors mentioned above. Consequently, cross-reactivity of receptors with ligand binding within the steroid hormone superfamily may occur. RXRs serve primarily as cofactors affecting the DNA binding affinity of nuclear receptors associated through heterodimer formation [16].

Nonselective retinoids are associated with an increased incidence of adverse effects, whereas receptor subtype-specific retinoids have a greater therapeutic index. Isotretinoin does not have any demonstrable affinity for retinoid nuclear receptors. Its mechanism of action is not entirely clear. Etretinate and acitretin have been shown to activate all three RAR subtypes [60]. Bexarotene is known as a "rexinoid" as it selectively activates only RXRs. Tazarotene belongs to the novel class of agents known as acetylenic retinoids. It binds all of the RAR receptor subtypes with selective affinity to RAR-β and RAR-γ [13].

The exact mechanism by which retinoids improve psoriasis is unclear. Current theories are based on findings suggesting psoriatic plaques have higher concentrations of retinoic acid compared to normal skin. RARs are believed to play the major role in mediating epithelial cell growth and proliferation, whereas RXRs are primarily involved in controlling apoptosis. It is suggested that because RAR-γ is predominantly expressed within the epidermis of humans, it is the major mediator of retinoid function within the skin [19]. Etretinate has been shown to increase degradation of endogenous retinoids, inhibit cytokine-induced retinoic acid formation, and increase levels of retinoic acid buffering proteins [60]. Through modulation of epidermal cell differentiation, a decrease in scaling, erythema, and thickness of psoriatic plaques occurs. Acitretin has been shown histologically to decrease stratum corneum thickness and psoriasis-associated epidermal and dermal inflammation [76].

Pharmacokinetics

Retinoids are absorbed in a manner similar to other fat-soluble molecules. Through formation of chylomicrons, retinoids are absorbed and transported through the circulation via lymphatic transport. Retinoids are transported within the circulation bound primarily by plasma proteins. It is presumed that naturally occurring vitamin A analogs are bound specifically to retinol binding protein, whereas synthetic retinoids bind nonspecifically to albumin, prealbumin, or lipoproteins [69]. The primary storage site for excess circulating retinoids occurs in the liver, either in parenchymal cells or in the fat-storing cells of Ito [24]. Approximately 90% of total body vitamin A stores are also found in the liver, primarily in the form of retinyl esters [56]. Metabolism of retinoids via oxidation to water-soluble byproducts also occurs mainly in the liver.

Lipid deposition is rare with most commercially available retinoids (isotretinoin, acitretin, bexarotene, tazarotene) as they are water soluble. Etretinate, however, is neutrally charged and consequently, extremely lipophilic. Etretinate readily accumulates within adipose tissue and undergoes very slow clearance. Its elimination half-life is approximately 120 days. Serum levels of etretinate are detectable up to 3 years after termination of therapy.

Hydrolysis of etretinate results in the formation of its *trans*-carboxylate metabolite, acitretin. Acitretin carries a negative charge, is approximately 50 times less lipophilic than etretinate, and does not accumulate in adipose tissue. Acitretin has an elimination half-life of 50 h [9]. Theoretically, it has less potential for long-term adverse effects.

Human studies have shown the presence of measurable etretinate levels in patients taking acitretin [35]. It has been demonstrated that varying amounts of alcohol consumption results in a proportional "reverse" ethylesterification of acitretin back into etretinate. The concentrations of etretinate produced were related to the amount of ethanol consumed, and not to plasma acitretin concentrations [25].

Tazarotene undergoes rapid hydrolysis within circulation to form tazarotenic acid. Tazarotenic acid becomes oxidized to an inactive sulfoxide metabolite by the CYP2C8 enzyme system. The estimated circulating half-life of tazarotenic acid is 7–12 h with once daily dosing of tazarotene (unpublished data).

Individual Agents

Isotretinoin

Isotretinoin is ineffective as monotherapy in the treatment of plaque psoriasis, but has displayed benefit in the treatment of pustular psoriasis. Moy et al. followed 11 patients with generalized pustular psoriasis and 10 patients with chronic plaque psoriasis who each received monotherapy with isotretinoin. The latter group was compared to 19 patients with chronic plaque psoriasis receiving etretinate monotherapy [49]. Most (10/11) patients with generalized pustular eruptions were successfully treated within 1 week, but relapsed upon withdrawal of isotretinoin. Patients with chronic plaque psoriasis demonstrated significantly greater clearance after a minimum of 8 weeks of therapy with etretinate (18/19) than with isotretinoin (4/10). The efficacy of isotretinoin when used in combination with phototherapy is enhanced, and is an improvement over either modality used alone (discussed below).

There are limited instances in which isotretinoin may play a role in the treatment of psoriasis. The advantage of isotretinoin over acitretin is its more rapid clearance from the body. This has particular significance in the treatment of women of childbearing potential. The recommended period for continued contraception after discontinuation of therapy with acitretin (3 years) may be difficult and often leads to noncompliance. In contrast, the recommended period for continued contraception after discontinuation of isotretinoin (1 month) is far more practical. However, with the development of newer agents with similar pharmacokinetic profiles (i.e., tazarotene), the role of isotretinoin in the treatment of psoriasis is nearing extinction.

Etretinate

Etretinate was the first systemic retinoid shown to be successful in the treatment of plaque psoriasis. Early studies with etretinate for the treatment of psoriasis were performed in Europe. Kaplan et al. performed a prospective trial in the United States in the early 1980s evaluating etretinate in 20 patients with recalcitrant psoriasis vulgaris [30]. The initial etretinate dose was 0.75 mg/kg per day with maintenance doses ranging from 0.4 to 1.25 mg/kg per day. Clinical improvement was seen for most patients (19/20) within 2 months and persisted through the treatment course. The average length of remission after discontinuation of therapy was 8 weeks.

The recommended starting dose for etretinate is 0.75–1.0 mg/kg per day divided twice daily, with a maximum dose of 1.5 mg/kg per day. Doses should be titrated according to patient response. The oral bioavailability of etretinate is enhanced with food intake. Despite the dramatic clinical improvement seen with etretinate, its use was ultimately discontinued due to its unfavorable pharmacokinetic profile. The prolonged systemic clearance rate of etretinate coupled with the toxicities associated with systemic retinoids (discussed below) led manufacturers to remove this drug from U.S. markets in 1998.

Acitretin

Acitretin is currently approved for use in recalcitrant, plaque, erythrodermic, and generalized pustular forms of psoriasis. It has also been reported effective for lichen planus [62], keratinization disorders such as Darier's disease, pityriasis rubra pilaris, and ichthyosiform disorders [15, 54], and as chemoprevention of cutaneous malignancies [45].

Acitretin is available in 10- and 25-mg capsules, with a recommended starting dose of 25–50 mg once daily [40]. Like etretinate, it is recommended that acitretin be administered with food as drug absorption is increased by 70% compared to fasting states [46]. Acitretin is contraindicated for patients allergic to parabens, a preservative in the capsule's shell [31].

Both efficacy and frequency of adverse effects with acitretin are dose-dependent [22]. It is recommended to start patients at lower doses to minimize adverse effects and increase the dose based upon response for each patient. Berbis et al studied varying dosing schedules (escalating, stable, and declining) in three groups of patients taking acitretin. They found no difference in efficacy between the three groups, but did note fewer side effects in the dose-escalation group [6].

Monotherapy with acitretin has been found to be most effective for pustular psoriasis. Generalized pustular psoriasis responds rapidly with acitretin, usually within 10 days of initiating therapy. Continued control can often be maintained with lower doses of acitretin. Some patients may relapse, though, or transition to plaque-type psoriasis. Erythrodermic psoriasis responds quickly with acitretin, as well. We recommend the liberal use of emollients and topical steroids (i.e. triamcinolone 0.1% ointment) along with cool baths for this condition.

Moderate to severe plaque-type psoriasis responds well to treatment with acitretin, especially when used in combination with topical anti-inflammatory agents and phototherapy (discussed below). Topical corticosteroids should be encouraged in all patients with plaque psoriasis requiring therapy with systemic retinoids. Topical calcipotriene has also been shown to augment the antipsoriatic effects of acitretin [4, 70].

Improvement of plaque psoriasis with acitretin occurs slowly; peak response is typically seen after a minimum of 3–6 months [21]. Patients should be cautioned that a flare of their psoriasis might occur within the first 1–2 - months of therapy, especially an increase in body surface area [40]. The intensity of psoriatic plaques (erythema, scaling, induration) is often still decreased in these instances [23].

Bexarotene

Oral bexarotene has been shown to improve the lesions of patients with plaque psoriasis [41]. A small dose escalation study conducted in Europe evaluated 37 patients with varying doses of bexarotene: 0.5 mg/kg per day (13 patients), 1.0 mg/kg per day (12 patients), and 2.0 mg/kg per day (12 patients) [65]. A 50% reduction in PASI rating from baseline was noted in 31% (0.5 mg/kg per day), 25% (1.0 mg/kg per day), and 25% (2.0 mg/kg per day) of patients. Improvements in plaque elevation and physicians global assessment (PGA) were also seen for each group. Its cost and unfavorable toxicity profile in comparison to other systemic retinoids currently limit the use of bexarotene for the treatment of psoriasis.

Tazarotene

Tazarotene was initially approved as topical therapy for psoriasis in 1997. Both topical forms (cream, gel) have also been shown effective in the treatment of acne, fine wrinkles, verruca vulgaris, and facial hyperpigmentation.

Oral tazarotene has recently been studied in the treatment of moderate to severe psoriasis with promising results. Two phase III clinical studies were recently completed comparing oral tazarotene (n=340) to placebo (n=350) in the treatment of moderate to severe psoriasis. Patients were administered 12 weeks of therapy (tazarotene 4.5 mg or placebo once daily) followed by a 12-week follow-up period. Over half of the patients (53.8%) experienced a 50% improvement in the overall psoriasis lesion assessment (14.9% for placebo) and 29.7% experienced a 75% improvement (7.4% for placebo). Fewer than 5% of patients discontinued therapy due to side effects [77].

Tazarotene was submitted to the FDA in December 2003 for the treatment of psoriasis; the manufacturer anticipates approval by the end of 2004. Tazarotene has a greater therapeutic index than its predecessors, likely due to its selective binding of nuclear retinoid receptors. The enhanced clearance of this agent provides an additional advantage over earlier retinoids in the treatment of psoriasis. While not allowed during clinical trials, we anticipate combination therapy with topical anti-inflammatory agents or phototherapy would likely further enhance the effectiveness of tazarotene in the treatment of psoriasis.

Combination of Systemic Retinoid with Phototherapy

Patients with moderate to severe psoriasis benefit from the combination of systemic retinoids and phototherapy. Initial studies demonstrated benefit from combination therapy with PUVA (Re-PUVA), but subsequent studies have also shown benefit with UVB (Re-UVB) and commercial tanning beds (re-TBUV). Patients tend to improve quicker with the combination of systemic retinoid and phototherapy than with either therapy alone. Cumulative ultraviolet exposure is frequently decreased and the overall toxicity profile for each modality is also decreased. Retinoids have been shown to have a protective role against the development of premalignant and malignant skin lesions, as well, further emphasizing their utility in combination with phototherapy [45].

Etretinate and acitretin have been the primary agents studied in combination with phototherapy for the treatment of moderate to severe plaque psoriasis. An early study by Lauharanta et al. compared the efficacy of etretinate, PUVA, and combination etretinate-PUVA in 80 patients with severe psoriasis over 14 weeks [36]. Complete remission was seen in 65% of the etretinate-PUVA group compared to 20% and 10% for PUVA only and etretinate only groups, respectively. In addition, there were 40% fewer irradiations and approximately one-third of the total UVA dose administered to the etretinate-PUVA group compared to PUVA alone.

Acitretin has also been shown beneficial for patients with psoriasis in combination with either PUVA [61, 67] or UVB [26, 42, 59]. Tanew et al. compared the efficacy of PUVA monotherapy to acitretin-PUVA in 48 patients with plaque psoriasis. Marked or complete clearance occurred in 96% of patients (22/23) treated with combination acitretin-PUVA compared to 80% of patients (20/25) treated with PUVA alone [67]. Mean cumulative UVA exposure was also reduced by 42% in the acitretin-PUVA group compared to the PUVA only group.

The combination of acitretin with UVB has the advantage over combination with PUVA of not requiring concomitant therapy with oral psoralen. Ruzicka et al. followed 78 patients comparing the efficacy of UVB plus acitretin (40 patients) versus UVB plus placebo (38 patients) over a maximum of 8 weeks combination therapy [59]. The decrease in PASI was 79% for the UVB-acitretin group versus 35% for the UVB-placebo group. Another study involved 41 patients receiving therapy with acitretin, UVB, or acitretin-UVB [26]. Clearance of psoriatic lesions (defined as 80–100% improvement) was observed in 89% of acitretin-UVB patients, 62.5% of UVB only patients, and 23% of acitretin only patients. In addition, total UVB dosage was reduced by 20% and total patient visits were decreased (19.3 versus 24.9) for the acitretin-UVB group compared to the UVB only group.

Patients with psoriasis who do not have access to standardized phototherapy frequently self-treat with commercial tanning beds [68]. Carlin et al. evaluated combination acitretin and commercial tanning bed therapy for patients with moderate to severe plaque psoriasis [10]. Patients were treated with acitretin 25 mg daily and commercial tanning bed light (mean UVB output of 4.7%) 4 to 5 times per week over 12 weeks. Retrospective analysis (telephone survey) of 26 patients was combined with a prospective trial in 17 patients. Clearance or near-clearance was reported by 83% (19/23) of patients in the retrospective trial. A similar effect was seen prospectively, with patients demonstrating an average PASI reduction of 78.6% from baseline. Physicians typically do not advocate tanning beds as they have more variability than phototherapy administered within in the office. However, the combination of tanning beds with systemic retinoids may serve a role for patients with recalcitrant plaque psoriasis without access to more conventional forms of phototherapy when used with extreme caution.

There also appears to a benefit with the combination of systemic retinoids and topical phototherapy. An initial study by Muchenberger et al. involved the treatment of four patients with severe psoriasis with combination acitretin and bath PUVA [50]. All patients improved by at least 90% after 3–5 weeks of therapy. Lower cumulative doses of UVA were required and the efficacy of combination therapy exceeded that seen in monotherapy with bath PUVA for patients with similar PASI scores [66]. The decrease in desquamation and induration of psoriatic plaques induced by oral retinoids may be of particular significance in facilitating the effectiveness of topical PUVA.

Isotretinoin has been shown effective in the treatment of plaque psoriasis when used in combination with PUVA. As discussed earlier, isotretinoin may be of particular advantage over acitretin in the treatment of fertile women. Anstey and Hawk reported success in four women (age 22–26) with isotretinoin 0.6 mg/kg per day used in combination with PUVA [3]. A 30–40% reduction in the number of treatments and cumulative UVA exposure was noted compared to prior phototherapy courses in the same patients without the use of a concomitant oral retinoid.

Systemic retinoids should be initiated 2 weeks prior to beginning phototherapy. Patients have an increased risk for developing radiation-induced erythema with ultraviolet therapy as all systemic retinoids can cause thinning of the stratum corneum. It is therefore recommended that both PUVA and UVB be escalated more gradually in these patients.

Toxicity

The syndrome of hypervitaminosis A occurs when the storage capacity of vitamin A is exceeded leading to increased levels of circulating retinol and retinyl esters. As a result, the nonphysiologic presentation of vitamin A compounds to otherwise retinoid-naïve peripheral tissue sites occurs. This syndrome was initially described over a century ago in Arctic explorers after they had consumed the livers of polar bears and huskies [7, 28], and serves as a template for understanding synthetic retinoid toxicity.

Table A3. Symptoms associated with acute hypervitaminosis A [47]

Gastrointestinal
Abdominal pain
Nausea
Vomiting
Anorexia
Hepatomegaly
Splenomegaly
Neurologic
Headache
Dizziness
Fatigue
Irritability
Increased intracranial pressure
Mucocutaneous
Generalized desquamation
Cheilitis
Hair loss
Petechiae
Epistaxis
Musculoskeletal
Long bone tenderness
Laboratory abnormalities
Elevated vitamin A
Elevated alkaline phosphatase
Elevated calcium
Elevated liver function assays

Acute hypervitaminosis A occurs following exposure from a single large dose. Symptoms (Table A3) are noted within approximately 4 hours and resolve within a few days. Chronic hypervitaminosis A has a much less specific clinical presentation (Table A4). The onset of symptoms, persistence of abnormal vitamin A levels, and resolution of disease displays considerable interpatient variability [64].

Teratogenicity

Naturally occurring retinoids play an important role in fetal development [16]. Increased in utero exposure to retinoids, though, leads to a variety of developmental abnormalities leading to the classification of all systemic retinoids as teratogens. All systemic retinoids are categorized as class X drugs in pregnancy.

Table A5 lists characteristic birth defects seen with *retinoic acid embryopathy* [34, 58]. First trimester exposure to retinoids, especially between weeks 3 and 6 of gestation, can lead to toxic effects upon neural crest development. Auditory, cardiovascular, ocular, skeletal, thymic, and central nervous system developmental abnormalities have also been associated with retinoids [34]. Spontaneous abortions have been reported to occur with isotretinoin in approximately one-third of exposed pregnancies. An increased rate of stillbirths has also been reported.

Women of childbearing potential are absolutely contraindicated from using systemic retinoids unless two acceptable forms of contraception are used. The makers of isotretinoin and tazarotene recommend women of childbearing potential continue two forms of contraception for at least 1 month after discontinuation of therapy. The presumed clearance of acitretin occurs within 3 weeks of discontinuation [23], but the FDA recommends 3 year post-therapy pregnancy avoidance for patients treated with acitretin [1]. This extension is due to the discovery of reverse metabolism of acitretin

IX

Table A4. Symptoms associated with chronic hypervitaminosis A [47]

Mucocutaneous	Psychiatric
Dry skin	Depression
Desquamation (generalized, fingertip, palm/sole)	Cyclothymia
Pruritus	Psychosis
Skin thinning	Irritability
Skin fragility	Musculoskeletal
Easy bruising	Muscle cramps
Cheilitis	Myalgia
Phototoxicity	Muscle stiffness
Granulation tissue	Stiff man syndrome
Dry nose	Arthralgia
Epistaxis	Bone pain
Sore mouth	Arthritis
Gingivitis	Backache
Hair loss	Isolated hyperostoses
Hair thinning	Diffuse idiopathic skeletal hyperostosis
Brittle nails	Renal
Ophthalmologic	Polyuria
Dry eyes	Dysuria
Blepharitis	Excessive thirst
Eyeball pain	Ankle edema
Papilledema	Hypercalcuria
Diplopia	Proteinuria
Blurred vision	Sterile pyuria
Exophthalmos	Endocrine
Gastrointestinal	Abnormal menses
Anorexia	Hypercalcemia
Weight loss	Laboratory test elevations
Nausea	Elevated triglyceride
Abdominal pain	Elevated cholesterol
Hepatomegaly	Elevated liver function assays
Cirrhosis	Elevated prothrombin time
Ascites	Relative lymphocytosis
Varices	Elevated erythrocyte sedimentation rate
Splenomegaly	Anemia
Neurologic	
Headache	
Fatigue	
Lethargy	
Hypersomnolence	
Insomnia	
Paresthesia	
Dysesthesia	

into etretinate with alcohol exposure, leading to measurable etretinate levels years after discontinuation of acitretin. In contrast to the FDA, a post-therapy pregnancy avoidance of 2 years is promoted in Europe [73]. Women of childbearing potential should avoid alcohol while taking acitretin and for 2 months following discontinuation of therapy.

Hyperlipidemia

Alteration of the blood lipid profile represents another major adverse effect associated with oral retinoids. Dose-dependent increases in serum levels of triglycerides and cholesterol result along with a decrease in high density lipoprotein cholesterol (HDL). The mechanism for

Table A5. Abnormalities seen with retinoid embryopathy [48, 49]

Auditory	Craniofacial
Microtia	Maxillary hypoplasia
Sensorineural hearing loss	Mandibular hypoplasia
Conductive hearing loss	Cleft palate
Absent auditory canals	Cleft lip
Vestibular dysfunction	Depressed midface
	Triangular microcephalic skull
Cardiovascular	Micrognathia
Abnormal origin of subclavian arteries	
Overriding aorta	Skeletal
Atrial septal defect	Absent clavicle
Aortic coarctation	Absent scapula
Ventricular septal defect	Short sternum
Hypoplastic aortic arch	Absent thumb
	Sternoumbilical raphe
Central nervous system	Long bone aplasia/hypoplasia
Hydrocephalus	Syndactyly
Microcephaly	
Meningomyelocele	Other
Abnormal cortical tract development	Anal atresia
Cerebellar vermis agenesis	Vaginal atresia
Leptomeningeal neuroglial heterotopias	Amastia
Spina bifida	Situs inversus
Posterior fossa cyst	Omphalocele
Motor retardation	Hydroureter
Facial nerve palsy	Tracheo-esophageal fistula
	Thymic aplasia/hypoplasia
Ocular	
Microphthalmia	
Exophthalmus	
Coloboma	
Blindness	
Strabismus	
Ptosis	
Optic nerve atrophy	

retinoid-induced hyperlipidemia is uncertain. It has been proposed to be related to alteration of hepatic lipoprotein metabolism.

Triglyceride levels may increase by 60% or more from baseline with acitretin [43]. While uncommon, pancreatitis may occur. Risk factors for developing hypertriglyceridemia with systemic retinoids include obesity, diabetes mellitus, family history of hyperlipidemia, and alcohol intake [31]. Total cholesterol elevations (>100%) occurred in 33% of 525 patients taking acitretin at doses ranging from 10 to 75 mg daily in clinical trials. HDL levels were also reported to decrease (>2 units) in 40% of patients [1]. Such abnormalities should be managed with reduction in dosage, dietary changes, and antihyperlipidemic therapy (e.g. genfibrozil, ferobibrate). Discontinuation of acitretin generally leads to normalization of lipid levels. No clinically significant alteration in the blood lipid profile was noted in phase III clinical studies with tazarotene [77].

Fish oil dietary supplementation with MaxEPA oil 15 ml/day (2.6 g eicosapentaneoic acid and 2.4 g docosohexaenoic acid) reduced triglyceride and cholesterol levels by 70% and 45%, respectively, in patients with isotretinoin-induced hyperlipidemia [44]. A similar reduction in triglycerides, but not cholesterol, was seen with the addition of MaxEPA oil for patients with etretinate-induced hyperlipidemia [44]. In addition, Frati et al reported clinical improvement in psoriatic lesions with omega-3 fish oil 1.5 g (0.9 g of eicosapentaenoic acid and 0.6 g of docosohexaenoic acid daily) in combination with etretinate [20].

Hepatic

Liver toxicity is relatively uncommon with acitretin and is presumed to be an idiosyncratic drug-induced hepatitis [71]. A study by Roenigk et al. compared pretreatment and post-treatment liver biopsies in 83 patients, with a mean daily acitretin dose of 46.2 g over a mean duration of 533 days. Only one patient in this study had progression to moderate to severe fibrosis, and no patients developed cirrhosis. Approximately 27% and 31% had elevated AST and ALT values, respectively, but these findings showed no correlation to changes in hepatic histology [57]. Previous studies have shown hepatic transaminase elevations of approximately 25%. These abnormalities usually are reversible after discontinuation of acitretin and occasionally resolve through continuation of therapy [14]. A cholestatic form of hepatitis has recently been reported secondary to acitretin [33], although there have been previous reports with etretinate [29, 32]. Patients at increased risk for hepatotoxicity with acitretin include alcoholics, diabetics, and obese individuals. These patients may require more frequent laboratory monitoring. Recent studies with tazarotene did not reveal any clinically significant elevations in liver function studies during treatment [77].

Mucocutaneous

Mucocutaneous side effects due to oral retinoids are commonly encountered and are often dose-related. Activation of RAR receptor subtypes is likely responsible for these adverse effects. The most commonly reported symptom is cheilitis. Dry skin, desquamation, rhinitis, pruritus, and vulvo-vaginal infections may also occur [2, 63]. Some patients may report a sensation of sticky hands or feet. Periungual pyogenic granulomas may also develop, but usually resolve with a reduction in dosage [37]. Alopecia secondary to acitretin may occur and can be quite pronounced. It is often distressing for patients, but generally resolves within 6–8 weeks after discontinuation of therapy. Studies with etretinate demonstrate that gradual shortening of the anagen phase leading to an increased telogen count is the primary mechanism involved, with a delay in the onset of anagen phase after normal shedding also playing a role [8].

Patients should avoid excessive sun exposure as they are likely to experience photosensitivity while taking oral retinoids [1]. All patients receiving systemic retinoids should be counseled on the importance of emollients and sunscreens in minimizing adverse effects. Some studies also propose vitamin E 800 IU daily to reduce the mucocutaneous adverse effects associated with systemic retinoids [37].

Ophthalmic

Conjunctivitis and dryness are the most common ophthalmic complaints, and can generally be alleviated with artificial lubricant eye drops. Patients frequently experience difficulty wearing contact lenses during therapy. Corneal erosions, corneal opacities, and iritis are less common adverse effects. Rarely, patients may develop persistent abnormal night vision. Ocular adverse effects unresponsive to lubricant eyedrops require prompt and thorough investigation by an ophthalmologist.

Musculoskeletal

Skeletal toxicity resulting from systemic retinoids mimics that seen with chronic hypervitaminosis A. Various changes such as premature epiphyseal closure, skeletal hyperostoses, extraspinal tendon and ligament calcification, and bone demineralization have each been observed.

Skeletal hyperostoses along the vertebrae and extraspinal tendon or ligament calcifications are well documented with etretinate and acitretin [17, 48]. Van Dooren-Greebe et al. reviewed 135 patients with a mean cumulative oral retinoid (etretinate and/or acitretin) dose of 31 g over a mean of 30 months and found no significant risk for increased skeletal abnormalities [72]. While some recommend baseline ankle films prior to oral retinoid therapy [52], there remain no clear guidelines for physicians regarding baseline and annual radiographic monitoring during long-term oral retinoid therapy.

Osteoporosis may also occur with certain systemic retinoids. It has been observed in patients treated with etretinate for long periods and also in patients with hypervitaminosis A. DiGiovanna et al. followed 24 patients over 2 years or more receiving a 50 g or more etretinate (15 patients) or isotretinoin (9 patients) [18]. Bone mineral density (BMD) testing was performed at five standard sites (lumbar spine, femoral neck, trochanter, radius, and Ward's triangle) and compared with age-, sex-, and weight-matched controls. BMD values were significantly decreased for the etretinate group but not for the isotretinoin group, implicating long-term etretinate as a risk factor for development of osteoporosis. A similar risk is likely present for acitretin, although has not yet been confirmed.

Isotretinoin was reported to cause premature epiphyseal closure in a 10-year-old boy. High-dose isotretinoin (3.5 mg/kg per day) was prescribed for over 4 years resulting in partial closure of the proximal epiphyses of the right tibia [47]. Another report by Prendiville et al. describes epiphyseal closure occurring in an 8-year-old boy and 11-year-old girl following 6 and 5 years, respectively, of etretinate therapy [55].

Arthralgias and myalgias have been reported with systemic retinoids. Muscle pain greater than expected is frequently reported with gymnasts, competitive ice skaters, ballet dancers, and long-distance joggers [39]. Elevated creatinine phosphokinase levels may also be present, especially in patients who undergo strenuous exercise or participate in contact sports. Typically, symptoms of pain respond well to rest and therapy with nonsteroidal anti-inflammatory drugs [16].

Pseudotumor Cerebri

Rare cases of pseudotumor cerebri (benign intracranial hypertension) have been reported with systemic retinoids, most often associated with concomitant administration of tetracyclines [38]. Headache, nausea, vomiting, and visual changes are common presenting symptoms. If papilledema is noted on examination, retinoid therapy should be discontinued immediately followed by prompt referral to a neurologist.

Drug Interactions

Multiple drug interactions can occur while taking systemic retinoids. The reverse esterification of acitretin to etretinate with ethanol has already been discussed. In addition, both alcohol and methotrexate may cause additive hepatotoxicity with each of the systemic retinoids. Vitamin A supplements are contraindicated in patients taking retinoids, as potentiated RAR-activity may lead to symptoms of hypervitaminosis A. No more than 5000 IU of vitamin A should be consumed daily [51]. The risk of pseudotumor cerebri is increased with patients taking retinoids along with tetracycline, minocycline, or corticosteroids. In addition, photosensitivity may be increased with tetracycline or doxycycline administration.

Inducers of the cytochrome P450 3A4 (CYP 3A4) system such as rifampin, rifabutin, phenobarbital, or phenytoin may reduce levels of etretinate or acitretin. Conversely, macrolide antibiotics (i.e., erythromycin, clarithromycin) and azole antifungal medications may increase drug levels via CYP 3A4 inhibition. (Azithromycin is unique amongst macrolide antibiotics in that it displays minimal CYP 3A4 inhibition.) Due to competitive CYP 3A4 metabolism, cyclosporine levels may increase in patients concomitantly taking retinoids. The progestin "minipill" contraceptive has decreased efficacy with concomitant acitretin use [5]. Diabetic therapeutics should be administered cautiously to patients on retinoid therapy, as well, given that retinoids may predispose to hypoglycemia [11].

Monitoring

Careful laboratory monitoring is required to ensure safe administration of systemic retinoids in the treatment of psoriasis. Prior to initiating therapy, a baseline liver function and fasting lipid profile should be checked. These values should be followed monthly during therapy, and less frequently after consistent stable results are obtained. Ankle radiographs to evaluate skeletal hyperostosis, as discussed earlier, may be considered at baseline in predisposed patients. Routine radiographic monitoring, however, should be driven by patient symptoms only. All female patients of childbearing potential should have a negative pregnancy test at baseline and monthly during therapy. In addition, patients should be counseled against pregnancy for at least 1 month following discontinuation of isotretinoin or tazarotene. Women should avoid pregnancy for a minimum of 3 years following discontinuation of acitretin.

References

1. [No author] Soriatane [package insert] (1997) Roche Laboratories, Nutley, NJ
2. [No author] Two new retinoids for psoriasis (1997) Medical Letter on Drugs & Therapeutics 39(1013): 105–106
3. Anstey A, Hawk JLM (1997) Isotretinoin-PUVA in women with psoriasis. Br J Dermatol 136:798–799
4. Ashcroft DM, Li Wan Po A, Williams HC, Griffiths CE (2000) Combination regimens of topical calcipotriene in chronic plaque psoriasis: systematic review of efficacy and tolerability. Arch Dermatol 136: 1536–1543
5. Berbis P, Bun H, Geiger JM, et al. (1988) Acitretin (RO10-1670) and oral contraceptives: interaction study. Arch Dermatol Res 280:388–389
6. Berbis P, Geiger JM, Vaisse C, Rognin C, Privat Y (1989) Benefit of progressively increasing doses during the initial treatment with acitretin in psoriasis. Dermatologica 178:88–92
7. Bernstein RE (1984) Liver and hypervitaminosis. N Engl J Med 311:604
8. Berth-Jones J, Shuttleworth D, Hutchinson PE (1990) A study of etretinate alopecia. Br J Dermatol 122:751–755
9. Brindley C (1989) An overview of recent clinical pharmacokinetic studies with acitretin (Ro 10-1670, Etretin). Dermatologica 178:79–87
10. Carlin CS, Callis KP, Krueger GG (2003) Efficacy of acitretin and commercial tanning bed therapy for psoriasis. Arch Dermatol 139:436–442
11. Cesario RM, Klausing K, Razzaghi H, et al. (2001) The rexinoid LG100754 is a novel RXR:PPARgamma agonist and decreases glucose levels in vivo. Mol Endocrinol 15:1360–1369
12. Chandraratna RA (1998) Rational design of receptor-selective retinoids. J Am Acad Dermatol 39: S124–S128
13. Chandraratna RA (1996) Tazarotene – first of a new generation of receptor-selective retinoids. Br J Dermatol 135:S18–S25
14. Cunningham WJ (1991) Side effect profile of retinoids. In: Roenigk HH Jr, Maibach HI (eds) Psoriasis, 2nd edn. Marcel Dekker, New York, pp 769–774
15. Dicken CH (1994) Treatment of classic pityriasis rubra pilaris. J Am Acad Dermatol 31:997–999
16. DiGiovanna JJ (2001) Systemic retinoid therapy. Dermatol Clin 19:161–167
17. DiGiovanna JJ, Helfgott RK, Gerber LH, Peck GL (1986) Extraspinal tendon and ligament calcification associated with long-term therapy with etretinate. N Engl J Med 315:1177–1182
18. DiGiovanna JJ, Sollitto RB, Abangan DL, Steinberg SM, Reynolds JC (1995) Osteoporosis is a toxic effect of long-term etretinate therapy. Arch Dermatol 131: 1263–1267
19. Elder JT, Fisher GJ, Zhang Q-Y, et al. (1991) Retinoic acid receptor gene expression in human skin. J Invest Dermatol 96:425–433
20. Frati C, Bevilacqua L, Apostolico V (1994) Association of etretinate and fish oil in psoriasis therapy. Inhibition of hypertriglyceridemia resulting from retinoid therapy after fish oil supplementation. Acta Derma Venereol 186:S151–S153
21. Geiger JM, Czarnetzki BM (1988) Acitretin (RO10-1670, Etretin): overall evaluation of clinical studies. Dermatologica 176:182–190
22. Goldfarb MT, Ellis CN, Gupta AK, Tincoff T, Hamilton TA, Voorhees JJ (1988) Acitretin improves psoriasis in a dose-dependent fashion. J Am Acad Dermatol 18:S655–S662
23. Gollnick H, Bauer R, Brindley C, et al. (1988) Acitretin versus etretinate in psoriasis. Clinical and pharmacokinetic results of a German multicenter study. J Am Acad Dermatol 19:458–468
24. Goodman DS (1984) Vitamin A and retinoids in health and disease. N Engl J Med 310:1023–1031
25. Gronhoj Larsen F, Steinkjer B, Jakobsen P, Hjorter A, Brockhoff PB, Nielsen-Kudsk F (2000) Acitretin is converted to etretinate only during concomitant alcohol intake. Br J Dermatol 143:1164–1169
26. Iest J, Boer J (1989) Combined treatment of psoriasis with acitretin and UVB phototherapy compared with acitretin alone and UVB alone. Br J Dermatol 120:665–670
27. Jones PH, Burnett RD, Fainaru I, et al. (2003) A phase 1 study of tazarotene in adults with advanced cancer. Br J Cancer 89:808–815

28. Kane EK (1971) Arctic explorations in 1853, 1854, 1855. Arno Press and The New York Times, New York, vol 1, pp 392–393
29. Kano Y, Fukuda M, Shiohara T, Nagashima M (1994) Cholestatic hepatitis occurring shortly after etretinate therapy. J Am Acad Dermatol 31:133–134
30. Kaplan RP, Russell DH, Lowe NJ (1983) Etretinate therapy for psoriasis: Clinical responses, remission times, epidermal DNA and polyamine responses. J Am Acad Dermatol 8:95–102
31. Katz HI, Waalen J, Leach EE (1999) Acitretin in psoriasis: An overview of adverse effects. J Am Acad Dermatol 41:S7–S12
32. Khouri MR, Saul SH, Dlugosz AA, Soloway RD (1987) Hepatocanalicular injury associated with vitamin A derivative etretinate: An idiosyncratic hypersensitivity reaction. Dig Dis Sci 32:1207–1211
33. Kreiss C, Amin S, Nalesnik MA, Chopra K, Shakil AO (2002) Severe cholestatic hepatitis in a patient taking acitretin. Am J Gastroenterol 97:775–777
34. Lammer EJ, Chen CT, Hoar RM, et al. (1985) Retinoic acid embryopathy. N Engl J Med 313:837–841
35. Larsen FG, Jakobsen P, Knudsen J, Weismann K, Kragballe K, Nielsen-Kudsk F (1993) Conversion of acitretin to etretinate in psoriatic patients is influenced by ethanol. J Invest Dermatol 100:623–627
36. Lauharanta J, Juvakoski T, Lassus A (1981) A clinical evaluation of the effects of an aromatic retinoid (Tigason), combination of retinoid and PUVA, and PUVA alone in severe psoriasis. Br J Dermatol 104: 325–332
37. Lebwohl M, Ali S (2001) Treatment of psoriasis, part 2. Systemic therapies. J Am Acad Dermatol 45: 649–661
38. Lee AG (1995) Pseudotumor cerebri after treatment with tetracycline and isotretinoin for acne. Cutis 55: 165–168
39. Leyden JJ (1998) The role of isotretinoin in the treatment of acne: personal observations. J Am Acad Dermatol 39:S45–49
40. Ling MR (1999) Acitretin: Optimal dosing strategies. J Am Acad Dermatol 41:S13–S17
41. Lowe MN, Plosker GL (2000) Bexarotene. Am J Clin Dermatol 1:245–250
42. Lowe NJ, Prystowsky JH, Bourget T, Edelstein J, Nychay S, Armstrong R (1991) Acitretin plus UVB therapy for psoriasis. Comparisons with placebo plus UVB and acitretin alone. J Am Acad Dermatol 24: 591–594
43. Mantel-Teeuwise AK, Kloosterman JM, Maitland-van der Zee AH, Klungel OH, Porsius AJ, de Boer A (2001) Drug-induced lipid changes: a review of the unintended effects of some commonly used drugs on serum lipid levels. Drug Safety 34:443–456
44. Marsden JR (1987) Effect of dietary fish oil on hyperlipidaemia due to isotretinoin and etretinate. Hum Toxicol 6:219–222
45. McKenna DB, Murphy GM (1999) Skin cancer chemoprophylaxis in renal transplant recipients: 5 years of experience using low-dose acitretin. Br J Dermatol 140:656–660
46. McNamara PJ, Jewell RC, Jensen BK, Brindley CJ (1988) Food increases the bioavailability of acitretin. J Clin Pharmacol 28:1051–1055
47. Milstone LM, McGuire J, Ablow RC (1982) Premature epiphyseal closure in a child receiving oral 13-*cis*-retinoic acid. J Am Acad Dermatol 7:663–666
48. Mork N, Kolbenstvedt A, Austad J (1996) Skeletal side-effects of 5 years acitretin treatment. Br J Dermatol 134:1156–1157
49. Moy RL, Kingston TP, Lowe NJ (1985) Isotretinoin vs etretinate therapy in generalized pustular and chronic psoriasis. Arch Dermatol 121:1297–1301
50. Muchenberger S, Schopf E, Simon JC (1997) The combination of oral acitretin and bath PUVA for the treatment of severe psoriasis. Br J Dermatol 137: 587–589
51. Nguyen EQH, Wolverton SE (2002) Systemic Retinoids. In: Wolverton SE (ed) Comprehensive dermatologic drug therapy. WB Saunders, Philadelphia, pp 269–310
52. Orfanos CE, Zouboulis CC, Almond-Roesler B, Geilen CC (1997) Current use and future potential role of retinoids in dermatology. Drugs 53:358–388
53. Peck GL, DiGiovanna JJ (1999) The retinoids. In: Freedberg IM, Eisen AZ, Wolff K, et al. (eds) Dermatology in general medicine. McGraw-Hill, New York, pp 2810–2820
54. Peck GL, Yoder FW (1976) Treatment of lamellar ichthyosis and other keratinizing dermatoses with a synthetic retinoid. Lancet 2:1172–1174
55. Prendiville J, Bingham EA, Burrows D (1986) Premature epiphyseal closure – a complication of etretinate therapy in children. J Am Acad Dermatol 15: 1259–1262
56. Raica N Jr, Scot J, Lowry L, et al. (1972) Vitamin A concentration in human tissues collected in five areas in the United States. Am J Clin Nutr 25:291–296
57. Roenigk HH, Callen JP, Guzoo CA, et al. (1999) Effects of acitretin on the liver. J Am Acad Dermatol 41:584–588
58. Rosa FW, Wilk AL, Kelsey FO (1986) Teratogen update: Vitamin A congeners. Teratology 33:355–364
59. Ruzicka T, Sommerburg C, Braun-Falco O, et al. (1990) Efficiency of acitretin in combination with UV-B in the treatment of severe psoriasis. Arch Dermatol 126:482–486
60. Saurat JH (1999) Retinoids and psoriasis: Novel issues in retinoid pharmacology and implications for psoriasis treatment. J Am Acad Dermatol 41:S2–S6
61. Saurat JH, Geiger JM, Amblard P, et al. (1988) Randomized double-blind multicenter study comparing acitretin-PUVA, etretinate-PUVA, and placebo-PUVA in the treatment of severe psoriasis. Dermatologica 177:218–224
62. Schroder K, Zaun H, Holzmann H, et al. (1989) Pustulosis palmo-plantaris. Clinical and histological changes during etretin (acitretin). Acta Derm Venereol 146:S111–S116
63. Shukenboom M, Middelbeek A, De Jong-Van den Berg L, et al. (1995) Vulvo-vaginal candidiasis associated with acitretin. J Clin Epidemiol 48:991–997

64. Silverman AK, Ellis CN, Voorhees JJ (1987) Hypervitaminosis A syndrome: a paradigm of retinoid side effects. J Am Acad Dermatol 16:1027–1039
65. Smith J, de Jong E, van Hooijdonk C, et al. (2000) A multicentre phase ii clinical and immunohistochemical trial of systemic bexarotene (Targretin) in psoriasis. J Invest Derm 114:776
66. Streit V, Wiedow O, Christophers E (1996) Treatment of psoriasis with polyethylene sheet bath PUVA. J Am Acad Dermatol 35:208–210
67. Tanew A, Guggenbichler A, Honigsmann H, Geiger JM, Fritsch P (1991) Photochemotherapy for severe psoriasis without or in combination with acitretin: a randomized, double-blind comparison study. J Am Acad Dermatol 25:682–684
68. Turner RJ, Farr PM, Walshaw D (1998) Many patients with psoriasis use sunbeds. Br Med J 317:412
69. Vahlquist A, Rollman O (1987) Clinical pharmacology of 3 generations of retinoids. Dermatologica 175: S20–S27
70. van de Kerkhof PC, Cambazard F, Hutchinson PE, et al. (1998) The effect of addition of calcipotriol ointment (50 micrograms/g) to acitretin therapy in psoriasis. Br J Dermatol 138:84–89
71. van Dietzhujsen TJM, van Haelst UJGM, van Dooren-Greebe RJ, et al. (1990) Severe hepatotoxic reaction with progression to cirrhosis after use of a novel retinoid (acitretin). J Hepatol 11:185–188
72. van Dooren-Greebe RJ, Lemmens JA, De Boo T, Hangx NM, Kuijpers AL, van de Kerkhof PC (1996) Prolonged treatment with oral retinoids in adults: no influence on the frequency and severity of spinal abnormalities. Br J Dermatol 134:71–76
73. Wiegand UW, Chou RC (1998) Pharmacokinetics of acitretin and etretinate. J Am Acad Dermatol 39: S25–S33
74. Wolbach SB, Howe PR (1925) Tissue changes following deprivation of fat soluble A vitamin. J Exp Med 43:753–757
75. Wolverton SE (1991) Retinoids. In: Wolverton SE, Wilkin JK (eds) Systemic drugs for skin diseases. WB Saunders, Philadelphia, pp 187–218
76. Yamauchi PS, Rizk D, Kormeili T, Patnaik R, Lowe NJ (2003) Systemic retinoids. In: Weinstein GD, Gottlieb AB (eds) Therapy of moderate-to-severe psoriasis, 2nd edn. Marcel Dekker, New York, pp 137–150
77. http://www.allergan.com/site/investors/pr details. asp?id =104739. Mar 24, 2003, Business Wire Magazine

4 Methotrexate and Cyclosporine

Jennifer C. Cather, Alan Menter

Introduction

Methotrexate and cyclosporine have historically been the most reliable therapeutic agents for all types of psoriasis (plaque, pustular, erythrodermic, etc.) [63]. Methotrexate has been the cornerstone of treatment for patients with more severe forms of psoriasis since its introduction in the 1970s. Cyclosporine not only has been extremely effective as therapy for psoriasis, the discovery of its efficacy led to many of the changes in thinking of psoriasis as primarily an immune mediated disease. The use of methotrexate and cyclosporine, however, has been limited by concerns, both founded and unfounded, about potential side effects of these treatments. In this chapter, we will review the basis for the use of methotrexate and cyclosporine along with their efficacy and safety.

Methotrexate

In 1951 Gubner reported aminopterin, a systemic anti-metabolite immunosuppressant, improved the cutaneous and rheumatologic manifestations of psoriasis [27]. Methotrexate, a compound similar to aminopterin but with an improved safety and therapeutic index, was soon after developed and was used widely in psoriasis. Methotrexate was approved by the FDA for the treatment of psoriasis in 1971.

Methotrexate has a myriad of effects on both T lymphocytes and keratinocytes which make it useful in the treatment of psoriasis [55]. Methotrexate's mechanism can best be classified as anti-inflammatory though there are clearly effects on adaptive immunity and keratinocyte proliferation. The effects of methotrexate on activated T lymphocytes occur at concentrations approximately 100 times lower than keratinocytes [31]. Induction of activated T lymphocyte apoptosis [20] and alteration of the proportion of TH1 and TH2 lymphocytes and their respective cytokines [9, 12] are both important anti-inflammatory actions attributed to methotrexate. Another potentially significant anti-inflammatory effect of methotrexate involves accumulation of adenosine, which acts to suppress neutrophil migration into skin [11, 10]. Additionally, Weinstein demonstrated that methotrexate inhibits the proliferation of keratinocytes by blocking the synthesis of nucleic acids [73]. Thus, methotrexate has potentially important effects on multiple arms of the pathophysiology of psoriasis.

Efficacy

As with many medications approved before the growth of evidenced based medicine in the 1980s and 90s, the data on the efficacy of methotrexate is limited. No placebo-controlled studies have been performed with methotrexate for the treatment of psoriasis. There were multiple early studies of methotrexate that led to the development of the dosing guidelines that are used presently. In an early, open-label, dose ranging study, three doses of methotrexate which ranged between 2.5 to 7.5 mg every 12 h once per week resulted in clearance in 31% of patients after 8–12 weeks [72]. Multiple other studies reported that dosing with 25 mg/week for 3–4 weeks clears approximately 50% of patients and a 75% improvement is seen in approximately 90% at this dose [64, 54, 4]. In these studies, patients generally tolerated the medication well but close monitoring of side effects, including liver function abnormalities was required. A few patients in all of these studies required discontinuation due to side effects of therapy. All of these studies were limited by a number of factors. None of this research on methotrexate was controlled or blinded, making bias a significant concern. Also of importance, these studies were conducted prior to the advent of quantifiable numerical endpoints (e.g., PASI) making comparison of these results to newer trials very difficult.

Recently, there have been a few attempts to conduct research on methotrexate for psoriasis using more recently accepted clinical endpoints. A small, open label, study was conducted by Calis and Kreuger in patients with plaque psoriasis. These patients were started on 15 mg/week with their doses tritrated upward based on response to medication. This study, that attempted to mimic the common use pattern of methotrexate in the United States, produced a surprisingly low PASI75 response of 23% [5]. This response rate was the first using the PASI and is significantly lower than what would generally be considered to be an equivalent response in previously reported studies. A randomized, controlled trial of methotrexate in comparison to cyclosporine was also conducted by a large European cooperative group [28]. In this relatively small trial (n=88), the PASI 75 response at 16 weeks was 64%, significantly higher than that found in the earlier study. However, the protocol used for dosing methotrexate in this trial was significantly more aggressive and 11 of 43 (23%) of patients given methotrexate needed to stop therapy due to liver function test abnormalities. Though the total dose of methotrexate given to patients was not published with the study, it is clear that aggressive dosing with methotrexate can lead to great efficacy but tolerability with this drug is limited at high doses.

Safety and Tolerability

The most important toxicity associated with chronic methotrexate therapy is hepatic fibrosis and cirrhosis. The frequency of liver toxicity is somewhat controversial, with estimates of the rate of fibrosis between 1% and 50% and of cirrhosis of 0–25% [76, 53, 62, 79, 63, 46, 65]. The risk of hepatotoxicity increases with higher cumulative doses [74]. Interestingly, patients with rheumatoid arthritis have a significantly lower incidence of hepatoxicity compared to psoriatics when exposed to the same total doses [58]. Addition of folic acid may decrease the risk of hematologic and hepatotoxicity [48]. The rate of hepatic disease is related to other, co-morbid, conditions. The primary complicating factor is the use of alcohol [76]. Other conditions that increase the frequency of liver toxicity include advanced age, diabetes mellitus, obesity, and pre-existing liver disease [53, 41]. Investigators have demonstrated that excluding these higher risk patients results in a much lower rate of liver toxicity [46, 2, 14].

Unlike other medications in which liver toxicity is a concern, there is no reliable correlation between liver function test abnormalities and histologic evidence of hepatic fibrosis. Routine laboratories including liver function tests may miss liver toxicity induced by methotrexate [80]. As a result, the American Academy of Dermatology recommends periodic liver biopsies scheduled usually after a total cumulative dose of 1.5 g, based on the presence or absence of known risk factors for hepatic disease (see Table A6 [80]). Biopsies should be done at least 2 weeks after the last dose of methotrexate. Continuation of therapy is dictated by liver biopsy results (Table A7 [63]). The recommendations differ from those of the American College of Rheumatology where routine liver biopsies are not recommended [39], suggesting that there may indeed be inherent differences in liver responses to MTX in psoriasis patients versus rheumatoid arthritis patients.

In Europe, serum type 3 procollagen aminopeptide is under study as a marker for patients with liver fibrosis resulting from methotrexate [3] and could potentially replace secondary and subsequent liver biopsies if serial amino-terminal propeptide of type III procollagen levels are normal [77]. However, this marker is unrehable if arthritis is present.

Bone marrow suppression is a potential consequence of methotrexate therapy. Though extremely rare, pancytopenia can be potentially lethal. In general, anemia, leucopenia, and thrombocytopenia are reversible when methotrexate is stopped, though leucovorin rescue is sometimes necessary [63]. Acute toxicity may include hematologic abnormalities, specifically leucopenia and thrombocytopenia [6]. For leucopenia less than $3500/mm^3$ or thrombocytopenia $<100{,}000/mm^3$, one should consider suspending therapy and rechecking a CBC in two weeks [63]. Additionally, as macrocytic anemia may occur, folic acid supplementation 1–5 mg daily is traditionally added. The most important risk factors for bone marrow toxicity are increased methotrexate levels that can be brought on by renal insufficiency, functional folate deficiency, or decreased renal excretion brought on by drug interactions (see below).

Table A6. Methotrexate liver biopsy schedule

One or more risk factors present:
A baseline liver biopsy is recommended at or near start of therapy
Biopsies repeated every 1 g or sooner
If no risk factors are present:
Baseline biopsy at 1–1.5 g
Biopsies at every 1.5 g thereafter in patients with normal LFTs and not risk factors
Biopsies may not be warranted if:
Patients are elderly or those with limited life expectancy
Patients have a bleeding diathesis
Patients with cardiac instability
Patients with acute illness

Table A7. Liver biopsy histology and impact on therapy

	Grade I	Grade II	Grade IIIA	Grade IIIB	Grade IV
Fatty infiltration	Mild	Moderate/severe			
Nuclear variability	Mild	Moderate/severe			
Portal inflammation	Mild	Moderate/severe			
Necrosis		Moderate/severe			
Fibrosis			Mild	Moderate/severe	
Cirrhosis					Present
	Continue therapy		Continue therapy but rebiopsy in 6 months	Discontinue	Discontinue

Drugs that interfere with folate metabolism, like sulfa, trimethoprim, and dapsone can also lead to a rapid and dangerous pancytopenia when combined with methotrexate.

Though there have been a number of case reports, the potential increased incidence of lymphoma in patients taking low-dose methotrexate for psoriasis is controversial [56]. There are also reports of acute pneumonitis in association with methotrexate though this occurrence is extremely rare [60]. Pulmonary symptoms such as a dry cough or shortness of breath should be evaluated at each visit for possible methotrexate pneumonitis or pulmonary fibrosis.

Methotrexate is pregnancy category X; therefore, women who are of childbearing potential require special consideration. Women who are pregnant, actively trying to conceive, or breastfeeding are absolute exclusions from methotrexate therapy. Thus, after completing MTX therapy, a minimum of one ovulatory cycle is mandatory before considering conception. Additionally, since oligospermia and sperm abnormalities have been reported, men should ensure adequate contraception until they have been off methotrexate for 3 months [70, 51].

Concomitant medications, most notably trimethoprim-sulfamethoxazole antibiotics and numerous other nephrotoxic agents should be avoided. Of note, certain nonsteroidal anti-inflammatory agents (salicylate, naproxen, ibuprofen) may increase methotrexate levels [71]. Naproxen can be taken on days methotrexate is not taken. Other nonsteroidals, specifically piroxicam (Feldene), flurbiprofen (Ansaid), ketoprofen (Orudis), and the newer cyclooxygenase-2 (COX-2) inhibitors, especially celecoxib (Celebrex), rofecoxib (Vioxx), and meloxicam (Mobic), have little impact on methotrexate levels [71]. Traditionally, dermatologists have been more conservative than their rheumatology colleagues in following the exclusionary guidelines.

Gastrointestinal (nausea, vomiting) symptoms, fatigue, headaches, and hair loss are the most common patient complaints. Patients may experience less nausea if methotrexate is taken in two to three divided doses or if higher doses of folic acid are supplemented [15, 32]. Oftentimes, subcutaneous or intramuscular routes of administration may decrease the gastrointestinal symptoms. Erosions involving oral mucosa or cutaneous psoriatic lesions are uncommon and should prompt investigation for possible overdose. Folinic acid (leucovorin calcium or citrovorum factor) is the specific antidote for methotrexate overdose. If an overdose is suspected early empiric therapy with leucovorin 20 mg (10 mg/m^2) is advised without for the results of methotrexate blood levels.

Initiation and Continuation of Therapy

Prior to initiating methotrexate therapy, the following laboratory studies are undertaken: complete blood count with platelets (CBC), comprehensive metabolic panel [electrolytes, blood urea nitrogen (BUN), serum creatinine (Cr), liver transaminases (AST, ALT, GGT), albumin, and alkaline phosphatase], cholesterol, triglycerides, serum pregnancy test (HCG), and urinalysis. Additionally, testing for human immunodeficiency virus (HIV) and hepatitis panel (hepatitis B and C) are considered important additional tests. Since methotrexate is an immunosuppressant, questions regarding possible exposure to tuberculosis and even PPD testing are in order. Finally, investigation into ultraviolet exposure and resultant skin cancers, prior immunosuppressants, and general health maintenance issues regarding history of cervical dysplasia, abnormal mammograms, and results of regular screening tests (if applicable) for prostate and colon cancer are of importance prior to the administration of any immunosuppressant.

After reviewing concomitant medications (Table A8) and baseline laboratories, and the decision is made to commence methotrexate therapy, a test dose of 5 mg is given followed by a repeat CBC in approximately 7 days to assess for possible MTX idiosyncratic reactions and myelosuppression. Dosing, usually initially 10–15 mg/week, may be given in a variety of ways (see Table A9). For elderly patients or patients with known renal dysfunction, dosing should be started more conservatively (7.5 or 10 mg/week) to reduce the likelihood of toxicity. Pending clinical response, the dosage may

Table A8. Important methotrexate drug interactions

Antibiotics: cephalothin, penicillins ± probenacid, sulfonamides, tetracycline trimethoprim-sulfamethoxazole
Antiparasitic: pyrimethamine, *triamethamine*
Antiseizure: barbituates, phenytoin
Nuclear hormone analogs: retinoids (debated), steroids
Nonsteroidal anti-inflammatories: salicylates, phenylbutazone
Platelet antagonists: dipyridamole, salicylates
Uricosuric agents: probenacid, colchicines
Miscellaneous: cyclosporine (debated), ethanol, sulfonylureas

Table A9. Methotrexate formulations

Methotrexate pills: 2.5-mg pills given in a divided dose regimen every 12 h once a week or all pills taken at the same time once a week
Methotrexate solution: 25 mg/cc may be given subcutaneously, intramuscularly, or orally in a beverage once a week
Methotrexate sustained release: (Trexall 5, 7.5, 10, 15 mg)

IX

be increased up to a maximum of 30 mg a week. Failing significant improvement within 12 - weeks, alternative treatment modalities should be introduced.

Initially, laboratories, including LFTs and blood counts are obtained every other week and then monthly or every 6 weeks – the exact frequency of laboratories is determined by dose, renal function, and laboratory history. Additionally, full skin examinations are performed every 6 months for skin cancer surveillance.

Combination Therapy with Methotrexate

There are a number of possible combinations that may increase the efficacy of methotrexate, including both topical and systemic combinations. Traditional topical psoriasis medications (steroids, calcipotriene, tazarotene, and the immune modulators) have all been combined successfully with methotrexate. De Jong et al. recently reported that the addition of topical calcipotriol to MTX therapy reduced the cumulative doses of MTX required for efficacy and increased time to relapse after methotrexate was discontinuation (i.e. a MTX-sparing effect) [13].

Several combinations with MTX are not advised given the potential for increased toxicity. For example, both hydroxyurea and 6-thioguanine individually can cause bone marrow suppression [63, 42]. Additionally, combination with phototherapy must be carefully considered. Methotrexate may increase sensitivity to ultraviolet light and also increase the risk of skin cancers as with other immunosuppressants [68]; combination with PUVA must also be done with caution and only if the benefits outweigh the risks. Of note, combination with PUVA has resulted in a lower amount of UVA exposure to induce clearing [50]. Utility has also been seen in combinations with UVB – a pretreatment phase with methotrexate as monotherapy followed by combination with UVB [63].

Several combination regimens have been helpful and have an acceptable safety profile in certain patients. Combining methotrexate with retinoids has been cautioned by some due to the possibility of increased hepatotoxicity [75]; others have however found this combination helpful for refractory disease [37]. Additionally, the safety of combination with cyclosporine has also been cautioned [37]; however, we personally have found this combination safe, especially for short 2–3 month cycles – as have several authors in certain cases of refractory RA [50] and psoriasis ± arthritis (M. Lebwohl, personal communication) [8], allowing for lower dosages of each of the agents to be used.

Additionally, regarding combination with the biologics, there is a significant amount of data supporting the combination of methotrexate with either etanercept [49] or infliximab [33] in psoriasis, psoriatic arthritis, or other autoimmune diseases such as Crohn's disease or rheumatoid arthritis. A smaller number of patients ($n<50$) have been treated with methotrexate and alefacept (Biogen, data on file). Additionally, combination trials are ongoing at this time with efalizumab for psoriatic arthritis.

Cyclosporine

In 1978, Mueller and Herrmann observed and reported the incidental improvement of psoriasis with cyclosporine given for the purpose of preventing renal transplant rejection [52]. A formal study by Ellis et al. in 1991 proved the efficacy of cyclosporine for plaque psoriasis [18]. Thereafter, clinical trials led to the eventual FDA approval of cyclosporine for the treatment of psoriasis for one year of continuous therapy in the U.S. in 1997. In the U.K., two years of continuous dosing is considered acceptable.

Cyclosporine inhibits calcineurin mediated dephosphorylation of NF-AT (nuclear factor of activated T cells). As a result, the production of numerous cytokines (including IL-2), chemokines, and growth factors is inhibited. Additionally, antigen presentation by Langerhans cells or dermal dendritic cells is reduced [16, 19]. Finally, adhesion molecule expression, such as E-selectin and intracellular adhesion molecule-1 (ICAM-1), is inhibited [59]. These multiple effects result in a generalized T cell mediated suppression of the adaptive immune system that has been used in almost all T cell mediated diseases, including solid organ transplantation.

Cyclosporine is highly lipophilic and insoluble in water. Accordingly, cyclosporine absorption is dependent on the presence of a high-fat diet and bile salts and thus is quite variable day

Table A10. Cyclosporine interactions (full list on Novartis web site)

A. Increase levels	B. Decrease levels
Antibiotics	Antibiotics
Erythromycin	Rifampin
Norfloxacin	Nafcillin
Doxycycline	IV trimethoprim-sulfamethoxazole
Antifungals	Antifungals
Ketoconazole	Griseofulvin
Itraconazole	Anticonvulsants
Fluconazole	Carbamazepine
Calcium channel blockers	Phenytoin
Diltiazem	Phenobarbital
Nicardipine	
Verapamil	C. Increased nephrotoxicity (any agent that raises cyclosporine level may increase nephrotoxicity in addition):
Antidepressants	
Zoloft	NSAIDs
Antivirals	Aspirin
Indinavir	Indomethacin
Nelfinavir	Piroxicam
Ritonavir	Diclofenac
Acyclovir	Diuretics
Hormones	Furosemide
Androgens	Thiazides
Estrogens	Immunosuppressants
Steroids	Melphalan
Miscellaneous	Tacrolimus
Allopurinol	D. Special concerns
Amiodarone	Digoxin (nephrotoxicity)
	Lovastatin (rhabdomyolysis)
	Methotrexate (decreases renal clearance by 25%)

to day and person to person. The microemulsion formulations (Neoral and Gengraf) has higher and more predictable absorption profile. The dose conversion from Sandimmune to the microemulsion formulation Neoral or Gengraf is 1:1 [1]. The conversion can be made safely – some dose reductions may be required [1]. For the remainder of this chapter, we will only discuss cyclosporine in its microemulsion formulation.

The bioavailability of cyclosporine after oral administration is 30%. Peak plasma concentrations are reached after 1.5 h and the elimination half-life is approximately 15 h. Unlike methotrexate, cyclosporine undergoes extensive hepatic metabolism (including a prominent enterohepatic circuit) via the cytochrome p450 pathway and is excreted primarily (>80%) in the bile and feces. Therefore, medications that alter the CYP 450 pathway and those which decrease renal perfusion must be given with caution since the metabolism and excretion of cyclosporine will be altered (see Table A10).

IX

Efficacy

Cyclosporine was one of the first medications for psoriasis to be systematically tested in blinded, multi-center, placebo controlled trials. It has generally been considered to be the most efficacious of traditional, systemic treatments. In the first double-blind, placebo-controlled dose-finding study of cyclosporine, 85 patients with refractory psoriasis were randomized into four groups – either placebo, 3 mg, 5 mg, or 7.5 mg/kg per day. After 8 weeks, the PASI improvement from baseline was 0%, 39%, 58%, and 71% respectively [18]. Upon discontinuation, relapse occurred within a few months.

These results have been built upon by further placebo controlled trials. In a two-phase study, 181 patients were treated with cyclosporine for 5 mg/kg per day. Doses varied between 3–6 mg/kg per day to gain optimal clinical response while controlling for laboratory abnormalities. If subjects in this trial achieved a 70% reduction of involved body surface area at week 16, they were eligible for the maintenance phase in which patients were randomly assigned to placebo, 1.5 mg/kg per day or 3 mg/kg per day for an additional 24 weeks [67]. Over 80% of the patients (n=142) went on to the second phase of the study. The mean percentage decrease in PASI was 86% at the end of the induction phase. Maintenance therapy with 3 mg/kg per day was associated with a relapse rate (loss of 50% of baseline improvement) of 42%, while the 1.5 mg/ kg per day and placebo arms were associated with a relapse rate of 84% and a median time to relapse of 6 weeks. A study involving 251 patients with plaque psoriasis treated for 21 months with 2.5–5 mg kg per day demonstrated a PASI75 of 52% and 92% respectively [40]. Thus, it is clear that cyclosporine has significant efficacy in the treatment of psoriasis both in initial response to medication and maintenance of response in patients who continue to use the drug.

Safety and Tolerability

While cyclosporine is generally considered to be an extremely efficacious medication for psoriasis, its use has been limited by concerns for its safety in extended use. This medication is generally well tolerated by patients and can be used safely. However, cyclosporine has been associated with a number of potentially important side effects that need to be considered when using this therapy, including renal, cardiovascular, and malignant side effects. Moreover, there are a number of adverse effects of which physicians and patients should be aware.

Renal toxicity in patients taking cyclosporine can be acute or chronic. Acute nephrotoxicity can be induced by afferent arteriole vasoconstriction and a subsequent decrease in the glomerular filtration rate [78]. There are generally no permanent structural changes in the kidney associated with this reaction making these acute effects reversible. Chronic nephrotoxicity occurs from exposure to cyclosporine for more extended periods [66, 36]. Elevations in serum creatinine may occur in between 24% and 46% of patients treated with cyclosporine. Moreover, nearly all patients demonstrate histological abnormalities on kidney biopsy from

2.5 to 3.5 years of low-dose cyclosporine therapy [44].

Given the spectrum of renal toxicity seen with cyclosporine therapy, there is a definitive need for monitoring of kidney function. If the serum creatinine rises above 25% baseline values, dose reduction is mandatory and increased monitoring is required until renal function normalizes. The authors obtain a glomerular filtration rate study every 6 months while a patient is on cyclosporine since serum creatinine is an unpredictable indicator of toxicity in some patients [22]. Dose reduction is also warranted if blood pressure elevates on therapy. In some circumstances, addition of a calcium channel blocker such as amlodipine is necessary. Interestingly, there is data which supports the addition of calcium channel blockers (specifically amlodipine) since they may protect patients from cyclosporine induced nephrotoxicity [61].

Hypertension has been related to the use of cyclosporine and has been estimated to occur in between 8.5% to 27% of patients [21, 30]. This side effect generally occurs over months and is not associated with rapid increases in blood pressure [35]. The effects of cyclosporine on blood pressure are generally dose dependent but may require anti-hypertensive therapy along with dose reduction. As many of the adverse effects of cyclosporine on the kidney are mediated by calcium fluxes, it has been suggested that calcium channel blockers should be the anti-hypertensives of choice when treatment is required [21].

Other side effects are dose dependent and most commonly include headache, nausea, paresthesias, tremor, malaise, hypertrichosis and gingival hyperplasia [18]. The most common reason for discontinuation in the initial months is nausea while hypertension or decreased renal function accounts for discontinuations later in the course of therapy. While the risk of lymphoma in CyA treated transplant patients is well known, until recently, this has been hotly debated in psoriasis patients [57, 81]. A European prospective study did not, in fact, show any increased risk over its 5-year observational period [57]. The lymphoproliferative disorders are usually EBV-related and regress when the medication is withdrawn [45]. Solid tumors, including squamous cell carcinoma of the skin can occur in patients treated with cyclosporine [43, 29]. The risk for cutaneous SCC is most evident in patients who have received PUVA therapy in the past [47]. Lipids, particularly triglycerides, are frequently raised with this therapy; however, rarely is medical intervention necessary if a low-fat diet and increased exercise is initiated [25, 69].

Contraindications

Similar to methotrexate, concomitant active infections (including HIV or Hepatitis), noncompliance, and underlying active malignancy are considered contraindications. Additionally, uncontrolled hypertension and renal dysfunction excludes patients from this therapy. Unlike methotrexate, pregnancy is not a contraindication (category C); however cyclosporine should not be administered to women who are breastfeeding. Finally, patients who require live attenuated vaccination should avoid cyclosporine; and vaccinations in general may be less effective while on this therapy.

Therapy with Cyclosporine

Baseline evaluations for cyclosporine are essentially identical to methotrexate (see Table A11) with the addition of serum magnesium and blood pressure readings (two separate evaluations separated in time). A number of medications interact with cyclosporine and medications (prescription and over the counter) should be reviewed at each visit. Physical examination including blood pressure (two occasions) and evaluation of occult infection or malignancy (investigation into ultraviolet exposure and resultant skin cancers) is necessary. Finally, as with methotrexate, evaluation of general health issues regarding tuberculosis exposure, history of malignancies or prior immunosuppressants, and results of appropriate routine screening tests (specifically regarding cervical dysplasia, abnormal mammograms, prostate and colon) are also important.

Table A11. Methotrexate and cyclosporine evaluations. PPD, tuberculin skin test; HIV, human immunodeficiency virus antibody status; CMP, electrolytes + liver function tests (AST, ALT, albumin, total bilirubin) + serum creatinine + blood urea nitrogen; CBC, complete blood count; Chol, cholesterol; Tg, triglycerides; serum HCG, serum pregnancy; Mg, magnesium; UA, urinalysis; Glofil, glomerular filtration rate; skin exams: full skin examination for skin cancer surveillance

	Baseline		Follow-up	
	MTX	CyA	MTX	CyA
PPD	X	X		
Hepatitis B&C	X	X		
HIV	X	X		
CMP	X	X	Every 4–8 weeks	Every 4–6 weeks
CBC	X	X	2 weeks after full dose; 7 days after test dose; 4 weeks after full dose; if stable every 4–8 weeks	Every 4–6 weeks
CHOL	X	X	Every 4–6 weeks	Every 4–6 weeks
TG	X	X	Every 4–6 weeks	Every 4–6 weeks
Serum HCG	X	X	Monthly	Every 4–6 weeks
Mg		X		Every 4–6 weeks
UA		X		Every 4–6 weeks
Glofil		X		Every 6 months
Blood pressure		2 times		Daily for 2 weeks then weekly
Skin exam	X	X	Every 6 months	Every 6 months

Response of psoriasis to cyclosporine is dose dependent [17]. Initial doses may range from 2.5 to 5 mg/kg per day (given in divided doses) depending on the severity of the disease [1, 7]. Capsules are available in 25 mg or 100 mg while the solution is available as 100 mg of cyclosporine per 5 ml dispensed in 50 ml bottles. The microemulsion capsules should be taken with food. The solution is usually dispersed in apple or orange juice (not grapefruit since it has flavanoids which inhibit the CYP 450 pathway), and given in a glass (not plastic) container.

During therapy, laboratories are performed every 2 weeks for the first month and then monthly up to every 6 weeks if clinically indicated. It is important for patients to maintain this weekly blood pressure log as a gradual rise in baseline blood pressure readings usually predates changes in serum creatinine levels as an early indicator of CyA nephrotoxicity. As with methotrexate, full skin examinations are performed every 6 months for skin cancer surveillance.

Combination Therapy with Cyclosporine

As with methotrexate, numerous topicals have been used as concomitant therapy to reduce the amount or duration of cyclosporine required [24, 34, 23, 26]. As cyclosporine is a known cause of increased skin cancer risk in the transplant population, combination with ultraviolet therapy is contraindicated. An increased incidence of nonmelanoma skin cancer has been seen in patients who have had cyclosporine and PUVA therapy [57].

Combination with retinoids has been reported [38]; however, lipid levels must be followed more carefully since they are increased by both agents. We find this combination helpful in thick, hyperkeratotic plaque psoriasis that has not responded adequately to cyclosporine alone. Additionally, as mentioned above, combination with methotrexate in select patients has been useful, allowing for possible lower dosages. Regarding the biologics, less is known regarding the safety of cyclosporine based combinations. We have used the combination of cyclosporine with alefacept in a number of patients (especially when transitioning patients off CyA therapy) and have not noted any increased toxicity. A formal combination trial is currently underway. Regardless, the numbers of patients treated with cyclosporine and biologicals as combination therapy is small and it will take years to establish the safety profiles.

Conclusion

While much of the current literature on systemic therapy for psoriasis involves the new biologic agents, methotrexate and cyclosporine remain an important part of the psoriasis armamentarium. The long history of safe and effective usage of these agents, as well as the substantially lower cost than many newer medications, makes it likely that these two agents will continue to be used. Dermatologists have traditionally been more risk adverse than their rheumatology colleagues in using both cyclosporine A and methotrexate and in fact have only embraced cyclosporine A in very small numbers. The evident difference in liver responsiveness between the psoriasis and rheumatoid arthritis population and having recommendations for liver biopsies in psoriasis treated patients has also led to less than optimal adoption by a significant number of dermatologists. Despite these issues and with dermatologists penchant for optimizing therapies with combination drug schedules, methotrexate is particularly likely to play an important role in future psoriasis systemic therapy protocols, either as monotherapy, in combination therapy, particularly with biologicals, or in traditional sequential/rotational therapy.

References

1. Berth-Jones J, Voorhees JJ (1996) Consensus conference on cyclosporin A microemulsion for psoriasis, June 1996. Br J Dermatol 135:775–777
2. Boffa MJ, Chalmers RJ, Haboubi NY, Shomaf M, Mitchell DM (1995) Sequential liver biopsies during long-term methotrexate treatment for psoriasis: a reappraisal. Br J Dermatol 133:774–778
3. Boffa MJ, Smith A, Chalmers RJ, Mitchell DM, Rowan B, Warnes TW, Shomaf M, Haboubi NY (1996) Serum type III procollagen aminopeptide for assessing liver damage in methotrexate-treated psoriatic patients. Br J Dermatol 135:538–544
4. Callaway JL, McAfee WC, Finlayson GR (1966) Management of psoriasis using methotrexate orally in a single weekly dose. South Med J 59:424–426
5. Carlin CS, Feldman SR, Krueger JG, Menter A, Krueger CG (2003) A 50% reduction in the Psoriasis Area and Severity Index (PASI 50) is a clinically significant endpoint. J Invest Dermatol 121(1): 0393 (Abstract)
6. Casserly CM, Stange KC, Chren MM (1993) Severe megaloblastic anemia in a patient receiving low-dose methotrexate for psoriasis. J Am Acad Dermatol 29:477–480
7. Cather JC, Abramovits W, Menter A (2001) Cyclosporine and tacrolimus in dermatology. Dermatol Clin 19:119–137, ix
8. Clark CM, Kirby B, Morris AD, Davison S, Zaki I, Emerson R, Saihan EM, Chalmers RJ, Barker JN, Allen BR, Griffiths CE (1999) Combination treatment with methotrexate and cyclosporin for severe recalcitrant psoriasis. Br J Dermatol 141:279–282
9. Constantin A, Loubet-Lescoulie P, Lambert N, Yassine-Diab B, Abbal M, Mazieres B, de Preval C, Cantagrel A (1998) Antiinflammatory and immunoregulatory action of methotrexate in the treatment of rheumatoid arthritis: evidence of increased interleukin-4 and interleukin-10 gene expression demonstrated in vitro by competitive reverse transcriptase-polymerase chain reaction. Arthritis Rheum 41:48–57
10. Cronstein BN (1997) The mechanism of action of methotrexate. Rheum Dis Clin North Am 23: 739–755
11. Cronstein BN, Eberle MA, Gruber HE, Levin RI (1991) Methotrexate inhibits neutrophil function by stimulating adenosine release from connective tissue cells. Proc Natl Acad Sci U S A 88:2441–2445
12. Dayan M, Segal R, Mozes E (1997) Cytokine manipulation by methotrexate treatment in murine experimental systemic lupus erythematosus. J Rheumatol 24:1075–1082
13. de Jong EM, Mork NJ, Seijger MM, De La BM, Lauharanta J, Jansen CT, Guilhou JJ, Guillot B, Ostrojic A, Souteyrand P, Vaillant L, Barnes L, Rogers S, Klaber MR, van de Kerkhof PC (2003) The combination of calcipotriol and methotrexate compared with methotrexate and vehicle in psoriasis: results of a

multicentre placebo-controlled randomized trial. Br J Dermatol 148:318–325

14. Dooren-Greebe RJ, Kuijpers AL, Mulder J, De Boo T, van de Kerkhof PC (1994) Methotrexate revisited: effects of long-term treatment in psoriasis. Br J Dermatol 130:204–210
15. Duhra P (1993) Treatment of gastrointestinal symptoms associated with methotrexate therapy for psoriasis. J Am Acad Dermatol 28:466–469
16. Dupuy P, Bagot M, Michel L, Descourt B, Dubertret L (1991) Cyclosporin A inhibits the antigen-presenting functions of freshly isolated human Langerhans cells in vitro. J Invest Dermatol 96:408–413
17. Ellis CN, Fradin MS, Hamilton TA, Voorhees JJ (1995) Duration of remission during maintenance cyclosporine therapy for psoriasis. Relationship to maintenance dose and degree of improvement during initial therapy. Arch Dermatol 131:791–795
18. Ellis CN, Fradin MS, Messana JM, Brown MD, Siegel MT, Hartley AH, Rocher LL, Wheeler S, Hamilton TA, Parish TG (1991) Cyclosporine for plaque-type psoriasis. Results of a multidose, double-blind trial. N Engl J Med 324:277–284
19. Furue M, Katz SI (1988) The effect of cyclosporine on epidermal cells. I. Cyclosporine inhibits accessory cell functions of epidermal Langerhans cells in vitro. J Immunol 140:4139–4143
20. Genestier L, Paillot R, Fournel S, Ferraro C, Miossec P, Revillard JP (1998) Immunosuppressive properties of methotrexate: apoptosis and clonal deletion of activated peripheral T cells. J Clin Invest 102: 322–328
21. Georgouras KE, Zagarella SS, Cains GD, Brown PJ (1997) Systemic treatment of severe psoriasis. Australas J Dermatol 38:171–180
22. Gilbert SC, Emmett M, Menter A, Silverman A, Klintmalm G (1989) Cyclosporine therapy for psoriasis: serum creatinine measurements are an unreliable predictor of decreased renal function. J Am Acad Dermatol 21:470–474
23. Gottlieb SL, Heftler NS, Gilleaudeau P, Johnson R, Vallat VP, Wolfe J, Gottlieb AB, Krueger JG (1995) Short-contact anthralin treatment augments therapeutic efficacy of cyclosporine in psoriasis: a clinical and pathologic study. J Am Acad Dermatol 33: 637–645
24. Griffiths CE, Powles AV, Baker BS, Fry L, Valdimarsson H (1988) Combination of cyclosporine A and topical corticosteroid in the treatment of psoriasis. Transplant Proc 20:50–52
25. Grossman RM, Delaney RJ, Brinton EA, Carter DM, Gottlieb AB (1991) Hypertriglyceridemia in patients with psoriasis treated with cyclosporine. J Am Acad Dermatol 25:648–651
26. Grossman RM, Thivolet J, Claudy A, Souteyrand P, Guilhou JJ, Thomas P, Amblard P, Belaich S, de Belilovsky C, de la BM (1994) A novel therapeutic approach to psoriasis with combination calcipotriol ointment and very low-dose cyclosporine: results of a multicenter placebo-controlled study. J Am Acad Dermatol 31:68–74
27. Gubner R (1951) Effect of aminopterin on epithelial tissues. AMA. Arch Derm Syphilol 64:688–699
28. Heydendael VM, Spuls PI, Opmeer BC, de Borgie CA, Reitsma JB, Goldschmidt WF, Bossuyt PM, Bos JD, de Rie MA (2003) Methotrexate versus cyclosporine in moderate-to-severe chronic plaque psoriasis. N Engl J Med 349:658–665
29. Hiesse C, Larue JR, Kriaa F, Blanchet P, Bellamy J, Benoit G, Charpentier B (1995) Incidence and type of malignancies occurring after renal transplantation in conventionally and in cyclosporine-treated recipients: single-center analysis of a 20-year period in 1600 patients. Transplant Proc 27:2450–2451
30. Ho VC, Griffiths CE, Berth-Jones J, Papp KA, Vanaclocha F, Dauden E, Beard A, Puvanarajan L, Paul C (2001) Intermittent short courses of cyclosporine microemulsion for the long-term management of psoriasis: a 2-year cohort study. J Am Acad Dermatol 44:643–651
31. Jeffes EW III, McCullough JL, Pittelkow MR, McCormick A, Almanzor J, Liu G, Dang M, Voss K, Voss J, Schlotzhauer A (1995) Methotrexate therapy of psoriasis: differential sensitivity of proliferating lymphoid and epithelial cells to the cytotoxic and growth-inhibitory effects of methotrexate. J Invest Dermatol 104:183–188
32. Kirby B, Lyon CC, Griffiths CE, Chalmers RJ (2000) The use of folic acid supplementation in psoriasis patients receiving methotrexate: a survey in the United Kingdom. Clin Exp Dermatol 25:265–268
33. Kirby B, Marsland AM, Carmichael AJ, Griffiths CE (2001) Successful treatment of severe recalcitrant psoriasis with combination infliximab and methotrexate. Clin Exp Dermatol 26:27–29
34. Kokelj F, Torsello P, Plozzer C (1998) Calcipotriol improves the efficacy of cyclosporine in the treatment of psoriasis vulgaris. J Eur Acad Dermatol Venereol 10:143–146
35. Koo J (1999) Systemic sequential therapy of psoriasis: a new paradigm for improved therapeutic results. J Am Acad Dermatol 41:S25–S28
36. Kopp JB, Klotman PE (1990) Cellular and molecular mechanisms of cyclosporin nephrotoxicity. J Am Soc Nephrol 1:162–179
37. Korstanje MJ, Breda Vriesman CJ, van de Staak WJ (1990) Cyclosporine and methotrexate: a dangerous combination. J Am Acad Dermatol 23:320–321
38. Korstanje MJ, van de Staak WJ (1990) Combination-therapy cyclosporin-A – etretinate for psoriasis. Clin Exp Dermatol 15:172–173
39. Kremer JM, Alarcon GS, Lightfoot RW Jr, Willkens RF, Furst DE, Williams HJ, Dent PB, Weinblatt ME (1994) Methotrexate for rheumatoid arthritis. Suggested guidelines for monitoring liver toxicity. American College of Rheumatology. Arthritis Rheum 37:316–328
40. Laburte C, Grossman R, Abi-Rached J, Abeywickrama KH, Dubertret L (1994) Efficacy and safety of oral cyclosporin A (CyA; Sandimmun) for long-term treatment of chronic severe plaque psoriasis. Br J Dermatol 130:366–375

41. Lanse SB, Arnold GL, Gowans JD, Kaplan MM (1985) Low incidence of hepatotoxicity associated with long-term, low-dose oral methotrexate in treatment of refractory psoriasis, psoriatic arthritis, and rheumatoid arthritis. An acceptable risk/benefit ratio. Dig Dis Sci 30: 104–109
42. Lebwohl M, Ali S (2001) Treatment of psoriasis, part 2. Systemic therapies. J Am Acad Dermatol 45: 649–661
43. London NJ, Farmery SM, Will EJ, Davison AM, Lodge JP (1995) Risk of neoplasia in renal transplant patients. Lancet 346: 403–406
44. Lowe NJ, Wieder JM, Rosenbach A, Johnson K, Kunkel R, Bainbridge C, Bourget T, Dimov I, Simpson K, Glass E, Grabie MT (1996) Long-term low-dose cyclosporine therapy for severe psoriasis: effects on renal function and structure. J Am Acad Dermatol 35: 710–719
45. Mahe E, Descamps V, Grossin M, Fraitag S, Crickx B (2003) CD30+ T-cell lymphoma in a patient with psoriasis treated with ciclosporin and infliximab. Br J Dermatol 149: 170–173
46. Malatjalian DA, Ross JB, Williams CN, Colwell SJ, Eastwood BJ (1996) Methotrexate hepatotoxicity in psoriatics: report of 104 patients from Nova Scotia, with analysis of risks from obesity, diabetes and alcohol consumption during long term follow-up. Can J Gastroenterol 10: 369–375
47. Marcil I, Stern RS (2001) Squamous-cell cancer of the skin in patients given PUVA and ciclosporin: nested cohort crossover study. Lancet 358: 1042–1045
48. McClure SL, Valentine J, Gordon KB (2002) Comparative tolerability of systemic treatments for plaque-type psoriasis. Drug Saf 25: 913–927
49. Mease PJ, Goffe BS, Metz J, VanderStoep A, Finck B, Burge DJ (2000) Etanercept in the treatment of psoriatic arthritis and psoriasis: a randomised trial. Lancet 356: 385–390
50. Morison WL, Momtaz K, Parrish JA, Fitzpatrick TB (1982) Combined methotrexate-PUVA therapy in the treatment of psoriasis. J Am Acad Dermatol 6: 46–51
51. Morris LF, Harrod MJ, Menter MA, Silverman AK (1993) Methotrexate and reproduction in men: case report and recommendations. J Am Acad Dermatol 29: 913–916
52. Mueller W, Herrmann B (1979) Cyclosporin A for psoriasis. N Engl J Med 301: 555
53. Nyfors A (1977) Liver biopsies from psoriatics related to methotrexate therapy. 3. Findings in post-methotrexate liver biopsies from 160 psoriatics. Acta Pathol Microbiol Scand [A] 85: 511–518
54. Nyfors A (1978) Benefits and adverse drug experiences during long-term methotrexate treatment of 248 psoriatics. Dan Med Bull 25: 208–211
55. Olsen EA (1991) The pharmacology of methotrexate. J Am Acad Dermatol 25: 306–318
56. Paul C, Le Tourneau A, Cayuela JM, Devidas A, Robert C, Molinie V, Dubertret L (1997) Epstein-Barr virus-associated lymphoproliferative disease during methotrexate therapy for psoriasis. Arch Dermatol 133: 867–871
57. Paul CF, Ho VC, McGeown C, Christophers E, Schmidtmann B, Guillaume JC, Lamarque V, Dubertret L (2003) Risk of malignancies in psoriasis patients treated with cyclosporine: a 5 y cohort study. J Invest Dermatol 120: 211–216
58. Petrazzuoli M, Rothe MJ, Grin-Jorgensen C, Ramsey WH, Grant-Kels JM (1994) Monitoring patients taking methotrexate for hepatotoxicity. Does the standard of care match published guidelines? J Am Acad Dermatol 31: 969–977
59. Petzelbauer P, Stingl G, Wolff K, Volc-Platzer B (1991) Cyclosporin A suppresses ICAM-1 expression by papillary endothelium in healing psoriatic plaques. J Invest Dermatol 96: 362–369
60. Phillips TJ, Jones DH, Baker H (1987) Pulmonary complications following methotrexate therapy. J Am Acad Dermatol 16: 373–375
61. Raman GV, Campbell SK, Farrer A, Albano JD, Cook J (1998) Modifying effects of amlodipine on cyclosporin A-induced changes in renal function in patients with psoriasis. J Hypertens Suppl 16: S39–S41
62. Robinson JK, Baughman RD, Auerbach R, Cimis RJ (1980) Methotrexate hepatotoxicity in psoriasis. Consideration of liver biopsies at regular intervals. Arch Dermatol 116: 413–415
63. Roenigk HH Jr, Auerbach R, Maibach H, Weinstein G, Lebwohl M (1998) Methotrexate in psoriasis: consensus conference. J Am Acad Dermatol 38: 478–485
64. Roenigk HH Jr, Fowler-Bergfeld W, Curtis GH (1969) Methotrexate for psoriasis in weekly oral doses. Arch Dermatol 99: 86–93
65. Roenigk HH Jr, Maibach HI, Weinstein GP (1973) Methotrexate therapy for psoriasis. Guideline revisions. Arch Dermatol 108: 35
66. Ruiz P, Kolbeck PC, Scroggs MW, Bollinger RR, Sanfilippo F (1988) Cyclosporine therapy and the development of interstitial fibrosis in renal allografts. Transplant Proc 20: 807–811
67. Shupack J, Abel E, Bauer E, Brown M, Drake L, Freinkel R, Guzzo C, Koo J, Levine N, Lowe N, McDonald C, Margolis D, Stiller M, Wintroub B, Bainbridge C, Evans S, Hilss S, Mietlowski W, Winslow C, Birnbaum JE (1997) Cyclosporine as maintenance therapy in patients with severe psoriasis. J Am Acad Dermatol 36: 423–432
68. Stern RS, Laird N (1994) The carcinogenic risk of treatments for severe psoriasis. Photochemotherapy Follow-up Study. Cancer 73: 2759–2764
69. Stiller MJ, Pak GH, Kenny C, Jondreau L, Davis I, Wachsman S, Shupack JL (1992) Elevation of fasting serum lipids in patients treated with low-dose cyclosporine for severe plaque-type psoriasis. An assessment of clinical significance when viewed as a risk factor for cardiovascular disease. J Am Acad Dermatol 27: 434–438
70. Sussman A, Leonard JM (1980) Psoriasis, methotrexate, and oligospermia. Arch Dermatol 116: 215–217

71. Tracy TS, Krohn K, Jones DR, Bradley JD, Hall SD, Brater DC (1992) The effects of a salicylate, ibuprofen, and naproxen on the disposition of methotrexate in patients with rheumatoid arthritis. Eur J Clin Pharmacol 42:121–125
72. Weinstein GD, Frost P (1971) Methotrexate for psoriasis. A new therapeutic schedule. Arch Dermatol 103:33–38
73. Weinstein GD, Velasco J (1972) Selective action of methotrexate on psoriatic epidermal cells. J Invest Dermatol 59:121–127
74. Whiting-O'Keefe QE, Fye KH, Sack KD (1991) Methotrexate and histologic hepatic abnormalities: a meta-analysis. Am J Med 90:711–716
75. Zachariae H (1990) Methotrexate side-effects. Br J Dermatol 122 Suppl 36:127–133
76. Zachariae H, Grunnet E, Sogaard H (1975) Liver biopsy in methotrexate-treated psoriatics – a re-evaluation. Acta Derm Venereol 55:291–296
77. Zachariae H, Heickendorff L, Sogaard H (2001) The value of amino-terminal propeptide of type III procollagen in routine screening for methotrexate-induced liver fibrosis: a 10-year follow-up. Br J Dermatol 144:100–103
78. Zachariae H, Kragballe K, Hansen HE, Marcussen N, Olsen S (1997) Renal biopsy findings in long-term cyclosporin treatment of psoriasis. Br J Dermatol 136:531–535
79. Zachariae H, Sogaard H (1987) Methotrexate-induced liver cirrhosis. A follow-up. Dermatologica 175:178–182
80. Zachariae H, Sogaard H, Heickendorff L (1996) Methotrexate-induced liver cirrhosis. Clinical, histological and serological studies – a further 10-year follow-up. Dermatology 192:343–346
81. Zackheim HS, Koo J, LeBoit PE, McCalmont TH, Bowman PH, Kashani-Sabet M, Jones C, Zehnder J (2002) Psoriasiform mycosis fungoides with fatal outcome after treatment with cyclosporine. J Am Acad Dermatol 47:155–157

B Psoriatic Arthritis

Christopher G. Jackson,
Daniel O. Clegg

Contents

1 Introduction

Ideal therapy for psoriatic arthritis (PsA) should target both rash and joint disease including peripheral and axial presentations, dactylitis, and enthesitis. The significant impact of PsA on quality of life is increasingly evident and comparable in severity to that of rheumatoid arthritis [1, 2]. Therefore, essential aims of therapy must include not only symptomatic improvement but also treatment directed at potential disease modification/amelioration. However, traditional disease modifying antirheumatic drug (DMARD) therapy, as detailed below, has been poorly studied in PsA. Uncontrolled experience has suggested modest efficacy for some DMARDs but these observations are especially difficult to interpret given the consistently high placebo response rates (three times as high as in RA) present in controlled PsA trials. Few well-designed, adequately-controlled randomized trials with traditional DMARDs have been performed, and the overall efficacy observed to date has been disappointing. Problematic trial design such as the difficulty in defining different disease PsA subgroups and the uncertain distribution of these subgroups between placebo and treatment arms additionally complicates the extrapolation of available data to clinical decision-making for the individual patient (see Chap. IV.B. for a discussion of disease subgroups in PsA). The latest advances in therapy for PsA appear promising and will be detailed in Chap. X.B.2; the important development of more reliable outcome measures incorporating symptomatic, functional, and radiologic end points are described in Chap. VI.B.

2 NSAIDs

Non-steroidal anti-inflammatory drugs (NSAIDs) are commonly prescribed as the initial therapy for both peripheral and axial disease. Placebo-controlled studies assessing efficacy are limited but confirm NSAID superiority in reducing tender/swollen joint counts and pain scores. No beneficial effect on rash (assessed by PASI score) or on ESR has been demonstrated to suggest that NSAIDs have a disease modifying effect [3]. Worsening of skin disease with initiation of NSAID therapy has been observed for both non-specific and COX2-specific NSAIDs [4–6], perhaps due to shunting of arachidonic acid metabolites down the leukotriene pathway; however, other controlled studies suggest this is not a major clinical issue [3]. No unusual toxicity associated with the use of NSAIDs in PsA has been reported.

3 Glucocorticoids

Periodic intra-articular injection of corticosteroid can be of particular value in patients with oligoarticular disease or those having well-controlled polyarticular disease except for one or two persistently active joints. In recently-devised guidelines, two failed injections are considered sufficient evidence of aggressive disease as to warrant consideration of anti-TNF therapy [7]. In general, systemic use of glucocorticoids should be used judiciously because of the risk of provoking a pustular flare in the skin disease on withdrawal [8].

4 Conventional DMARDS

Sulfasalazine

IX

The efficacy of sulfasalazine in RA and other seronegative arthritides led to its initial use in PsA. Benefit was suggested in a number of pilot studies, and several early controlled trials documented a modest degree of clinical improvement. Typical of these early controlled trials [9] is a 24-week double-blind placebo-controlled study of 30 patients using a dose of 2 g/day. Significant improvement was observed in morning stiffness, number of painful joints, articular index, clinical score, and pain score, with the favorable response being more pronounced in patients with polyarticular disease [10]. Clinical benefit was observed as early as 4 weeks in one study [11] and was associated with a reduction in ESR in another [12].

Three further trials involving considerably larger numbers of patients reached similar conclusions, with efficacy being primarily observed in patient-reported measures. A study of 91 patients treated with a dose of 3 g/day over 24 weeks revealed significant improvement in patient global assessment [13] whereas a study of 120 patients treated for a similar period demonstrated significant improvement only in reduction of pain [14]. In the largest and longest controlled trial, which evaluated 221 patients treated with 2 g/day over 36 weeks, patient global assessment was the only efficacy parameter to achieve statistically significant improvement [15]. Benefit with sulfasalazine appears to be confined to peripheral PsA as no improvement in axial disease has been demonstrated [16]. Only rare reports exist of either improvement or exacerbation in cutaneous disease activity with sulfasalazine therapy.

Methotrexate

The efficacy of methotrexate in PsA was first demonstrated in 1964 in a double-blind placebo-controlled study of 21 patients with active skin disease and peripheral arthritis [17]. Three doses of parenteral methotrexate (1–3 mg/kg) were administered at 10-day intervals and patients followed for approximately 3 months. Significant improvement in joint tenderness, joint range of motion, extent of skin involvement, and erythrocyte sedimentation rate was documented, but the majority of patients experienced a recurrence of skin and joint disease within 1–4 months following therapy. Adverse events were not infrequent but were not judged severe enough to interrupt treatment.

A subsequent randomized, double-blind, placebo-controlled trial with methotrexate administered in an oral low-dose pulse regimen (7.5–15 mg/week) over 12 weeks showed better patient tolerance. However, the only response measure to attain statistical significance was the physician assessment of arthritis activity [18]. In a retrospective report of 40 patients treated over 12 years with a mean methotrexate dose of 11.2 mg/week, 38 patients had an excellent or good articular response, 36 had cutaneous resolution, and only two withdrew due to toxicity (leukopenia and stomatitis) [19]. Seven patients underwent 11 liver biopsies during the study period, with one patient found to have micronodular cirrhosis at a cumulative methotrexate dose of 400 mg (with an unchanged biopsy at a cumulative dose of 1080 mg). Whether the use of methotrexate in PsA patients results in more frequent or severe toxicity compared with RA patients remains uncertain but no increase in adverse events was suggested in a retrospective study of 104 patients followed over 2 decades [20]. No consensus exists as to the indications for liver biopsy in methotrexate-treated PsA patients. In a 24-month study of 38 patients, no improvement in radiographic progression was seen with methotrexate compared to matched controls [21].

Oral and Parenteral Gold

Improvement in some clinical parameters has been observed following treatment with both oral and parenteral gold in PsA. In a 6-month double-blind placebo-controlled study of auranofin (6 mg/day) involving 238 patients, the auranofin-treated group showed modest but significant improvement in physician's global assessment as well as in occupational and daily function scores compared with the placebo group. No significant difference was seen in either morning stiffness or joint tenderness/swelling [22]. The rate of withdrawal from auranofin due to adverse drug reactions was 10%.

An uncontrolled study of parenteral gold reported remission or 50% reduction in number of inflamed joints in 10 of 14 patients [23] with toxicity similar to that observed in RA. A double-blind comparison of auranofin (6 mg/day), intramuscular gold sodium thiomalate (50 mg/week), and placebo demonstrated significant improvement in the Ritchie articular index, the visual analog pain score, and the erythrocyte sedimentation rate (ESR) over 24 weeks for the parenteral gold group while the auranofin group was comparable to placebo [24]. No improvement in radiographic disease progression was seen in a small controlled 2-year study of parenteral gold. Neither oral nor parenteral gold has been associated with significant flare or improvement in cutaneous psoriasis.

When comparisons have been made retrospectively [25] and prospectively [26] between gold and methotrexate therapy, PsA patients treated with methotrexate appear to be 9 times more likely to respond and 5 times less likely to discontinue therapy compared to gold-treated patients. The observed mean treatment survival with methotrexate was 16 months compared to 6 months with gold therapy.

Leflunomide

Leflunomide is a selective pyrimidine synthesis inhibitor that targets activated T cells unable to rely solely on a salvage pathway for expansion [27]. An open-label study of six patients with psoriatic polyarthritis showed a significant decrease in CRP level as well as in the tender and swollen joint count but not in the extent of psoriasis after 3 months of therapy [28]. Another study conducted in 12 patients with polyarticular PsA who had failed at least one DMARD confirmed the clinical efficacy of leflunomide in the 8 patients available for follow-up after 2 years [29]. Psoriatic rash improved in two-thirds of the patients.

These promising results led to a randomized double blind placebo controlled study of 6 months duration in 188 patients with active psoriatic arthritis (>3 tender and swollen joints) and active rash (>3% body surface area). More than half of the patients had been inadequately controlled by prior DMARD therapy including methotrexate. Fifty-nine percent (59%) of leflunomide treated patients met the primary efficacy endpoint (psoriatic arthritis response criteria; PsARC) compared with 29.7% of placebo treated patients. Additionally, 24% of leflunomide-treated patients (compared with 0% placebo-treated) had significant PASI score improvements. Treatment was relatively well tolerated with adverse effects similar to the RA experience and no unusual toxicity was reported [30]. Leflunomide is a teratogen and should be used with care in women of childbearing potential.

Azathioprine and 6-Mercaptopurine

Reports of benefit with the purine analog, azathioprine, and its derivative, 6-mercaptopurine, exist for both psoriasis and PsA; however, the study populations are small and no placebo-controlled data are available. Eleven of 13 patients treated with 6-mercaptopurine (20–50 mg/kg per day) showed improvement in both joint and skin disease within 3 weeks of initiation of therapy, with maintenance of this improvement on a dose of 1 mg/kg per day which produced only minimal adverse effects [31]. A 12-month double-blind crossover study of azathioprine (3 mg/kg per day) in six patients demonstrated moderate or marked joint improvement in all six patients with cutaneous improvement in four but patient tolerance was poor with the dose of azathioprine having to be reduced in five patients because of leukopenia.

Cyclosporine A

Cyclosporine A has been reported to be of possible benefit in both cutaneous psoriasis and PsA. A small 6-month open study of PsA patients (seven of whom were refractory to methotrexate) treated with a starting dose of 3.5 mg/kg per day produced marked improvement in joint and skin disease in seven of eight patients after 2 months [32]. There was one withdrawal from the study because of lack of efficacy, while three patients required a 25% reduction in the cyclosporine A dose due to a 50% increase in serum creatinine. A prospective controlled trial comparing cyclosporine A (3 mg/kg per day) with methotrexate (7.5 mg weekly) over a 1-year period reported equivalent efficacy in 35 patients but combined withdrawals due lack of efficacy and toxicity were greater in the cyclosporine A group [33].

A single 6-month pilot trial of cyclosporine A (3–5 mg/kg per day) in combination with methotrexate (10–15 mg/week) in eight patients who had failed prior second-line therapy demonstrated significant improvement in all patients during the first month of therapy and persistent benefit for five throughout the study period [34]. Further studies are needed to define the benefit and toxicity of combination therapy in PsA.

Antimalarial Agents

Chloroquine (250 mg/day) and hydroxychloroquine (200–400 mg/day) appear to produce some clinical benefit in approximately 75% of PsA patients who have been studied but may be associated with a significant adverse effect on the skin disease. The spectrum of suspected cutaneous toxicity includes exacerbation of plaques, photosensitivity, generalized erythroderma, evolution to pustular psoriasis, and/or the development of an exfoliative dermatitis. The reported incidence of these reactions has ranged from 0% to 100%. It is important to note that more frequent reactions were observed in early trials that had fewer patients and primarily utilized regimens with quinacrine, while much less toxicity has been seen in more recent trials involving larger numbers of patients treated with chloroquine or hydroxychloroquine [35].

D-Penicillamine

A favorable effect on psoriatic arthritis has been observed with the use of D-penicillamine, but the available information is anecdotal and very limited. Eleven patients (two with spondylitis, four with asymmetric oligoarthritis, and five with symmetric polyarthritis) were randomized to an initial phase consisting of treatment with either D-penicillamine or placebo for 4 months [36], followed by 4 months of treatment with D-penicillamine for all patients. The maximum dose of D-penicillamine was 750 mg/ day, and no unusual toxicity was observed. Clinical benefit was seen only during D-penicillamine treatment; however, no efficacy measure attained statistically significant improvement.

Colchicine

Colchicine is an alkaloid known to attenuate inflammatory activity by interfering with neutrophil chemotaxis. A pilot study reported that 11 of 22 patients with psoriasis treated with colchicine (0.02 mg/kg/day) had significant cutaneous clearing with four of eight patients with arthralgias being symptomatically improved [37]. A subsequent 16-week, double-blind placebo-controlled crossover study of 15 PsA patients treated with colchicine 1.5 mg/day demonstrated efficacy in 10 of the 12 patients (83%)

[38]. Statistical improvement was seen in grip strength, Ritchie index, joint pain, joint swelling, and patient global assessment with colchicine treatment. Gastrointestinal symptoms required the withdrawal of two patients from the study and a temporary dose reduction in five other patients. No unanticipated clinical or laboratory toxicity was seen.

Mycophenolate Mofetil

Mycophenolate mofetil reversibly inhibits the *de novo* pathway of purine synthesis, resulting in suppression of B and T lymphocyte activation [39]. The primary use of mycophenolate mofetil at present is in organ transplantation, although a preliminary investigation in RA has suggested benefit [40]. A potential role in PsA has also been suggested from an open trial in which three of six patients with refractory disease experienced significant improvement [41]. No corresponding improvement in skin disease was seen. There were no withdrawals due to toxicity, and no serious adverse reactions were reported. Further study will be needed to confirm and extend these preliminary observations of benefit.

Retinoids

Etretinate, a vitamin A derivative, is the most commonly used retinoid in the treatment of psoriasis, and limited experience with this agent in PsA has suggested a beneficial effect. In a pilot study of 40 patients treated with etretinate (50 mg/day) for a mean of 21.9 weeks, significant improvement in the number of tender joints, the duration of morning stiffness, and the erythrocyte sedimentation rate was observed [42] with maximal improvement for most efficacy measurements observed at 12–16 weeks. Mucocutaneous reactions consisting of dried and cracked lips, mouth soreness, and nosebleeds were common (39 of 40 patients) and required cessation of treatment in nine patients. Other relatively frequent adverse effects were alopecia, hyperlipidemia, myalgias, and elevated transaminase levels. Etretinate is a teratogen and should not be used in women of child-bearing potential.

Photochemotherapy

The most commonly used form of photochemotherapy involves the oral administration of 8-methoxypsoralen followed by exposure to long-wave ultraviolet-A light (PUVA). A prospective study of 27 patients treated with PUVA found a favorable response in 49% of patients with peripheral arthritis whereas no benefit was seen in patients with spondylitis [43]. In responders, improvement in the peripheral arthritis seemed to correlate with clearing of the skin disease, but no such relationship was observed in patients with axial disease. Extracorporeal photochemotherapy, also known as photopheresis, is associated with a decrease in the in vitro viability, proliferation, and mitogen response of lymphocytes but clinical improvement in arthritis symptoms is variable and no improvement in skin disease has been observed [44, 45].

Somatostatin

Somatostatin may benefit some PsA patients but requires prolonged intravenous infusion (48 h) and is poorly tolerated because of nausea. In one study, patients having more extensive skin lesions and polyarticular joint disease appeared more responsive [46].

Miscellaneous

Very preliminary reports of benefit in patients with PsA exist, mostly in the form of case reports, for a number of other therapies with agents have immunomodulating therapies common to traditional DMARDs. Excluding the cytokine inhibitors and other biologic therapies which are discussed in Chap. X.B, these include bromocriptine, cimetidine, fumaric acid, 2-chlorodeoxyadenosine, parenteral nitrogen mustard, peptide T, radiation synovectomy with yttrium-90, dietary supplements, total lymph node irradiation, and autologous stem cell transplantation. Further study is needed to define what role, if any, these regimens might have in patient management.

5 Conclusion

For a disease as prevalent as PsA, the evidence base supporting the efficacy of traditional DMARDs is very limited. Marginal benefit with sulfasalazine and, perhaps, gold has been demonstrated for peripheral PsA but the rationale for methotrexate and cyclosporin remains largely empiric despite their common use and established efficacy in cutaneous disease. No traditional DMARD has been shown to prevent radiographic progression nor has any significant impact on dactylitis, enthesitis, or axial disease been evident. Renewed interest in PsA clinical research has highlighted the need for better definition, standardization and validation of disease-specific outcome measures. With improved methodology, more rigorous clinical investigation will be possible to better define the proper place of conventional DMARDs in the treatment of PsA, whether as monotherapy, in combination with each other, or with newer biologic agents.

References

1. Husted JA, et al. (2001) Health-related quality of life of patients with psoriatic arthritis: a comparison with patients with rheumatoid arthritis. Arthritis Rheum 45:151–158
2. Rahman P, et al. (2001) Comparison of radiological severity in psoriatic arthritis and rheumatoid arthritis. J Rheumatol 28:1041–1044
3. Sarzi-Puttini P, et al. (2001) The role of NSAIDs in psoriatic arthritis: evidence from a controlled study with nimesulide. Clin Exp Rheumatol 19 (1 Suppl 22):S17–S20
4. Meyerhoff JO (1983) Exacerbation of psoriasis with meclofenamate. N Engl J Med 309:496
5. Clark DW, Coulter DM (2003) Psoriasis associated with rofecoxib. Arch Dermatol 139:1223
6. Ben-Chetrit E, Rubinow A (1986) Exacerbation of psoriasis by ibuprofen. Cutis 38:45
7. Maksymowych WP, et al. (2003) Canadian Rheumatology Association Consensus on the use of anti-tumor necrosis factor-alpha directed therapies in the treatment of spondyloarthritis. J Rheumatol 30:1356–1363
8. Baker H, Ryan TJ (1968) Generalized pustular psoriasis. A clinical and epidemiological study of 104 cases. Br J Dermatol 80:771–793
9. Farr M, et al. (1990) Sulphasalazine in psoriatic arthritis: a double-blind placebo-controlled study. Br J Rheumatol 29:46–49
10. Gupta AK, et al. (1995) Sulfasalazine therapy for psoriatic arthritis: a double blind, placebo controlled trial. J Rheumatol 22:894–898
11. Fraser SM, et al. (1993) Sulphasalazine in the management of psoriatic arthritis. Br J Rheumatol 32:923–925
12. Dougados M, et al. (1995) Sulfasalazine in the treatment of spondylarthropathy. A randomized, multicenter, double-blind, placebo-controlled study. Arthritis Rheum 38:618–627
13. Combe B, et al. (1996) Sulphasalazine in psoriatic arthritis: a randomized, multicentre, placebo-controlled study. Br J Rheumatol 35:664–668
14. Rahman P, et al. (1998) The use of sulfasalazine in psoriatic arthritis: a clinic experience. J Rheumatol 25:1957–1961
15. Clegg DO, et al. (1996) Comparison of sulfasalazine and placebo in the treatment of psoriatic arthritis. A Department of Veterans Affairs Cooperative Study. Arthritis Rheum 39:2013–2020
16. Clegg DO, Reda DJ, Abdellatif M (1999) Comparison of sulfasalazine and placebo for the treatment of axial and peripheral articular manifestations of the seronegative spondylarthropathies: a Department of Veterans Affairs cooperative study. Arthritis Rheum 42:2325–2329
17. Black RL, O'Brien WM, Van Scott EJ, et al. (1964) Methotrexate therapy in psoriatic arthritis. JAMA 189:141
18. Willkens RF, et al. 1984 Randomized, double-blind, placebo controlled trial of low-dose pulse methotrexate in psoriatic arthritis. Arthritis Rheum 27:376–381
19. Espinoza LR, et al. (1992) Psoriatic arthritis: clinical response and side effects to methotrexate therapy. J Rheumatol 19:872–877
20. Wollina U, Stander K, Barta U (2001) Toxicity of methotrexate treatment in psoriasis and psoriatic arthritis – short- and long-term toxicity in 104 patients. Clin Rheumatol 20:406–410
21. Abu-Shakra M, et al. (1995) Longterm methotrexate therapy in psoriatic arthritis: clinical and radiological outcome. J Rheumatol 22:241–245
22. Carette S, et al. (1989) A double-blind placebo-controlled study of auranofin in patients with psoriatic arthritis. Arthritis Rheum 32:158–165

23. Dorwart BB, et al. (1978) Chrysotherapy in psoriatic arthritis. Efficacy and toxicity compared to rheumatoid arthritis. Arthritis Rheum 21:513–515
24. Palit J, et al. (1990) A multicentre double-blind comparison of auranofin, intramuscular gold thiomalate and placebo in patients with psoriatic arthritis. Br J Rheumatol 29:280–283
25. Lacaille D, et al. (2000) Longterm therapy of psoriatic arthritis: intramuscular gold or methotrexate? J Rheumatol 27:1922–1927
26. Gomez-Vaquero C, et al. (1996) Termination of disease-modifying drugs in psoriatic arthritis: study of 109 courses of treatment. Br J Rheumatol 35: 564–567
27. Fox R (1998) Mechanism of action of leflunomide in rheumatoid arthritis. J Rheumatol 25(Suppl 53): 20–26
28. Manguso F, Oriente A, Peluso R, Oriente P (2001) Leflunomide in psoriatic polyarthritis: an Italian pilot study. Arthritis Rheum 44(9S):S121
29. Liang GC, Barr WG (2001) Open trial of leflunomide for refractory psoriasis and psoriatic arthritis. J Clin Rheumatol 7:366–370
30. Kaltwasser JP, Nash P, Gladman D, Rosen CF, Behrens F, Jones P, Wollenhaupt J, Falk FG, Mease P, for the TOPAS Study Group (2004) Efficacy and safety of leflunomide in the treatment of psoriatic arthritis and psoriasis. Arthritis Rheum 50(6): 1939–1950
31. Baum J, et al. (1973) Treatment of psoriatic arthritis with 6-mercaptopurine. Arthritis Rheum 16: 139–147
32. Steinsson K, Jonsdottir I, Valdimarsson H (1990) Cyclosporin A in psoriatic arthritis: an open study. Ann Rheum Dis 49:603–606
33. Spadaro A, et al. (1995) Comparison of cyclosporin A and methotrexate in the treatment of psoriatic arthritis: a one-year prospective study. Clin Exp Rheumatol 13:589–593
34. Mazzanti G, et al. (1994) Methotrexate and cyclosporin combined therapy in severe psoriatic arthritis. A pilot study. Acta Derm Venereol Suppl (Stockh) 186:116–117
35. Gladman DD, et al. (1992) Chloroquine therapy in psoriatic arthritis. J Rheumatol 19:1724–1726
36. Price R, Gibson T (1986) D-Penicillamine and psoriatic arthropathy. Br J Rheumatol 25:228
37. Wahba A, Cohen H (1980) Therapeutic trials with oral colchicine in psoriasis. Acta Derm Venereol 60: 515–520
38. Seideman P, Fjellner B, Johannesson A (1987) Psoriatic arthritis treated with oral colchicine. J Rheumatol 14:777–779
39. Lipsky JJ (1996) Mycophenolate mofetil. Lancet 348: 1357–1359
40. Schiff MH, Goldblum R, Rees MMC (1991) New DMARD, mycophenolate mofetil, effectively treats rheumatoid arthritis patients for 1 year. Arthritis Rheum 34(Suppl):S89
41. Grundmann-Kollmann M, et al. (2000) Treatment of chronic plaque-stage psoriasis and psoriatic arthritis with mycophenolate mofetil. J Am Acad Dermatol 42:835–837
42. Klinkhoff AV, et al. (1989) Pilot study of etretinate in psoriatic arthritis. J Rheumatol 16:789–791
43. Goupille P, Soutif D, Valat JP (1992) Treatment of psoriatic arthropathy. Semin Arthritis Rheum 21: 355–367
44. Wilfert H, et al. (1990) Treatment of psoriatic arthritis by extracorporeal photochemotherapy. Br J Dermatol 122:225–232
45. Vahlquist C, et al. (1996) Treatment of psoriatic arthritis with extracorporeal photochemotherapy and conventional psoralen-ultraviolet A irradiation. Arthritis Rheum 39:1519–1523
46. Matucci-Cerinic M, et al. (1988) Somatostatin treatment of psoriatic arthritis. Int J Dermatol 27:56–58

Biologic Therapy

X

A Psoriasis

Contents

1 Anti-T-Cell Agents

Richard G.B. Langley, Christa L. Doherty, Scott J. Murray

Introduction

Compelling laboratory and clinical evidence indicates that T cells play a cardinal role in the pathogenesis of psoriasis [32]. This information has provided a rationale and coupled with advances in immunology and molecular biology has permitted the development of novel biologic therapies for psoriasis and psoriatic arthritis [13, 32, 38, 41]. Strictly speaking, this has resulted in four basic strategies that involve: reducing pathogenic T cells; inhibiting T-cell activation and trafficking of T cells from the circulation into the dermis and epidermis; modifying the abnormal cytokine profile or immune deviation; and blocking the release or neutralizing pro-inflammatory cytokines [43, 17]. The focus of this chapter is on biologic agents that reduce or inhibit T-cell activation, and/or trafficking of T cells. In addition, we will concentrate on those molecules that are in late stage clinical development and will briefly review promising, but preliminary, biologic therapies that are in phase I/II stages of development.

Early Anti-T-Cell Biologics

Anti-T-cell biologic therapies were introduced for the treatment of psoriasis in the early 1990s. Some of these early agents have not been fully developed for this indication but set the initial basis for using T-cell selective molecules for immunotherapy. While these agents are not in general use at this time, they are instructive in identifying the mechanisms on which available therapy is based.

Denileukin Diftitox (DAB 389- IL-2; ONTAK, Ligand Pharm, La Jolla, CA)

Activated pathogenic T cells in psoriatic lesions express the IL-2 receptor (CD25) [11]. Denileukin diftitox is a fusion protein composed of human interleukin-2 and the amino acid sequence for diphtheria toxin. IL-2 diptheria toxin binds, and is specifically toxic to, the high affinity IL-2 receptor expressed on the activated T cell, thus causing selective cell death. To further clarify the role of the activated T cell in the pathogenesis of psoriasis, denileukin diftitox was systemically administered to ten patients with psoriasis. Clinical improvement was associated with decreased intraepidermal CD3+ and CD8+ T cells. This provided critical evidence to support the immunological basis of psoriasis, which was not firmly established at the time [25]. Phase II studies further supported the antipsoriatic activity of Denileukin diftitox. However, increased side effects were reported at higher doses with 10 of the 41 subjects being discontinued as a result of adverse events. Flu like symptoms were the most commonly reported adverse event, but multiple other side effects have been identified. One serious adverse event was reported in which a patient developed a coagulopathy and arterial thrombosis. Such potential serious side-effects have restricted the development of this therapy for psoriasis, and it has been subsequently utilized in the treatment of cutaneous T-cell lymphoma for which it is approved in the United States [50].

CTLA4Ig

The contact between B7 (CD80 and CD86) molecules on antigen presenting cells with CD28 on T cells is an important costimulatory signal for T-cell activation. Cytotoxic T-lymphocyte associated antigen (CTLA-4) is a secondary receptor for the B7 molecules that inhibits the activation response. CTLA4Ig is a soluble chimeric protein that binds CD80 (B7–1) and CD86 (B7–2) on antigen presenting cells, thereby blocking interaction with the receptors on the T cell (CD28 and CD152), preventing the costimulatory signal necessary for activation of the T cell [1, 2]. Thus, this agent was used under the theory that it could block the development of activation of T cells in psoriasis. In a phase I, open label, dose escalated trial, 43 psoriasis patients received 4 infusions of CTLA4Ig. In this study, 46% (19/41) of evaluable patients achieved a 50% or greater reduction in Physicians Global Assessment (PGA) compared to baseline. Clinical improvement was associated with reduced epidermal hyperplasia and lesional T cells without increased T-cell apoptosis, indicating the mechanism involves inhibition of T-cell proliferation, T-cell recruitment, and/or proliferation [2]. Although the initial studies were promising, this molecule is no longer being investigated for the treatment of psoriasis.

Anti-T-Cell Biologics Approved for Use in the United States

Alefacept (Amevive, Biogen, Cambridge, MA)

■ **Structure and Mechanism.** Alefacept is a dimeric recombinant fusion protein composed of the CD2 binding portion of the first extracellular domain of LFA-3 fused to the Fc portion of human IgG1 hinge, CH2 and CH3 domains [49]. It is a novel biologic agent designed to block the interaction between LFA-3 and CD2 on T lymphocytes. Alefacept has two different mechanisms that impact on the generation of an inflammatory response by T cells:

- 1. Alefacept blocks lymphocyte activation because the LFA-3 portion of the molecule binds directly to the T-cell CD2 receptor. For T-cell activation, two signals are required: a primary signal involving the interaction of the T-cell receptor with the major histocompatibility complex and antigen on antigen presenting cells (APC); and a second signal involving costimulatory receptor ligand interaction at the T cell and APC, such as the LFA–CD2 signal [6]. The LFA-3–CD2 signal is important in T-cell evolution, proliferation and cytotoxic effector functions. By preventing the interaction between LFA-3 and CD2 alefacept can interfere with the activation of T lymphocytes [34, 8].
- 2. Alefacept can also cause reductions in CD45RO+ memory effector cells by bridging CD2 on T cells with the LFA-3 portion of alefacept and the IgG_1 portion of the molecule binds to the FcγR III receptor on accessory cells, including natural killer cells and macrophages. This in turn leads to T-cell apoptosis primarily in cells that express high levels of CD2 [42]. Memory-effector T cells (CD45RO+) that exhibit an upregulation of CD2 are therefore specifically bound and depleted by this mechanism. The apoptosis is selective, in that naïve (CD4+, CD45RA+, and CD8+, CD45RA+) T cells are left relatively intact [9].

Pharmacokinetics and Pharmacodynamics. Although studied in intravenous and intramuscular modes of delivery, the intramuscular form is the only marketed form available. Once absorption from the intramuscular injection is complete, alefacept elimination from the serum is consistent with the infusion half-life of approximately 12 days. This data has supported the administration of alefacept by IV bolus or by IM injection [55].

In phase II studies, flow cytometry was performed to quantify populations of CD4+, CD8+, CD45RO+ and CD45RA+ lymphocytes as well as CD19+ B cells, CD16+ and CD56+ natural killer cells, all cells that express varying amounts of CD2 on their surface. A dose dependent reduction in peripheral blood memory effector cells (CD4+CD45RO+ and CD8+CD45RO+) was noted. This reduction of CD4+ cells was selective to the activated memory effector (CD45RO+) population as the naïve (CD45RA+) cells did not change appreciably, providing a targeted reduction of pathogenic T cells (Fig. A1). The reduction in the number of memory effector T cells was correlated with improvement in psoriasis on an overall but not an individual basis.

Clinical Trials. There have been multiple randomized placebo controlled trials of alefacept given both IV and IM. Ellis and Krueger [9] reported the results of alefacept in 229 patients with chronic plaque psoriasis in a phase II, multi-center, double-blind, placebo-controlled trial. Alefacept was given weekly in doses of 0.025, 0.075 or 0.15 mg/kg or placebo for 12 weeks with 12 weeks of follow-up. The primary and secondary efficacy endpoints are summarized in Table A1. The primary efficacy endpoint was ≥75% reduction in PASI 2 weeks after treatment; 14%, 33% and 31% of the patients that received 0.025, 0.075, or 0.15 mg/kg respectively attained this endpoint compared to 10% of patients receiving placebo. A ≥50% PASI reduction was attained in 36%, 60% and 56% for those patients receiving 0.025, 0.075 or 0.15 mg/kg per week of alefacept and 27% for placebo patients 2 weeks after treatment. The mean reduction in PASI measured 2 weeks after

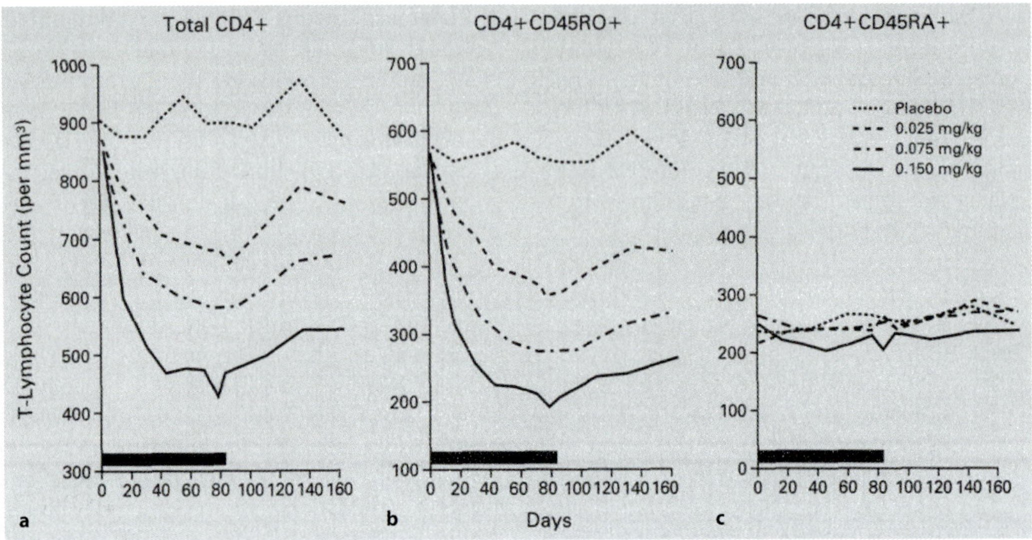

Fig. A1a–c. Peripheral-Blood T-Lymphocyte Counts. Mean counts of CD4+ T lymphocytes (Panel A), CD4+CD45RO+ memory effector T lymphocytes (Panel B), and CD4+CD45RA+ naive T lymphocytes (Panel C) are shown according to treatment group. The bars represent the treatment period. Data for all patients who could be evaluated in the intention-to-treat analysis, including those who received concomitant medications in the follow-up period, are shown. The results for CD8+ memory effector and naive T lymphocytes in the four groups of patients were nearly identical to the results for CD4+ cells

treatment was 38%, 53%, and 53% in patients receiving 0.025, 0.075, and 0.15 mg/kg per week compared to 21% in the placebo group (≤0.001).

In a phase III study, 553 patients were randomized to once weekly intravenous alefacept (7.5 mg or placebo) in a double blind, controlled study in patients with chronic plaque psoriasis. This study also examined the effect of one or two consecutive 12-week courses of intravenous alefacept [29]. Cohort 1 (n=183) was treated with two alefacept courses, whereas cohort 2 (n=184) was treated with an initial alefacept course followed by placebo, and the third cohort (n=186) received an initial placebo course followed by alefacept. In all three groups there was a treatment free 12-week period between the two treatment courses.

Table A1. Percentage of patients responding to the first course treatment in the intravenous study and the intramuscular study 2 weeks post-dosing

Treatment response (reduction in disease activity from baseline)	Placebo (n=186)	Alefacept (Amevive) 7.5 mg IV (n=367)[a]	Placebo (n=168)	Alefacept (Amevive) 15 mg IM (n=166)
≥75% reduction PASI	4%	14%	5%	21%
≥50% reduction PASI	10%	38%	18%	42%
PGA "almost clear" or "clear"	4%	11%	5%	14%
≥75% reduction PASI at any time	8%	28%	13%	33%
≥50% reduction PASI at any time	24%	56%	35%	57%

[a] Cohorts 1 and 2 are combined

In both courses, active treatment with alefacept produced a mean decrease in PASI which peaked 8 weeks after the course of active treatment. The primary end point was a 75% reduction in the PASI 2 weeks after the treatment course, and 14% (53/367) of the alefacept 7.5 mg and 4% (7/186) of the placebo treated patients achieved this result ($p \leq 0.001$). After course 1, the mean reduction in PASI from baseline was 47% in the alefacept treated group compared to 20% in the placebo treated group. A 50% reduction in PASI, 2 weeks after treatment, was noted in 38% (139/367) and 10% (18/186) of the 7.5 mg intravenous and placebo group, respectively ($p \leq 0.001$).

In the initial phase II studies, it was noted that the response to alefacept could be delayed, and that the peak response of patients could be observed during the post-dosing period and beyond the set primary end point of 2 weeks post-dosing. Because patients could continue to improve weeks or months after treatment, an analysis of achieving the outcome measures at any time throughout the study was pre-specified. A ≥75% or ≥50% improvement in PASI at any time throughout the study was reached in course 1 in 28% and 56% of alefacept treated patients compared to 8% and 24% respectively for those receiving placebo ($p \leq 0.001$).

An additional course of alefacept resulted in an incremental improvement in the outcome measures studied. A second course of alefacept (7.5 mg IV) resulted in 26% (47/183) and 55% (100/183) of patients achieving a 75% and 50% reduction of PASI 2 weeks after treatment. A 75% and 50% reduction in PASI at any time was attained by 40% (73/183) and 71% (130/183) of patients that received two courses of alefacept (7.5 mg IV). Additionally, the clinical response to alefacept was durable following a single course of alefacept being in the order of 7 months (216 days). The duration of response was defined as the median duration of a ≥50% reduction in PASI, and was determined from the responding population (those that achieved a 75% reduction in PASI). Menter and Cather recently reported the safety and efficacy of patients with multiple courses of IV alefacept [46]. Each additional course of alefacept showed an incremental benefit with repeat courses. Safety and efficacy were consistent with prior phase II and III results.

The safety and efficacy of intramuscular alefacept was demonstrated in a pivotal phase III international randomized, double blind, placebo-controlled study in which 507 patients were randomized into one of three 12-week arms: placebo (n=168); alefacept 10 mg IM weekly (n=173); or alefacept 15 mg (n=166) followed by 12 weeks of observation [36]. The efficacy results of this study are summarized in Table A1. A dose related improvement was noted in PASI scores and the decrease in mean PASI scores continued after the 12-week treatment period. The primary efficacy end point was a 75% reduction in PASI 2 weeks after therapy, and 21%, 14%, and 5% of alefacept 15 mg, 10 mg, and placebo met this endpoint, respectively ($p \leq 0.001$ between alefacept 15 mg and placebo). A 50% reduction in PASI was reached in 42% of alefacept 15 mg and 18% of placebo (Fig. A2) ($p \leq 0.001$ between alefacept 15 mg and placebo). Mean reduction in PASI was 46%, 41% and 25% in the 15 mg alefacept, 10 mg alefacept, and placebo group, respectively, which peaked at 6 weeks post-dosing.

Because of the delayed effect of alefacept, the pre-specified analysis of the primary and several secondary endpoints was examined through-

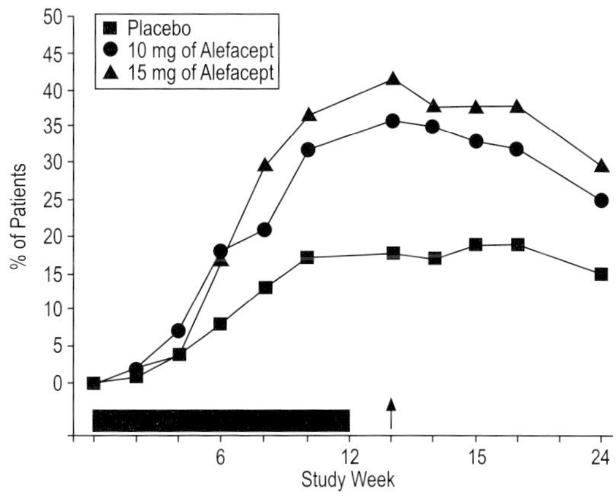

Fig. A2. Percentage of subjects reaching PASI 75 response in phase III clinical trial of alefacept for chronic plaque psoriasis. The arrow indicates the primary endpoint of the study, two weeks after the final dose of alefacept was given out the study period (at any time after the primary endpoint was reached). A 75% reduction in PASI from baseline was noted in 33%, 28%, and 13% of alefacept 15 mg, 10 mg, or placebo treated patients throughout the study period ($p \leq 0.001$). The percentage of patients reaching at least 50% reduction in PASI was significantly higher in the 15 mg alefacept ($p \leq 0.001$) and 10 mg alefacept ($p \leq 0.002$) compared to placebo, with 57%, 53%, and 35% of patients reaching the endpoint, throughout the study period.

Consistent with phase II and phase III intravenous studies, the clinical response to IM alefacept was durable. Of patients in the 15-mg alefacept group with a 75% reduction in PASI 2 weeks after the last dose, 74% maintained a reduction of at least 50% in their PASI throughout the 12-week follow-up. We subsequently reported an extension of the phase III intramuscular alefacept study in which patients that received alefacept 15 mg/week were given a second 12-week course, whereas those that received placebo or 10-mg alefacept were given a 12-week course of alefacept 10 mg. Of the patients who achieved a PASI 75% or greater following one course of alefacept 15 mg, the median duration of response (maintained a 50% PASI reduction) was 209 days. A second course of alefacept resulted in incremental benefit with an overall response of 43% of patients achieving PASI 75 and 69% attaining at least a PASI 50.

Recently, an extended 16-week course of alefacept was compared to the standard 12-week course and interim results were recently reported for 20 patients [27]. In each group 60% (6/10) of patients achieved PASI 50 at any time between weeks 12 and 24. PASI 75 was attained by 10% (1/10) in the 12-week course and 30% (3/10) in the extended 16-week group. No significant differences were seen in the frequency of adverse events between the two groups. This was consistent with the profile observed in phase III studies. Although preliminary, and involving only small numbers of patients, the interim analysis suggests incremental benefit to extended dosing. There was a significant improvement in PASI at week 20 and 24 favoring the 16-week treatment group. Studies are still ongoing to look at the potential benefit of a longer 16-week course.

■ **Safety.** Alefacept has been well tolerated in clinical studies with over 1500 patients evaluated to date. Incidence of the most common adverse events such as headache, pharyngitis, accidental injuries, and infections are not significantly different than with placebo [37]. Adverse events occurring in greater than 10% of patients in the intramuscular trial conducted by Lebwohl et al. [36] are outlined in Table A2. In this trial, if patients had a CD4+ lymphocyte count below 250 µl, a placebo was substituted, and if the counts remained below this level for

Table A2. Adverse events reported in at least 10% of patients in either alefacept group [data are number (percentage) of patients]

Adverse event	Placebo (n=168)	10 mg of alefacept (n=173)	15 mg of alefacept (n=166)	Total alefacept (n=339)
Headache	26 (15)	34 (20)	30 (18)	64 (19)
Pruritus	16 (10)	24 (14)	30 (18)	54 (16)
Infection[a]	19 (11)	25 (14)	26 (16)	51 (15)
CD4+ cell count <250/µl[b]	0	1 (<1)	1 (<1)	2 (<1)
Pharyngitis	15 (9)	20 (12)	20 (12)	40 (12)
Accidental injury	19 (11)	22 (13)	16 (10)	38 (11)
Rhinitis	11 (7)	24 (14)	9 (5)	33 (10)
Asthenia	18 (11)	10 (6)	18 (11)	28 (8)

[a] Includes events coded to the COSTART (COSTART, Coding Symbols for *Thesaurus of Adverse Reaction Terms*) term *infection*; common cold was the most commonly used description in this category
[b] Includes infections that occurred after the onset of CD4+ cell count <250/µl

four visits, there was permanent placebo substitution. Less than 1% of patients in 10-mg and 15-mg intramuscular alefacept groups had CD4+ counts less than 250 µl, and there were no permanent placebo substitutions [36].

In the intravenous trial conducted by Krueger et al. [29], the only adverse event in the initial course that had a greater than 5% incidence in the combined alefacept group was chills (10% vs. 1%). Chills were generally mild and transient, lasting less than 24 h, occurring in only 4% of patients in the second course and decreasing with additional treatments.

Pivotal phase III intravenous and intramuscular studies have demonstrated similar rates of infection between the placebo and alefacept treated patients [29, 37]. No opportunistic infections have been reported in the alefacept clinical trial program to date [29]. In addition, there has been no association with lower CD4+ lymphocyte counts and infections.

Several studies have been conducted to assess the integrity of T-cell-dependent immune responses. In a phase II study, delayed-type hypersensitivity skin testing was performed and the immune response to recall antigen was similar between alefacept and placebo treated patients. In addition, no cases of TB infection have been reported in patients treated with alefacept, even in PPD positive (X-ray negative) subjects [47].

A randomized, nonblinded, parallel group, phase 2 study with 46 patients affected by chronic psoriasis was evaluated for primary and secondary responses to a neoantigen (ϕX174) and acquired immunity to a recall antigen (tetanus toxin) [19]. The mean anti-ϕX174 titers were comparable between patients treated with 7.5 mg IV alefacept once weekly for 12 - weeks and untreated psoriatic control patients. In addition, antibody titers rose rapidly in alefacept treated control patients, and anti-tetanus antibody titers were similar (Fig. A3).

Injection site reactions were seen in 16% of patients treated with intramuscular alefacept and 8% of placebo treated patients. Injection site reactions were typically mild and transient, not recurring with subsequent doses [4, 36]. Approximately 1–4% of patients develop anti-alefacept antibodies [30], but levels are low

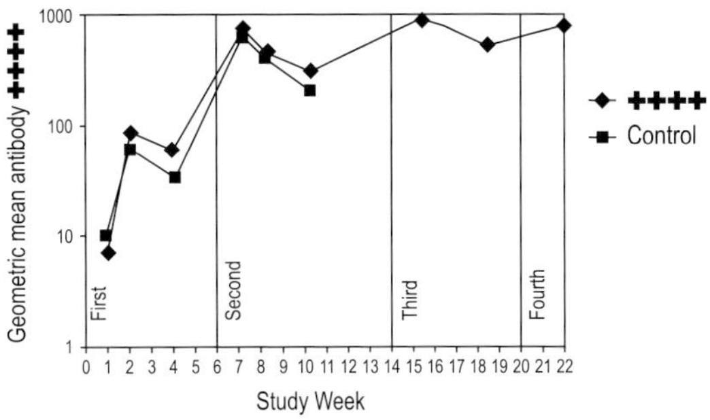

Fig. A3. Total anti- X174 antibody titers in alefacept and control groups after each X174 immunization. Solid squares, Control group; solid diamonds, alefacept group. There is no statistical difference between subjects treated with alefacept and those with psoriasis on no immunosuppressive therapy in response to this novel antigen

(<1:40), did not cause hypersensitivity reactions or interfere with alefacept efficacy [36, 48].

The rate of malignancies in alefacept treated patients to date has been low, and not increased beyond that seen in placebo treated patients in clinical trials, nor that expected in age and sex matched controls. Of 1357 patients that received at least one course of alefacept reported in the biologics license application to the FDA, 25 patients were diagnosed with 35 malignancies. Of these, 66% (23/35) were non-melanoma skin cancer (17 squamous cell carcinoma; 6 basal cell carcinomas) [4]. In addition, there were three cases of lymphoma, two of which were Hodgkin's disease and one non-Hodgkin's lymphoma (follicular center cell) [5].

During treatment, dose-dependent reductions in peripheral blood CD4+ memory effector cells (CD45RO+) have been noted [9]. Consistent with phase II studies, memory effector cells are preferentially affected, as naïve cells (CD45RA+) were not reduced. Improvement in psoriasis has been correlated with reductions in CD4+ (CD45RO+) cells, although not on an individual basis [9]. We reported biweekly measurement of CD4 counts provide adequate safety monitoring in alefacept recipients [35]. Incidence of adverse events was similar to that in patients with weekly monitoring.

Krueger et al. [31] examined the safety profile of alefacept given in multiple courses combined with MTX, cyclosporine, systemic retinoids, mid or high potency topical steroids and UVB. There was no increase in adverse events or opportunistic infections in any combination group. MTX induced hepatotoxicity and cyclosporine induced renal changes were not increased.

■ **Concomitant Therapy.** Alefacept has a relatively slow onset of action compared to other biologic agents [37], peaking at 16 weeks after the first of 12 weekly injections. Therefore, there may be a role for other, more rapidly acting systemic agents, or ultraviolet therapy in inducing a more rapid initial remission. Krueger theorizes that a shared common mechanism of action (selective apoptosis of activated T cells) for phototherapy (UVB, narrow band UVB, and PUVA) and alefacept make an additive or synergistic relationship for these modalities possible [28]. Gordon studied the effect of IM alefacept given in multiple courses in patients with stable disease at baseline being treated with MTX, cyclosporine, systemic retinoids, mid or high potency topical steroids and UVB [14]. Across all groups 61% of alefacept patients had PGA improvements of one category and 32% improved by two categories. The largest benefit was found in patients with the most severe disease at baseline. The efficacy of using alefacept to transition patients safely off MTX therapy has been demonstrated by Menter et al. [45] in a group of 12 patients. A smaller study (n=3) demonstrated similar success and safety transitioning patients off cyclosporine [18].

■ **Summary.** Alefacept has been shown to be an effective treatment for chronic psoriasis, with a slow onset but a durable response. Currently a treatment course is given of 12 weeks with a repeat weekly course if needed after 12 weeks, although new regimens are currently being studied. Laboratory monitoring of lymphocyte counts is recommended although we have recently determined that reduced monitoring is safe [35]. A representative patient demonstrating photographic improvement is shown

X

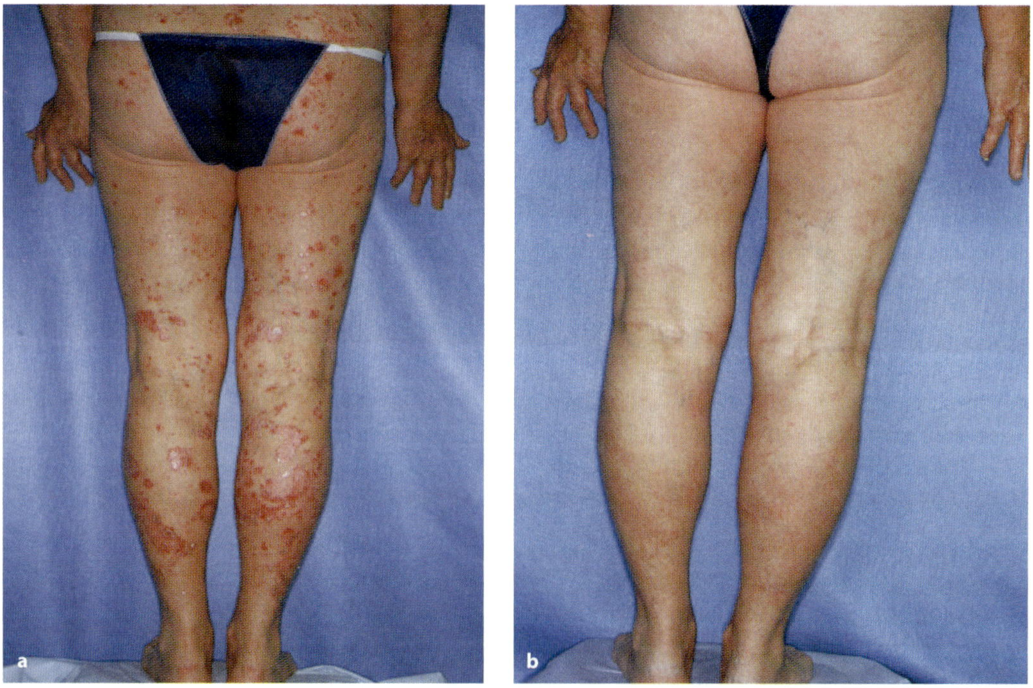

Fig. A4a, b. Response to alefacept. Subject treated with IM alefacept two weeks after his final dose in phase III trial. The change respresents at least a 75% improvement in the subject's PASI

in Fig. A4. Ongoing studies are still establishing the ideal treatment parameters and systemic treatment combinations for this novel agent.

Efalizumab (Raptiva, Anti CD11a, Genentech, South San Francisco, CA)

Structure and Mechanism. Efalizumab (anti-CD11a, hu1124) is a recombinant humanized monoclonal IgG1 antibody directed against the alpha subunit (CD11a) of the leukocyte function associated antigen-1 (LFA-1) [16, 20, 39–41, 51, 56]. Located on the surface of the T cell, LFA-1 is an adhesion molecule that binds to intercellular adhesion molecule-1 (ICAM-1) that is expressed by the antigen presenting cell, and on the surface of vascular endothelium [32, 39]. Efalizumab inhibits the binding between LFA-1 and ICAM-1, disrupting several key T-cell mediated events that are important in the pathogenesis of psoriasis including: initial T-cell activation; trafficking of T cells from the circulation into sites of inflammation (dermis and epidermis); and the secondary reactivation of memory T cells [20, 38, 39, 41]. Additionally, 1 or 2 days after administering a dose of efalizumab of 1 mg/kg per week subcutaneously, CD11a expression on circulating T lymphocyte was reduced 15–25% [12]. This data suggests that efalizumab may induce intracellular signaling events that can alter T-cell processes.

Pharmacokinetics and Pharmacodynamics. A pharmacokinetic study in patients with moderate to severe plaque psoriasis indicated serum concentrations reached a steady state at 4 weeks, and the bioavailability was 50%. The mean time to eliminate efalizumab after the last steady-state dose was 25 days (range = 13–35 days in 17 patients) [12]. In a phase III clinical trial, efalizumab treatment of psoriasis led to approximately a twofold increase of circulating lymphocytes [12]. The increase in circulating lymphocytes is expected, as efalizumab inhibits the binding between LFA-1 and ICAM-1 inhibiting the trafficking of T cells from the circulation into sites of inflammation.

Clinical Trials. In the phase I and phase II development program for efalizumab, multiple immunohistological parameters were measured. In the phase I study of intravenous dosing of efalizumab, decreases in dermal and epidermal T cells were noted as well as decreases in markers of keratinocyte response including ICAM expression and Ki-67 [21]. In a later study, keratinocyte expression of K16 was negative at day 56 in 30–40% of patients receiving at least 0.3 mg/kg per week. Epidermal thickness was measured in the different dose groups, with decreasing epidermal thickness noted in progressively higher dose groups. The improvements in the histologic, immunohistologic, and clinical improvements correlated with serum efalizumab levels and CD11a downmodulation, supporting the hypothesized mechanism of action of efalizumab [22]. A dose dependent response was observed in the pharmacokinetic and pharmacodynamic analyses. At doses of at least 0.3 mg/kg per week CD11a downmodulation was achieved and maintained between doses, on circulating and lesional T cells.

These early studies, along with the clinical results of early IV and sub-cutaneous dosing of efalizumab [51, 24], indicated subcutaneous administration of efalizumab was potentially efficacious in psoriasis. There have been several large, well designed *phase III* trials conducted to further assess the efficacy, safety and tolerability of subcutaneously administered efalizumab.

Lebwohl et al. [38] reported a double blind, placebo controlled, parallel group, multicenter study consisting of three phases: weeks 0–12 (first treatment phase); weeks 13–24 (extended treatment phase); and weeks 25–36 (follow-up). A total of 597 patients were randomized in a ratio of 2 : 2 : 1 to receive 1 mg/kg per week (n=232) or 2 mg/kg per week (n=243) of efalizumab, or placebo (n=122) for the first 12 weeks. Treatment assignment for the next 12 weeks was dependent upon each patient's PASI response to the first 12 weeks of treatment. Patients who achieved a reduction in their PASI score of ≥50% at week 12 were rerandomized to receive 2 mg/kg of efalizumab every week or every other week or placebo in a 1 : 1 : 1 ratio. Patients who achieved a reduction in their PASI score of <50% were rerandomized to receive 4 mg/kg per week or placebo in a ratio of 2:1.

During the first treatment phase, patients who received active treatment with efalizumab at either dose had a significantly better response than those who received placebo as measured by a reduction in PASI scores. At week 12, 28% (69/243), 22% (52/232), and 5% (6/122) of efalizumab 2 mg/kg per week, 1 mg/kg per week, and placebo treated patients attained a 75% reduction in PASI, respectively ($p \leq 0.001$). At week 12, 57% (138/243), 52% (120/232) and 16% (19/122) of efalizumab 2 mg/kg per week, 1 mg/kg per week, and placebo achieved a 50% reduction in PASI, respectively ($p \leq 0.001$). A mean improvement in PASI of 51% in the 1 mg/kg per week efalizumab group, 52% in the 2 mg/kg per week efalizumab group, and 17% in the placebo group was observed during the first treatment phase ($p \leq 0.001$) (Fig. A5). A representative patient demonstrating photographic improvement is shown in Fig. A6 [38].

In the extended treatment phase, patients that achieved a 75% reduction in PASI (n=121) were re-randomized (n=119) to efalizumab 2 mg/kg per week, 2 mg/kg every other week, or placebo. A ≥75% reduction in PASI was maintained in 77% (30/39), 78% (31/40), and 20% (8/40) of the 2 mg/kg per week, 2 mg/kg every other week, and placebo ($p \leq 0.001$) [38].

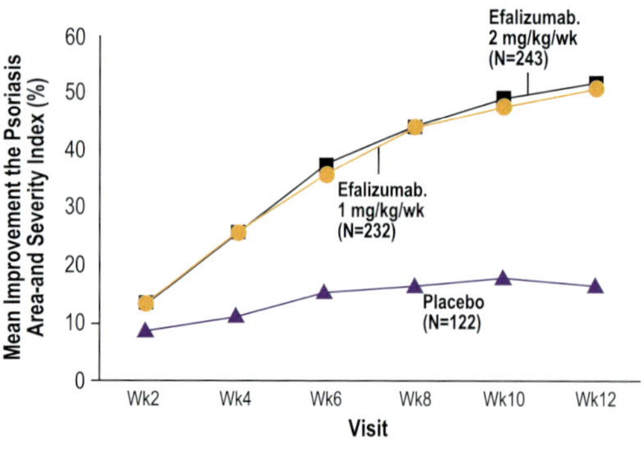

Fig. A5. Mean Improvements in the Psoriasis Area-and-Severity Index during the First-Treatment Period. The psoriasis area-and-severity index, based on skin-surface involvement and the severity of erythema, desquamation, and plaque induration, ranges from 0 to 72, with higher scores indicating more severe disease and a reduction in the scores indicating improvement

In the follow-up phase, 12 weeks after efalizumab was discontinued, approximately one-third of the subjects that received continuous efalizumab therapy for 24 weeks maintained at least 50% of the improvement. The time to relapse, defined as loss of 50% of improvement in PASI, in patients who had at least 75% improvement at week 24, was approximately 84 days. This indicated that efalizumab is a suppressive therapy, and requires continued use to maintain clinical improvement in most patients. It is important when stopping efalizumab to consider alternate therapies to maintain clinical improvements, and prevent rapid recurrence of disease. Currently, ongoing clinical trials are defining optimal tapering regimens, and regimens that include transitioning to alternate systemic agents.

Patients who had achieved PASI 50 but not PASI 75 during the first 12 weeks of treatment and who continued treatment with efalizumab achieved PASI 75 in significantly more people than those receiving placebo. 53% (25/47), 29% (13/45) and 4% (2/46) of 2 mg/ kg per week, 1 mg/kg per week, and placebo, respectively, achieved a PASI 75 or better by week 24. This indicated that continued treatment with efalizumab provided an incremental benefit. Lastly, 13% (15/118) of patients who had not achieved PASI 50 during the first treatment phase and who continued efalizumab treatment at an escalated dose of 4 mg/kg per week subcutaneously also achieved PASI 75 in significantly more people than those who received placebo, indicating that dose escalation may be beneficial to subjects who initially have a limited response to efalizumab treatment [38].

Safety was monitored through the review of adverse events and laboratory assessments. The injections were well tolerated and most adverse events were acute and mild to moderate in severity. Acute adverse events were defined as those occurring within 2 days of administration of study drug and were most likely to occur after the first dose of study medication and decreased in frequency over time. Common adverse drug related events were headache, chills, fever, nausea and myalgia.

The incidence of infection was not increased and there was no evidence of end organ toxic-

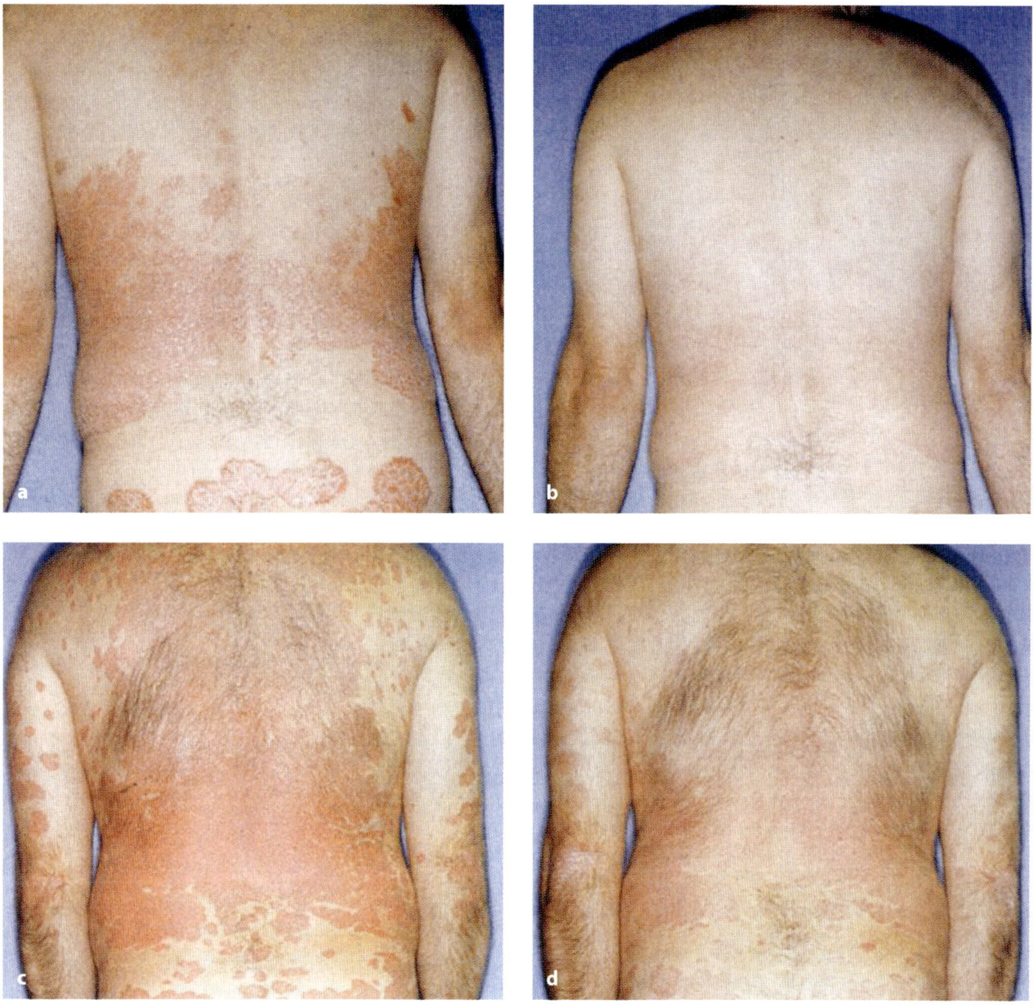

Fig. A6a–d. Representative Responses to Efalizumab. Panels **a** and **b** show the same subject at base line and at day 84 of efalizumab theray, respectively: the change reflects an improvement of at least 75 percent in the psoriasis area-and-severity index. Panels **c** and **d** show a different subject at base line and at day 84 of efalizumab therapy; the change in this subject reflects an improvement of 50 to 74 percent in the psoriasis area-and-severity index

ity. Adverse events occurring in at least 10% of patients, during the first course, are summarized in Table A3.

Gordon et al. reported a second pivotal, phase III randomized, double blind, parallel-group, placebo controlled study with efalizumab [16]. In this study, 556 adult patients were randomized to a 12-week course of subcutaneous efalizumab at 1 mg/kg (n=369) or placebo (n=187). At the end of the 12-week treatment course, 27% (98/369) of patients receiving 1 mg/kg weekly attained a 75% reduction in PASI compared to 4% (8/187) of placebo treated patients ($p\leq0.001$). A PASI 50 was attained in 59% (216/369) and 14% (26/187) of efalizumab and placebo treated patients, respectively ($p\leq0.001$). The response to treatment with efalizumab was rapid, with a significant difference in mean PASI changes between treatment and placebo groups noted as early as week 4 [16].

The main clinical endpoints for the two major phase III trials are summarized in the Table

Table A3. Adverse events during the first treatment phase

Type of adverse event	Placebo (n=122)	Efalizumab (1 mg/kg per week) (n=232)	Efalizumab (2 mg/kg per week) (n=243)	p value[a]
Headache	29 (24)	71 (31)	93 (38)	0.02
Infection	19 (16)	27 (12)	43 (18)	0.78
Nausea	11 (9)	34 (15)	35 (14)	0.14
Chills	3 (2)	38 (16)	31 (13)	<0.001
Pain	4 (3)	35 (15)	29 (12)	<0.001
Fever	6 (5)	26 (11)	29 (12)	0.03
Asthenia	7 (6)	17 (7)	27 (11)	0.28
Arthralgia	6 (5)	24 (10)	12 (5)	0.43

[a] P values are for the comparisons between the combined efalizumab groups and the placebo group and were calculated with the use of post hoc, two-sided Fisher's exact tests, without adjustment for multiple comparisons

Table A4. Percentage of patients responding to efalizumab at week 12: a pivotal phase III trial (Lebwohl/Gordon et al.). N/A, not applicable: This dose was not studied in the second pivotal study reported by Gordon et al.

Treatment response (reduction in disease activity from baseline)	Placebo (n=186)	Efalizumab (1 mg/kg per week)	Efalizumab (2 mg/kg per week)
≥75% reduction PASI	5%/4%	22%/27%	28%/NA
≥50% reduction PASI	16%/14%	52%/59%	57%/NA
Mean PASI improvement at week 12	17%/19%	51%/52%	52%/NA

p<0.001 for the comparison with the placebo group

A4 below. Significant improvements were also noted for other clinical endpoints including overall lesion severity, physician global assessment and patient reported outcomes (Dermatology Quality of Life Index; Visual Analog Scale for Itching, and Psoriasis Symptom Assessment).

■ **Safety.** We have recently reported pooled safety data on 2325 patients treated in phase III clinical trials for 12 weeks. In these studies patients were randomized to receive 12 weeks of either efalizumab 1 mg/kg per week or 2 mg/kg per week, or placebo. Data was pooled for this safety analysis to provide the largest patient cohort and to increase the probability of detecting rare events. The majority of adverse events were mild-moderate in intensity. The most common adverse events, occurring in greater than 5% of patients, included headache, nonspecific infection, chills, nausea, pain, myalgia, flu-like symptoms, asthenia, and back pain. These adverse events and the associated frequencies compared to placebo are listed in Table A5 below. Consistent with phase I/II studies, acute adverse events (headache, fever, chills, nausea, vomiting) were generally mild-moderate, transient, and self-limited, often resolving by the second or third injection. Thrombocytopenia has been reported in 0.3% (8/2762) of patients in the clinical trial program, requiring regular monitoring of platelets [12].

In clinical trials with efalizumab serious adverse events have been uncommon and similar between efalizumab and placebo treated patients. The incidences of general and serious infections were similar between efalizumab and placebo treated patients. There was no indication of hepatotoxicity or nephrotoxicity nor were there any reported cases of tuberculosis, or opportunistic infections such as *Pneumocystis carinii* pneumonia, histoplasmosis, toxo-

Table A5. Adverse events occurring in ≥5% of patients in either group and ≥1% more frequently in one treatment group compared to the other during weeks 1–12 in four randomized, placebo-controlled trials

Adverse event[a]	Placebo (*n*=715)	Efalizumab all patients (*n*=1620)
Headache	159 (22%)	542 (34%)
Nonspecific infection[b]	110 (15%)	225 (14%)
Chills	32 (5%)	207 (13%)
Nausea	51 (7%)	184 (11%)
Generalized pain	38 (5%)	167 (10%)
Myalgia	35 (5%)	134 (8%)
Fever	24 (3%)	126 (8%)
Asthenia	37 (5%)	119 (7%)
Flu syndrome	29 (4%)	102 (6%)
Back pain	14 (2%)	75 (5%)

[a] Multiple occurrences of the same event for a patient were counted once in the overall incidence

[b] Generally colds or upper respiratory tract infection

plasmosis, or *Mycobacterium avium* complex. Moreover, the overall incidence of malignancy in efalizumab treated patients was low and similar to patients treated with placebo [41].

Following discontinuation of treatment with efalizumab, psoriasis will generally recur in the order of 80 days. "Flare" or "rebound" of psoriasis (flaring or rebound of psoriasis >125% PASI from baseline) and new morphologies of psoriaisis (inflammatory plaques; pustular lesions) were also reported [41]. While uncommon, clinical trials and clinical experience suggest that these occur most frequently in patients who have not had a satisfactory clinical response to efalizumab. Thus, it is important to use caution and have a definitive treatment plan in place for patients whose disease does not respond to efalizumab or for patients for whom therapy is being discontinued.

■ **Extended Treatment.** Long-term studies are clearly required for all biologic agents to confirm the safety of the short-term studies. Ongoing long-term phase III studies are currently evaluating the safety, efficacy and tolerability of efalizumab treatment beyond 12 weeks [20]. Available data for 182 patients receiving up to 24 months of efalizumab treatment was recently examined. Overall, treatment was well tolerated over 24 months. The incidence of adverse events did not increase over time and the types of common adverse events did not change with time. There was no evidence of end organ toxicity or accumulation of efalizumab in the serum.

Conclusion

Advances in understanding the key pathogenic steps of psoriasis, and particularly the key role of T cells, has permitted the development of novel biologic therapies for psoriasis and psoriatic arthritis. The highly targeted nature of biologic agents is in contrast to the nonspecific mechanism of conventional systemic agents for psoriasis which also have potential for acute and cumulative end organ toxicity. Such specificity of biologic agents is providing new choices for patients and physicians, with efficacious but safer agents with less end organ toxicity. This chapter has reviewed some of the key advances in the area of biologic agents which impact T-cell number, proliferation or trafficking. The initial efficacy and safety data are promising, and the longer term data on safety will be of importance in evaluating the relative role of these agents in the management of psoriasis.

References

1. Abrams JR, Kelley SL, Hayes E, Kikuchi T, Brown MJ, Kang S, Lebwohl MG, Guzzo CA, Jegasothy BV, Linsley PS, Krueger JG (2000) Blockade of T lymphocyte costimulation with cytotoxic T lymphocyte-associated antigen 4-immunoglobin (CTLA4Ig) reverses the cellular pathology of psoriatic plaques, including the activation of keratinocytes, dendritic cells, and endothelial cells. J Exp Med 192:681–694
2. Abrams JR, Lebwohl MG, Guzzo CA, Jegasothy BV, Goldfarb MT, Goffe BS, Menter A, Lowe NJ, Krueger

G, Brown MJ, Weiner RS, Birkhofer MJ, Warner GL, Berry KK, Linsley PS, Krueger JG, Ochs HD, Kelley SL, Kang S (1999) CTLA41g-medicated blockade of T-cell costimulation in patients with psoriasis vulgaris. J Clin Invest 103:1243–1252
3. Bagel J, Garland WT, Breneman D, Holick M, Littlejohn TW, Crosby D, Faust H, Fivenson D, Nichols J (1998) Administration of DAB3891L-2 to patients with recalcitrant psoriasis: a double blind, phase II multicenter trial. J Am Acad Dermatol 38:938–944
4. Biogen, Inc. Amevive (Alefacept) Briefing Document. Dermatologic and Ophthalmic Drugs Advisory Meeting. Available at: http://www.fda.gov/ohrms/dockets/ac/02/briefing.3865B1_Biogen.pdf
5. Biogen Inc. Amevive (Alefacept) US Product Monograph. Available at: http://www.Amevive.com/en_US/fragment/portlet/FINAL_Amevive_Label.pdf
6. Danielian S, Fagard R, Alcover A, Acuto O, Fischer S (1991) The Tyrosine kinase activity of p56lck is increased in human T-cells activated via CD2. Eur J Immunol 21:1967–1970
7. Deckert F, Legay F (1999) Development and validation of an immunoreceptor assay for simulect based on surface plasmon resonance. Anal Biochem 274:81–89
8. Dustin ML, Springer TA (1988) Lymphocyte function-associated antigen-1 (LFA-1) interaction with intercellular adhesion molecule-1 (ICAM-1) is one of at least three mechanisms for lymphocyte adhesion to cultured endothelial cells. J Cell Biol 107:321–331
9. Ellis CN, Krueger GG (2001) Treatment of chronic plaque psoriasis by selective targeting of memory effector T lymphocytes. N Engl J Med 345:248–255
10. Ellis CN, Mordin MM, Adler EY (2003) Effects of Alefacept on health-related quality of life in patients with psoriasis. Am J Clin Dermatol 4:131–139
11. Ferenczi K, Burack L, Pope M, Krueger JG, Austin LM (2000) CD69, HLA-DR and the IL-2R identify persistency activated T cells in psoriasis vulgaris lesional skin: blood and skin comparison by flow cytometry. J Autoimmun 14:63–78
12. Genentech Inc. Raptiva (Efalizumab) US Product Monograph Available at: http://www.gene.com/gene/products/information/immunological/raptiva/insert.jsp
13. Gniadecki R, Zachariae C, Calverley M (2002) Trends and developments in the pharmacological treatment of psoriasis. Acta Derm Venereol 82:401–410
14. Gordon KB (2004) Efficacy of multiple courses of alefacept in combination with other psoriasis therapies: a study that reflects the clinical practice setting. Poster presented at: 62nd Annual American Academy of Dermatology Meeting; February 6–11; Washington, DC
15. Gordon KB, Langley RG (2003) Remittive effects of intramuscular Alefacept in psoriasis. J Drugs Dermatol 2:624–628
16. Gordon KB, Papp KA, Hamilton RTC, Vilieke PA, Dunner W, Li N, Bresnahan BW, Merter A (2003) Efalizumb for patients with moderate to severe plaque psoriasis: a randomized controlled trial. Jama 290:3073–3080
17. Gordon KB, West DP (2001) Biologic therapy in dermatology. In: Wolverton SE (ed) Comprehensive dermatologic drug therapy. WB Saunders, Philadelphia, pp 928–942
18. Gottlieb A (2004) Alefacept in combination with tapering doses of cyclosporine in patients with psoriasis. Poster presented at: 62nd Annual American Academy of Dermatology Meeting; February 6–11; Washington, DC
19. Gottlieb AB, Casale TB, Frankel E, Goffe B, Lowe N, Ochs HD, Roberts JL, Washenik K, Vaishnaw AK, Gordon KB (2003) CD4+ T-cell-directed antibody responses are maintained in patients with psoriasis receiving alefacept: results of a randomized study. J Am Acad Dermatol 49:816–825
20. Gottlieb AB, Gordon K, Caro I, Li N, Chastain RL, Leonardi CL (2004) Long-term Efalizumab therapy safely maintains psoriasis area and severity index improvement: preliminary results from an open-label trial. Poster presented at: 62nd Annual American Academy of Dermatology Meeting; February 6–11; Washington, DC
21. Gottlieb A, Krueger JG, Bright R, Ling M, Lebwohl M, Kang S, Feldman S, Spellman M, Wittkowski K, Ochs HD, Jardieu P, Bauer R, White M, Dedrick R, Garavoy M (2000) Effects of administration of a single dose of a humanized monoclonal antibody to CD11a on the immunobiology and clinical activity of psoriasis. J Am Acad Dermatol 42:428–435
22. Gottlieb AB, Krueger JG, Wittkowski K, Dedrick R, Walicke PA, Garovoy M (2002) Psoriasis as a model for T-cell-mediated disease: immunobiologic and clinical effects of treatment with multiple doses of efalizaumab, an anti-CD11a antibody. Arch Dermatol 138:591–600
23. Gottlieb AB, Lebwohl M, Shirin S, Sherr A, Gilleaudeau P, Singer G, Solodkina G, Grossman R, Gisoldi E, Phillips S, Neisler HM, Krueger JG (2000) Anti-CD4 monoclonal antibody treatment of moderate to severe psoriasis vulgaris: results of a pilot, multicenter, multiple-dose, placebo-controlled study. J Am Acad Dermatol 43:595–604
24. Gottlieb AB, Miller B, Lowe N, Shapiro W, Hudson C, Bright R, Ling M, Magee A, McCall CO, Rist T, Dummer W, Walicke P, Bauer RF, White M, Garovoy M (2003) Subcutaneously administered efalizumab (anti-CD11a) improves signs and symptoms of moderate to severe plaque psoriasis. J Cutan Med Surg 198–207
25. Gottlieb SL, Gilleaudeau P, Johnson R, Estes L, Woodworth TG, Gottlieb AB, Krueger JG (1995) Response of psoriasis to a lymphocyte-selective toxin (DAB3891L-2) suggests a primary immune, but not keratinocyte, pathogenic basis. Nat Med 1:442–447
26. Grassberger M, Baumruker T, Enz A, Hiestand P, Hultsch T, Kalthoff F, Schuler W, Schulz M, Werner

X

FJ, Winiski A, Wolff B, Zenke G (1999) A novel anti-inflammatory drug, SDZ ASM 981, for the treatment of skin diseases: in vitro pharmacology. Br J Dermatol 141: 264–273

27. Gribetz CH, Blum R, Brady C, Cohen S, Lebwohl M (2004) Safety and efficacy of an extended 16-week course of alefacept in the treatment of chronic plaque psoriasis: an interim analysis. Poster presented at: 62nd Annual American Academy of Dermatology Meeting; February 6–11; Washington, DC
28. Krueger GG, Callis KP (2003) Development and use of alefacept to treat psoriasis. J Am Acad Dermatol 49: S87–97
29. Krueger GG, Papp KA, Stough DB, Loven KH, Gulliver WP, Ellis CN (2002) A randomized, double blind, placebo-controlled phase III study evaluating efficacy and tolerability of 2 courses of alefacept in patients with chronic plaque psoriasis. J Am Acad Dermatol 47: 821–833
30. Krueger GG, Vaishnaw A, Gordon K (2002) Alefacept (LFA-3/IgG1), a fully human fusion protein, is non-immunogenic in patients with chronic psoriasis (poster #P583). Presented at the 60th Annual Meeting of the American Academy of Dermatology; February 22–27; New Orleans, LA
31. Krueger GG, Van de Kerkhof P (2004) Safety of multiple courses of alefacept in combination with other psoriasis therapies: a study that reflects the clinical practice setting. Poster presented at: 62nd Annual American Academy of Dermatology Meeting; February 6–11; Washington, DC
32. Krueger JG (2002) The immunologic basis for the treatment of psoriasis with new biologic agents. J Am Acad Dermatol 46: 1–23
33. Krueger JG, Walters IB, Miyazawa M, Gilleaudeau P, Hakimi J, Light S, Sherr A, Gottlieb AB (2000) Successful in vivo blockade of CD25 (high-affinity interleukin 2 receptor) on T cells by administration of humanized anti-Tac antibody to patients with psoriasis. J Am Acad Dermatol 43: 448–458
34. Kuypers TW, Roos D (1989) Leukocyte membrane adhesion proteins LFA-1, CR3 and p150,95: a review of functional and regulatory aspects. Res Immunol 140: 461–486
35. Langley R, Baker D, Roberts J (2004) The safety of alefacept using a reduced schedule for monitoring T cells. Poster presented at: 62nd Annual American Academy of Dermatology Meeting; February 6–11; Washington, DC
36. Lebwohl M, Christophers E, Langley R, Ortonne JP, Griffiths CE (2003) An international, randomized, double-blind, placebo-controlled phase 3 trial of intramuscular alefacept in patients with chronic plaque psoriasis. Arch Dermatol 139: 791–793
37. Lebwohl M, Gordon K, Lowe N, et al. (2002) Safety profile of alefacept: pooled results of placebo-controlled trials (abstract no. P1993) Ann Dermatol Venereol 129 (Suppl): 1S761
38. Lebwohl M, Tyring SK, Hamilton TK, Toth D, Glazer S, Tawfik NH, Walicke P, Dummer W, Wang X, Garovoy M, Pariser D (2003) A novel targeted T-cell modulator, efalizumab, for plaque psoriasis. N Engl J Med 349: 2004–2013
39. Leonardi C (2004) Efalizumab (Raptiva): A new therapeutic option for the long-term management of plaque psoriasis. Psoriasis Forum: Spring
40. Leonardi CL (2003) Efalizumab: an overview. J Am Acad Dermatol 49: S98–104
41. Leonardi CL, Goffe B, Sobell J, Caro I, Wang X, Papp KA (2004) The safety of Efalizumab in patients with moderate to severe plaque psoriasis: summary of clinical trial experience. Poster presented at: 62nd Annual American Academy of Dermatology Meeting; February 6–11; Washington, DC
42. Majeau GR, Meier B, Jimmo D, Kioussis PS (1994) Mechanism of lymphocyte function-associated molecule 3-Ig fusion proteins inhibition of T cell responses: structure/function analysis in vitro and in human CD2 transgenic mice. J Immunol 152: 2753
43. Mehlis SL, Gordon KB (2003) The immunology of psoriasis and biologic immunotherapy. J Am Acad Dermatol 49: S44–50
44. Meingassner JG, Grassberger M, Fahrngruber H, Moore HD, Schuurman H, Stutz A (1997) A novel anti-inflammatory drug, SDZ ASM 981, for the topical and oral treatment of skin diseases: in vitro pharmacology. Br J Dermatol 137: 568–576
45. Menter A, Abramovits W, Cather JC (2004) Alefacept in combination with tapering doses of methotrexate in patients with psoriasis. Poster presented at: 62nd Annual American Academy of Dermatology Meeting; February 6–11; Washington, DC
46. Menter A, Cather JC (2004) Long term use of alefacept: safety and off-treatment responses in patients who have received multiple courses of therapy. Poster presented at: 62nd Annual American Academy of Dermatology Meeting; February 6–11; Washington, DC
47. Menter A, Cather JC, Abramovits W (2004) Tuberculosis testing and the use of biologic therapies for the treatment of psoriasis. Poster presented at: 62nd Annual American Academy of Dermatology Meeting; February 6–11; Washington, DC
48. Poole R (2002) Alefacept: An effective therapy for psoriasis. Inpharma 1328: 9–11
49. Miller GT, Hochman PS, Meier W, Tizard R, Bixler SA, Rosa M D, Wallner BP (1993) Specific interaction of lymphocyte function-associated antigen 3 with CD2 can inhibit T cell responses. J Exp Med 178: 211
50. Owen CM, Harrison PV (2000) Successful treatment of severe psoriasis with basiliximab, an interleukin-2 receptor monoclonal antibody. Clin Exp Dermatol 25: 195–197
51. Papp K, Bissonnette R, Krueger JG, Carey W, Gratton D, Gulliver WP, Lui Lynde CW, Magee A, Minier D, Ouellet JP, Patel P, Shapiro J, Shear NH, Kramer S, Walicke P, Bauer R, Dedrick RL, Kim SS, White M,

Garovoy MR (2001) The treatment of moderate to severe psoriasis with a new anti-CD11a monoclonal antibody. J Am Acad Dermatol 45:665–674
52. Papp K, Ellis C, Menter A, et al. (2002) Alefacept improves psoriasis and quality of life: results of a multiple-course trial (abstract no. P2012). Anal Dermatol Venereol 129 (Suppl): S764
53. Poulin YP, Lynde C, Lauzon G, Gupta AK, Barber K, Hull PR, Gilliver WP, Toth D, Gratton D, Langley RGB, Yatscoff R (2004) A randomized, multicenter, double blind, placebo controlled phase 2 trial of ISA247 in patients with chronic plaque psoriasis. J Cutan Med Surg (in press)
54. Rappersberger K, Komar M, Ebelin ME, Scott G, Burtin P, Greig G, Kehren J, Chibout SD, Cordier A, Holter W, Richter L, Oberhauer R, Stuetz A, Wolff K (2002) Pimecrolimus identifies a common genomic anti-inflammatory profile, is clinically highly effective in psoriasis and is well tolerated. J Invest Dermatol 119:876–887
55. Vaishnaw AK (2002) Pharmacokinetics, biologic activity, and tolerability of Alefacept by intravenous and intramuscular administration. J Pharmatokinet Pharmacodyn 29:415–426
56. Weinberg JM, Tutrone WD (2003) Biologic therapy for psoriasis: the T-cell targeted therapies – efalizumab and alefacept Cutis 71:4

X

2 TNF Antagonist Therapy

Bruce E. Strober

Introduction

Tumor necrosis factor alpha (TNF-α) inhibition indisputably treats psoriasis. But long before this fact was confirmed by a variety of clinical trials and case reports multiple avenues of investigation hinted at the fundamental importance of TNF-α in the pathogenesis of psoriasis. For example, when compared to normal skin, psoriasis plaques show increased levels of TNF-α focused on dermal dendrocytes of the papillary dermis, around blood vessels, and at the dermo-epidermal junction. Surrogate markers of TNF-α expression, such as ICAM-1, are also upregulated [35]. In fact, similar to lesions of other inflammatory diseases responsive to TNF-α inhibition (such as rheumatoid arthritis), psoriasis plaques have a T-helper type 1 profile of cytokines including not only TNF-α, but also interleukin-2 (IL-2) and interferon-gamma (IFN-γ) [46]. Other investigations showed that psoriatic plaques contains higher levels of TNF-α relative to both uninvolved skin from the same patient and skin from normal volunteers without psoriasis. Furthermore, lesional and serum TNF-α levels correlate directly with the psoriasis area and severity (PASI) score of the patient, with effective anti-psoriatic therapy (ultraviolet phototherapy and topical corticosteroids) resulting in a reduction of TNF-α levels in the serum and both involved and uninvolved skin of patients with psoriasis [2, 6, 12, 39]. From this perspective, TNF-α inhibition using the newer biologic therapies represents a rational, targeted therapy that effectively neutralizes a central mediator of psoriatic disease. This chapter reviews three different biologic drugs – etanercept, infliximab, and adalimumab (Table A6) – and the safety and efficacy data that support their use in patients with moderate to severe psoriasis.

Etanercept

Etanercept Structure, Pharmacokinetics, and Pharmacodynamics

Etanercept is a dimeric human fusion protein consisting of two extracellular ligand-binding domains of the p75 TNFR fused to the Fc por-

Table A6. Anti-TNF therapies for psoriasis

Generic name	Brand name	Structure	Method of delivery
Etanercept	Enbrel	Human, TNF receptor fusion protein	Subcutaneous, twice weekly or once weekly
Infliximab	Remicade	Chimeric monoclonal antibody	Intravenous infusion, 2–8 week intervals
Adalimumab	Humira	Human monoclonal antibody	Subcutaneous, every other week

tion of human IgG1. The drug is self-administered as a 25 mg subcutaneous injection (pediatric patients are dosed by weight, and a 50 mg dose will be available during 2005). Etanercept has a molecular weight of 150 kDa. The dimeric structure of etanercept allows the molecule to bind simultaneously to two molecules of TNF-α, and thus neutralizes the pro-inflammatory behavior of this cytokine by preventing its binding to the TNFR. Etanercept also can bind to lymphotoxin-α (LT-α, or TNF-β), theoretically also neutralizing the biologic behavior of this molecule. Essentially, etanercept is a soluble version of the TNFR, similar to the endogenous soluble TNF receptors (formed by the cleavage of the extracellular domain of the TNFR) that naturally regulate TNF activity in vivo. But, owing to its dimeric structure, etanercept possesses 50–1000 fold higher affinity for TNF-α than the naturally-occurring monomeric soluble receptor [34]. Furthermore, the immunoglobulin-like structure of etanercept significantly lengthens the in vivo terminal half-life of the drug, which is approximately 100 h. The pharmacokinetics of the drug do not vary significantly between patients with either rheumatoid arthritis or plaque psoriasis, nor do these values vary with either the gender or age of the patient. The effects of either renal or hepatic failure on the metabolism of etanercept have not been formally evaluated [11].

The Efficacy of Etanercept in the Treatment of Plaque Psoriasis

To date, etanercept has been formally evaluated for the treatment of plaque psoriasis in four placebo-controlled studies, one in the context of a larger study evaluating psoriatic arthritis, and the other three studies strictly evaluating psoriasis regardless of the presence of psoriatic arthritis. The first study was a rheumatologic evaluation of the efficacy of etanercept in treating psoriatic arthritis. Of course, most patients in this study had plaque psoriasis, and therefore the drug's ability to clear psoriasis simultaneously could be evaluated. Unlike most trials of biologics for psoriasis, in this study, slightly less than half the patients enrolled were receiving methotrexate at a stable dose, as opposed to using etanercept as monotherapy. Importantly, the presence or absence of concomitant methotrexate did not positively or negatively alter the efficacy of etanercept. In this subanalysis, 38 patients had more than 3% of their body surface area (BSA) covered with psoriasis, and 19 of these patients received etanercept 25 mg twice weekly (the remaining 19 patients received placebo). After 12 weeks of continuous etanercept therapy, the percent of patients achieving a PASI 75 (75% reduction in the PASI score) was 26%, versus 0% of the patients in the placebo arm [30].

The first randomized, placebo-controlled study exclusively evaluating etanercept as a monotherapy treatment for plaque psoriasis enrolled 112 patients, all of whom had moderate to severe psoriasis. The mean PASI score in this group of patients was approximately 18, defining this study – as opposed to the previous – as examining patients with more extensive cutaneous disease. After 12 weeks of etanercept 25 mg twice weekly as monotherapy 30% of patients achieved a PASI 75 (compared to 2% of the placebo group), and after 24 weeks of continuous therapy 56% of patients achieved a PASI 75 (compared to 5% of the placebo group). These differences between the etanercept-receiving group and the placebo group were statistically significant [19]. An important point demonstrated by this study is that etanercept can provide increasing benefit to patients for up to 24 weeks of therapy. Nevertheless, from this and other studies, it is clear that patients as a group generally see their maximum PASI reduction within 20 weeks of initiating etanercept therapy.

After the previous two small studies clearly illustrated the potential of etanercept as monotherapy to treat psoriasis, two larger studies were initiated. The first was carried out in the United States, and enrolled 652 patients. Similar to the smaller study by Gottlieb et al., only patients with moderate to severe psoriasis and not receiving any other therapies (systemic therapy, phototherapy, or effective topical therapy) were enrolled. The mean PASI score for this group of patients was approximately 18. The study design was unique for etanercept in two major aspects: (1) a placebo group was followed for only 12 weeks of analysis, and subsequently (at the 13th week) "crossed over" into an active treatment cohort that received etanercept 25 mg twice weekly; (2) three different doses of etanercept were evaluated: 25 mg once weekly, 25 mg twice weekly, and 50 mg twice weekly. The highest dose represented a departure from the standard "rheumatologic" dosing, and was based on the assumption that a higher dose would translate into a better PASI response. This assumption was proven correct across all treatment arms, as the percentage of patients achieving a PASI 75 after 12 weeks of continuous therapy was 4% in the placebo group, 14% in the low dose (25 mg once weekly) group, 34% in the rheumatologic dose (25 mg twice weekly) group, and 49% in the high dose (50 mg twice weekly) group. After 24 weeks of continuous therapy the percentage of patients achieving PASI 75 was 25% in the low dose group, 44% in the rheumatologic dose group, and 59% in the high dose group, further supporting the belief that patients often continue to benefit from longer term therapy with etanercept. Interestingly, the placebo group that was crossed over at the 13th week to the 25 mg twice weekly dose achieved after 12 weeks a PASI 75 in 33% of patients, and thus corroborated the efficacy data of the other distinct cohort of patients that had received the same dose during the first 12 weeks of the study [25].

Another phase of the U.S. study evaluated the ability to abruptly discontinue treatment with etanercept, allow relapse of psoriasis, and then commence re-treatment with etanercept at the same dose as used previously. This analysis focused only on responders to etanercept (defined as achieving a PASI 50 response during the first 24 weeks of the study) and had two primary questions: (1) What is the median time to relapse (as defined as the loss of 50% of the PASI improvement from baseline) after abrupt discontinuation of etanercept? (2) Does re-treatment after a hiatus from treatment allow for a similar level of efficacy when compared to the initial treatment period? This analysis revealed that after the discontinuation of etanercept the median duration of time to relapse of plaque psoriasis was 85 days. Subsequently, relapsed patients were re-treated with etanercept at the same dose they had received previously. The re-treatment portion of the study was not perfect, as it involved smaller numbers of patients analyzed, and patients with less stable psoriasis (they were worsening, by definition). Nevertheless, after 12 weeks of re-treatment patients achieved comparable control – i.e., achievement of their lowest PASI score after the initial 24 week treatment period [18, 24].

Importantly, in the context of the U.S. study no patients displayed a rebound flare (worsening of their psoriasis to 125% of their baseline PASI within 12 weeks) or morphological change of their psoriasis (to pustular or erythrodermic forms, for example) while either receiving or after abrupt withdrawal of drug. The distillation of these clinical trial data indicates that patients can be safely withdrawn from and restarted with etanercept therapy without concern for either rebound flare of their disease or tachyphylaxis. The lack of tachyphylaxis demonstrated by etanercept is consistent with the observation that etanercept demonstrates low immunogenicity in the clinical trials for psoriasis and its other indications, where no patients displayed the formation of neutralizing antibodies to the drug [11]. But, it should be noted that there are isolated instances in clinical practice where etanercept – like other modalities and medications for psoriasis (i.e., phototherapy, methotrexate, or cyclosporine) – loses efficacy and patients will need either a higher dose of the drug, or a second modality added to better control the disease exacerbation. One must remember that psoriasis is a waxing and waning illness that may show episodic flares in severity not easily controlled by standard doses of any given medication or modality.

The second large study evaluating etanercept enrolled 580 patients and was conducted in Europe, Canada, and a few sites in the United States. Again, only patients with moderate to severe psoriasis (mean baseline PASI approximately 19) and not receiving any other therapies (systemic therapy, phototherapy, or topical therapy) were enrolled. The study design involved three groups of patients during the first 12 weeks: one group receiving a placebo, and the other two groups receiving either etanercept 25 mg twice weekly or 50 mg twice weekly as monotherapy. After the 12th week, all three groups were continued on etanercept 25 mg twice weekly for 12 more weeks. For the first 12 weeks, the data from this study were nearly identical to that of the U.S. study, as the percentage of patients achieving PASI 75 was 34% of the patients in the 25 mg twice weekly group and 49% of the patients in the 50 mg twice weekly group (versus 3% in the placebo group). After the second 12-week period where all three groups received the same dose of etanercept at 25 mg twice weekly, the placebo group, as expected, showed a response to the study drug with 28% of patients achieving PASI 75. The group of patients that started on etanercept 25 mg twice weekly for 12 weeks continued to improve for the second 12 weeks at the same dose, with 45% achieving a PASI 75 by the end of week 24. Finally, the high dose group that received etanercept 50 mg twice weekly for the first 12 weeks was "stepped down" to the lower dose of 25 mg twice weekly for the following 12 weeks. Interestingly, 54% of patients in that arm had achieved PASI 75 by week 24, in essence, demonstrating that induction with high dose etanercept for 12 weeks followed by maintenance with the lower rheumatologic dose allowed a retention of the PASI 75 response from week 12. Further, 77% of patients who achieved PASI 75 after 12 weeks of the high dose etanercept retained their PASI 75 response after stepping down to the lower dose for another 12 weeks. Conversely, 33% of the patients who did *not* achieve a PASI 75 response after 12 weeks of the high dose eventually achieved PASI 75 during the subsequent 12 weeks while on the *lower* rheumatologic dose [10]. Such data indicate that (1) some patients (23% of the responders to high dose etanercept) will need more than the etanercept 25 mg twice weekly dose (perhaps either 75 or 100 mg of a total weekly dose) to maintain a robust clearance of their psoriasis; (2) some patients may achieve PASI 75 later than the 12-week time point (in other words, "late responders"); and (3) etanercept given as an "induction" high dose rapidly clears many patients, and this clearance can be maintained after 3 months using the lower rheumatologic dose as "maintenance".

Taken together, and considering the good safety profile for the high dose group (to be discussed later), these data combined with the author's experience indicate that all patients with moderate to severe plaque psoriasis who are appropriate patients for etanercept should be treated for 3 months on the high dose (50 mg twice weekly) etanercept and then "stepped down" to the lower dose (either 25 mg twice weekly or 50 mg once weekly) as maintenance for at least 1 month. After this 4-month period, it should be obvious which patients are responding adequately to etanercept monotherapy, and which should be considered for either combination therapy (with a second systemic modality, for example) or another modality entirely (a different biologic therapy, for example). In other words, the "step down" approach allows the practitioner to identify etanercept non-responders within a 4-month period of time. In practice, approximately two-thirds of patients who go through the "step down" regimen achieve favorable clearance of their psoriasis by the 24th week of continuous therapy (as defined by those who reach PASI 50, or as defined by the patient, and keeping in mind that "favorable response" may be less than a PASI 75 response for many patients).

Etanercept Safety and Tolerability Data from the Psoriasis Studies

Etanercept was a well-tolerated medication during its psoriasis clinical trial experience. Overwhelming, the most common adverse event associated with etanercept is an injection site reaction (ISR) that occurred in approximately 14% of all patients in the psoriasis studies. Most commonly, this reaction is asymptomatic and undetectable by the patient, but the occasional patient will manifest an erythematous patch or plaque at the site of injection that may be pruritic or tender. The ISR often appears after the second injection of drug, and might be displayed simultaneously at not only the most recent but also the previously injected site. The histologic features of the ISR show a superficial, perivascular or "cuffing" infiltrate comprised predominantly of lymphocytes with eosinophils. Neutrophils and macrophages are also noted. Most of the infiltrating cells are of an activated, mature cytotoxic T-lymphocyte lineage [52]. The ISR is thus thought to be a T-lymphocyte-mediated delayed type hypersensitivity reaction that also wanes over time – specifically, continued use of etanercept over 4 weeks lessens the incidence and severity of the reaction – suggesting a progressive desensitization (acquired tolerance) to the allergen. The ISR takes several hours to develop after injection and may last 3–5 days. Anaphylactoid or IgE-mediated hypersensitivity is not a common feature of etanercept administration, with one patient experiencing angioedema in the clinical trials [11].

In general, other adverse events or serious adverse events were infrequent and not biased toward any of the different treatment groups, regardless of whether patients received placebo for 12 weeks followed by 12 weeks of etanercept 25 mg twice weekly, etanercept 25 mg twice weekly for 24 weeks, or etanercept 50 mg twice weekly for 24 weeks. Similarly, serious infectious adverse events were infrequent and did not arise with a greater frequency in the high dose group of patients when compared to the placebo-crossover group or the lower dose groups [25]. In summary, 24 weeks of therapy with etanercept is well-tolerated and displays a similar safety profile regardless of dose used (up to the 50 mg twice weekly dose).

X

Infliximab

Infliximab Structure, Pharmacokinetics, and Pharmacodynamics

Infliximab is a chimeric IgG1κ monoclonal antibody directed against TNF-α that consists of both murine and human amino acid sequence. The drug is administered as an intravenous infusion over approximately 2–3 h, and is dosed by the weight of the patient. Infliximab has a molecular weight of approximately 149 kDa, and binds specifically to both the soluble and transmembrane forms of TNF-α, neutralizing the pro-inflammatory behavior of TNF-α by preventing its binding to the TNFR. Infliximab does not bind to or neutralize lymphotoxin-α (LT-α, or TNF-β). Cells expressing transmembrane TNF-α bound by infliximab can be lysed both in vitro and in vivo. The terminal half-life of infliximab after infusion at both low (3 mg/kg) and high (10 mg/kg) doses is approximately 10 days. The effects of either renal or hepatic failure on the metabolism of infliximab have not been formally evaluated [20].

The Efficacy of Infliximab in the Treatment of Plaque Psoriasis

The efficacy of infliximab in treating psoriasis has been firmly established by case reports, initially, and later by two double blind, placebo-controlled studies. The case reports hinted at infliximab's high potency in clearing psoriatic patients: a 57-year-old woman with severe psoriasis and Crohn's disease who after receiving one dose of infliximab demonstrated a lessened need for prednisone (to control her Crohn's disease) and a reduction in her PASI score from 34.1 to 12.1 [37]; six patients with longstanding psoriasis and psoriatic arthritis who after three doses of infliximab showed significant improvement in their skin disease [36]; finally, two patients with psoriatic arthritis and psoriasis – one erythrodermic – who demonstrated complete clearing of their psoriasis and improvement in their joint symptoms after one infusion of infliximab [38].

Subsequently, a single-site, blinded study evaluating infliximab versus placebo was conducted. In this study 33 patients were randomized to three groups: 11 received placebo, 11 received infliximab at 5 mg/kg, and 11 received infliximab at 10 mg/kg. Each group received 3 infusions over 6 weeks. All patients had moderate to severe psoriasis with mean PASI scores greater than 20. In short, the results were dramatic, with 82% of the patients receiving infliximab at 5 mg/kg and 73% of the patients receiving infliximab at 10 mg/kg groups achieving PASI 75 (versus 18% of the placebo group) [7].

A larger multicenter, double-blind, placebo-controlled study was then initiated. Like all typical studies evaluating biologic agents for psoriasis, this study only included patients with moderate to severe disease (mean baseline PASI approximately 18–20) and not receiving any other therapies. Two different doses (either 3 mg/kg or 5 mg/kg) of infliximab given as three separate infusions or placebo were administered over 6 weeks to 249 patients, 99 in each active treatment group receiving infliximab, and 51 in the placebo group. Ten weeks after the first infusion, 72% of the 3 mg/kg group, 88% of the 5 mg/kg group, and 6% of the placebo group had achieved PASI 75 reduction in their psoriasis. Interestingly, approximately one-half of the patients achieved a PASI 90 (essentially, cleared) response. Furthermore, patients receiving infliximab maintained their PASI 75 response off drug for approximately 3–4 months after the last infusion, indicating that, in theory, after a course of three infusions with infliximab long-term remission can be achieved [17].

The aforementioned study defined conclusively that infliximab is a powerful agent for the treatment of psoriasis, perhaps more efficacious than cyclosporine, a drug believed previously to be unrivaled in its anti-psoriatic efficacy. Nevertheless, use of infliximab in both psoriasis patients and for its other indications (rheumatoid arthritis and Crohn's disease) has established that in some patients infliximab – when used as monotherapy – has waning efficacy over time, eventually showing no efficacy even at very high doses. Infliximab, consisting of both human and murine amino acid sequences, is a chimeric monoclonal antibody that induces the formation of neutralizing human antichimeric antibodies (HACAs) in some patients receiving the drug. These antibodies may account for the loss of therapeutic efficacy of infliximab over many treatment courses for a variety of indications. Concomitant methotrexate tends to reduce the formation of these neutralizing antibodies, and likely prolongs the efficacy of infliximab [9, 28, 43]. In fact, in the study of monotherapy infliximab for the treatment of psoriasis described above patients after the 3rd dose were followed off drug until their psoriasis had relapsed, and at 26 weeks after the first infusion 23% of patients had developed antibodies (at varying titers) to infliximab [17]. Whether all of these newly formed antibodies were, in fact, neutralizing and, more importantly, associated with reduced infliximab efficacy is unclear. Further, it is unclear whether a long hiatus between infusions – as a part of this study – increases the likelihood of neutralizing antibody formation. Regardless, given the antigenicity of the drug the optimum manner with which infliximab is administered to patients with psoriasis is uncertain. Many practitioners will not administer infliximab as monotherapy, instead mandating that another immunomodulatory drug such as methotrexate be given concomitantly. In the very least, if not an ideal long-term monotherapy, infliximab certainly is an ideal "induction" therapy that rapidly clears most patients with moderate to severe psoriasis. One option is to transition patients cleared by infliximab after three infusions (with or without low dose methotrexate) to another modality – perhaps, another TNF-α inhibitor. Of course, long-term use of infliximab in combination with methotrexate represents another viable option.

Infliximab Safety and Tolerability Data from the Psoriasis Studies

In the smaller 33 patient, single-site trial evaluating infliximab for psoriasis, there were no reported serious adverse events through a 10-week period of evaluation. Headache was the only adverse event that occurred with greater frequency in the infliximab-treated patients. No infusion reactions were noted in this trial [7].

The larger, multi-site study of 249 patients revealed a greater number of adverse events, but also evaluated patients over a longer period of 30 weeks. Seventy-eight percent of patients receiving either the 3 mg/kg or 5 mg/kg dose of infliximab reported at least one adverse event during approximately 30 weeks of follow-up. This is compared to 63% of the placebo group over a shorter 20 weeks of follow-up. Adverse events that occurred in at least 5% of patients and that were notably more frequent in the infliximab-treated population were headache, pruritus, sinusitis, pain, arthralgia, pharyngitis, rhinitis, nausea, back pain, myalgia, fatigue, diarrhea, and flushing. There were four "reasonably-related to infliximab" serious adverse events including squamous cell carcinoma, cholecystitis with cholelithiasis, diverticulitis, and sepsis deriving from pyelonephritis [17].

Infusion reactions are well-documented feature of infliximab administration in some patients. An infusion reaction was defined in this study as any adverse event occurring during infusion and up to 1 h post-infusion. The most common symptoms and signs associated with infusions reactions are fever, chills, chest pain, hypotension, hypertension, dyspnea, urticaria, and pruritus. In the large psoriasis study, after 26 weeks, 6.6% of infliximab infusions were associated with infusion reactions (versus 0.7% of the placebo infusions). Of the infliximab-associated infusion reactions 65% (or 4.2% of all infusions) were mild in intensity, 30% (or 2.0% of all infusions) were moderate in intensity, and 5% (or 0.3% of all infusions) were severe. No serious infusion reactions (involving anaphylaxis, convulsion, erythematous rash, and hypotension) were noted [17].

X

Adalimumab

Adalimumab Structure, Pharmacokinetics, and Pharmacodynamics

Adalimumab is the third TNF-α inhibitor that has been formally evaluated for the treatment of psoriasis. Adalimumab is a human IgG1κ monoclonal antibody directed against TNF-α. Adalimumab contains no murine amino acid sequence. The drug is administered as a subcutaneous injection of 40 mg either once every other week or once weekly. Adalimumab has a molecular weight of approximately 148 kDa, and binds specifically to both the soluble and transmembrane forms of TNF-α, neutralizing the pro-inflammatory behavior of TNF-α by preventing its binding to the TNFR. Adalimumab does not bind to or neutralize lymphotoxin-α (LT-α, or TNF-β). Cells expressing transmembrane TNF-α bound by adalimumab can be lysed in vitro in the presence of complement. The approximate terminal half-life of infliximab is 2 weeks. In the presence of anti-adalimumab antibodies the drug is cleared more efficiently, while in patients over the age of 40 adalimumab is cleared less efficiently. There are no gender-related differences in adalimumab clearance rates. Concomitantly administered methotrexate reduces adalimumab clearance by 29% after one dose and 44% after multiple doses of methotrexate. The effects of either renal or hepatic failure on the metabolism of adalimumab have not been formally evaluated [1].

The Efficacy of Adalimumab in the Treatment of Plaque Psoriasis

When compared to either etanercept of infliximab, there are fewer studies supporting the use of adalimumab for the treatment of plaque psoriasis. Nevertheless, the one placebo-controlled study presented indicates that adalimumab will be a potent option for the treatment of psoriasis. This was a phase II, double-blind, placebo-controlled analysis of monotherapy adalimumab involving 148 patients with moderate to severe plaque psoriasis. The entry criterion for the degree of psoriasis – 5% body surface area, with mean baseline PASI scores between 14 and 16.7 – was lower than the other studies discussed in this chapter (which mandated at least 10% body surface area of involvement and resulted in baseline mean PASI scores greater than or equal to 18), but certainly included patients who would be candidates for systemic therapy or phototherapy. The pool of patients was divided into three groups: one cohort was a placebo/crossover group (52 patients), and received a placebo injection for 12 weeks followed by a "loading dose" of 80 mg for the 13th week, and then 40 mg every other week through 24 weeks; a second cohort (46 patients) received an initial "loading dose" of adalimumab 80 mg followed by 40 mg injections every other week for a total of 24 weeks; and a third (50 patients) high dose group received *two* initial "loading" adalimumab injections of 80 mg given on consecutive weeks followed by weekly injections of adalimumab 40 mg for the following 22 weeks. The results indicated that adalimumab effectively treats psoriasis better than placebo and that higher doses of adalimumab provide greater efficacy. Specifically, at the end of the 24-week dosing period 64% of the 40 mg every other week dosing group had achieved a PASI 75, while 72% of the high dose, 40 mg weekly group achieved a PASI 75. Only 4% of the placebo group achieved a PASI 75 after 12 weeks (compared to 53% and 80% of the patients in the adalimumab-receiving cohorts after 12 weeks). The adverse event rates that occurred during this study were comparable between the placebo and active treatment arms, but the serious adverse event rates were higher in the adalimumab-treated groups relative to the placebo-adalimumab crossover cohort. Specifically, 6.7% and 10% of the lower-dose and higher-dose adalimumab-treated cohorts, respectively, had serious adverse events after 24 weeks of therapy (compared with 0% of the placebo/crossover cohort). The nature of these serious adverse events and their relationship to adalimumab treatment were not available at the time of this chapter's writing [48].

While adalimumab appears to be an effective therapy for psoriasis, the dosing of the drug for this indication has not been clearly defined. In rheumatoid arthritis, the standard dosing involves no loading dose, and an initial dosing of 40 mg every other week, with the option to increase to weekly dosing if response is inadequate and the patient is not taking concomitant methotrexate. Long term safety data on loading dosing and weekly dosing currently is not extensive. Further, at this time the durability of response after discontinuation of the drug has not been studied.

Adalimumab is a fully human monoclonal antibody, and thus would not be expected to display significant antigenicity in dosed patients. Nevertheless, approximately 5% of patients being treated for rheumatoid arthritis with adalimumab developed low-titer neutralizing antibodies at least once during therapy. Patients taking concomitant methotrexate had a significantly reduced rate of antibody formation. Further, rheumatoid arthritis patients with neutralizing antibodies to adalimumab achieved less benefit from the drug than patients who did not generate neutralizing antibodies [1, 31]. The long-term significance of these findings is unclear with regard to the efficacy of adalimumab in psoriasis therapy, and only will be learned through extensive use of the drug in both long term clinical trials and in clinical practice.

Long-Term Safety Data for the Anti-TNF Therapies

In both clinical trials and in postmarketing use TNF-α inhibitors have been shown to be generally safe. Most of the data regarding the safety of TNF-α inhibitors have been established from investigations of patients receiving these drugs for the treatment of rheumatoid arthritis (RA). However, regarding TNF-α-inhibitor safety in patients with psoriasis and psoriatic arthritis (PsA) the current body of evidence is growing.

Sources of Safety Data

Two primary methods are used to accumulate safety data for any given drug. The first of these is the clinical trial – either placebo-controlled or open-label extensions of placebo-controlled trials. In a clinical trial, each subject is seen regularly, and nearly every adverse event is recorded. The major drawback of clinical trials safety data is that it is not truly reflective of "real life" clinical experience, often being drawn from the treatment of healthy patients without concomitant medical illnesses (such illnesses – such as diabetes or immunodeficiency – generally exclude patients from study entry). The second method of gathering safety data is postmarketing surveillance. Although a large body of data are gathered once a drug has been FDA-approved and marketed, with far greater numbers of patients being treated when compared to clinical trials, the collection of such information is inexact and depends on the vigilance, accuracy, and interest of clinicians in the field. Therefore, postmarketing data suffer from underreporting and the problems inherent in anecdotal reports. Nevertheless, in combination, both types of data – clinical trials and postmarketing – are necessary to guide and suggest adaptations for ongoing use of any medication.

Clinical Trials and Postmarketing Data

A large body of evidence has been accumulated on etanercept. Because etanercept was first approved and used for patients with RA, most of the safety data are derived from the RA population. As of December 2003, clinical trials data had been collected on more than 5,100 patients, for a total of approximately 10,500 patient-years of evidence. In postmarketing use, more than 230,000 patients have received etanercept, equivalent to more than 423,000 patient-years. More than 1,000 patients are now in their fifth year of treatment, and some 425 patients have continued treatment into their sixth year.

Clinical studies of etanercept in psoriatic disease, specifically, have included approximately 2,500 patients enrolled in a variety of trials. These have involved studies of psoriasis and/or psoriatic arthritis, including the recently published 24-week, double-blind study involving 652 patients receiving various dosage regimens of etanercept [25]. Another study completed in Europe, Canada, and the United States will add approximately 580 more psoriasis patients. Ultimately, by end of 2004 controlled and open label data will be available on more than 5,500 patients with psoriatic disease who are receiving or have received etanercept. Of course, postmarketing safety data will also grow rapidly for the psoriasis population as currently etanercept is being used extensively in clinical practice in the United States for both psoriasis and psoriatic arthritis.

Similarly, a large amount of safety data has been gleaned from studies involving infliximab. Most of these safety data are derived from the RA and Crohn's disease populations. As of March of 2003, more than 1,650 patients representing approximately 3,500 patient-years of exposure have been enrolled in clinical trials for infliximab. Furthermore, in postmarketing use across all indications, more than 430,000 patients have received infliximab representing more than 750,000 patient-years of use. Infliximab is only used off-label for psoriasis and psoriatic arthritis, currently, and thus postmarketing surveillance for this group of patients is limited.

The safety data on infliximab discussed in this chapter is from the 54-week phase III study, the Anti-Tumor Necrosis Factor Trial in Rheumatoid Arthritis With Concomitant Therapy (ATTRACT), and from the package insert for infliximab [20, 26]. Long-term safety data for infliximab in the treatment of psoriasis is not currently available.

Reported Adverse Events for the TNF-Inhibiting Agents

An injection-site reaction (ISR) is the most predictable and consistent adverse event that occurs in patients who receive etanercept, and it has been seen in approximately 37% of those who receive this agent for rheumatoid arthritis (significantly higher than the incidence of 14% seen in the psoriasis studies). In placebo-controlled clinical trials for all indications for etanercept the most common type of adverse event was an upper respiratory tract infection, occurring in between 12% and 20% of patients, but not at an increased frequency when compared to the placebo groups [11].

In patients with RA treated with infliximab in the ATTRACT trial and other published clinical studies, the most commonly reported adverse events included upper respiratory infections, nausea, sinusitis, and diarrhea. In all cases, these were mild and did not interfere with therapy or prevent administration of the next dose of infliximab.

Infusion reactions are a well-documented feature of infliximab administration in some patients. Generally, an infusion reaction is defined as any adverse event occurring during infusion and up to 1–2 h post-infusion. The most common symptoms and signs associated with infusions reactions are fever, chills, chest pain, hypotension, hypertension, dyspnea, urticaria, and pruritus. In clinical studies, approximately 20% of patients receiving infliximab experience an infusion reaction, compared to 10% of control patients receiving a placebo. Most infusion reactions are mild, with fewer than 1% defined as serious, resulting in anaphylaxis, convulsion, erythematous rash, and hypotension. In clinical trials, approximately 3% of subjects discontinued infliximab because of infusion reactions. Patients who develop antibodies to infliximab have a two- to threefold increased risk of developing an infusion reaction. Concomitant use of another immunumodulatory medication (such as methotrexate) reduces the risk of both developing antibodies to infliximab and the infusion reaction [20].

TNF Inhibition And Infection Risk in Rheumatoid Arthritis Studies

When TNF-inhibiting treatment was introduced, there was great concern over a theoretical risk for serious infections such as pneumonia, severe urinary tract infections, tuberculosis (TB), and sepsis. When considering the infection risk of any drug, it is important to examine the results from two perspectives. First, if a patient has an infection and treatment with a particular agent is initiated, does a risk exist that the infection will be exacerbated or more difficult to treat? Second, if a patient does not have an infection and therapy is started, will there be a greater likelihood of infection developing? Importantly, is there potential for an increased risk for opportunistic infections, including TB?

With regard to long-term tolerability in patients receiving etanercept for RA in clinical trials, there does not seem to be an increased risk of serious infection with individuals receiving etanercept [49], regardless of whether they have early RA or advanced RA, when compared to their control populations. The lack of increased infection risk persists as patients receive this drug chronically [3, 33].

Patients who received infliximab in published RA clinical trials did have higher rates of serious infections compared with those in placebo groups, but the differences were not statistically significant. Further, sepsis is not an uncommon problem among patients with RA who are taking methotrexate, and subjects in many of the infliximab trials were given methotrexate with infliximab [20]. One large double-blind, placebo-controlled study evaluating infliximab with methotrexate for the treatment RA over 30 weeks showed that the frequency of any infection was significantly increased in patients receiving 10 mg/kg of infliximab, but not in those receiving 3 mg/kg. The number of infections classified as serious (life threatening or leading to hospital treatment) was no more frequent with infliximab (1–6%) than in patients receiving placebo (6%) [27].

Without long-term data for adalimumab in the treatment of psoriasis, the clinical trials data for rheumatoid arthritis is the only extensive resource. In clinical trials evaluating adalimumab for RA, the incidence of serious infections was 0.04 per patient-year in adalimumab-treated patients, compared to 0.02 per patient-year in placebo-treated patients [1]. A placebo-controlled study following RA patients treated over 24 weeks showed no apparent difference between serious infection risk in adalimumab-treated patients and placebo-treated patients (1.3% vs. 1.9%) [14]. A 24-week, placebo-controlled study evaluating adalimumab in patients with active RA receiving methotrexate showed a comparable rate of infections between the adalimumab-treated and placebo-treated groups (1.55/patient-year vs. 1.38/patient year) [50]. Another study involving a 26-week placebo-controlled examination of adalimumab for patients with RA for whom previous disease modifying antirheumatic drug (DMARD) treatment had failed, the drug showed rates of serious infections occurring more in adalimumab-treated patients (10/434; 2.3%) than in placebo treated patients (0/110; 0%). All cases of serious infection were treated and resolved during the course of the trial [47]. Finally, a recently published placebo-controlled, 52-week study of adalimumab for patients with active RA who had failed methotrexate showed a higher risk of serious infection in patients receiving adalimumab in combination with methotrexate when compared to patients receiving methotrexate alone (3.8% vs. 0.5%, $p \leq 0.02$) [21]. The disparate results of these studies, all placebo-controlled, emphasizes the difficulty in analyzing data across clinical trials studying different populations of patients with perhaps different risk factors for developing serious infection.

It should be noted that in postmarketing use of etanercept, infliximab, and adalimumab serious infections and sepsis have been reported. Most of these cases involved patients also receiving concomitant immunosuppressive therapy that, in addition to their underlying medical condition (such as RA), could predispose them to infection [1, 11, 20].

From the accumulated long-term tolerability data, it does not appear that TNF-inhibiting therapy greatly increases the risk of infection. However, given the theoretical risk of infection after TNF blockade, vigilance on this issue is warranted, and patients who do develop infections during a course of therapy with any of these agents should be monitored closely. Use of a TNF-inhibiting agent should be discontinued in the context of a febrile illness – especially bacterial or fungal – or if sepsis develops. The patient should be observed and the infection treated appropriately. Treatment with the TNF inhibitor may be restarted when the infection clears, especially if the clinical situation dictates the use of a TNF inhibitor as the best or only reasonable therapy. Local infection – such as either a herpes simplex virus or a human papilloma virus infection – do not require cessation of anti-TNF therapy. Importantly, patients should not be started on anti-TNF therapy if they have an active infection, or a history of recurrent bacterial or fungal infections requiring frequent antimicrobial treatment.

Tuberculosis (TB) reactivation has occurred subsequent to the initiation of anti-TNF therapy, often presenting as extrapulmonary or disseminated TB. Infliximab and adalimumab carry a boxed warning regarding tuberculosis in their labeling, and a purified protein derivative (PPD) test is required prior to initiation of therapy with these drugs. Owing to a lower postmarketing rate of TB reactivation, a PPD test is not required for patients to begin therapy with etanercept, but it may be advisable depending on geographic location. Performance of a PPD test may be a reasonable precaution for patients living in metropolitan areas with large populations of people derived from countries with high endemic rates of tuberculosis. The author's personal preference is to administer a PPD to any patient prior to receiving a TNF-inhibiting therapy. In all instances of detected latent TB effective anti-tuberculosis therapy should be initiated prior to starting anti-TNF therapy.

Malignancy Risk with TNF Inhibition

Investigators in clinical trials of anti-TNF biologic agents have been alert for any signs of an increased risk for malignancy. For all three anti-TNF agents both clinical trials data and postmarketing surveillance do not support the notion that TNF blockade increases the risk of malignancy. In fact, as of March of 2003, open label extension clinical trials of etanercept (involving over 8,300 patient-years of exposure), infliximab (over 2,400 patient-years of exposure), and adalimumab (involving over 4,800 patient-years of exposure) do not reveal an occurrence of malignancies (including lymphoreticular malignancy) that exceeds that which would be expected in a matched population not receiving these drugs [13].

Malignancy rates in the etanercept clinical trials for psoriasis and psoriatic arthritis are comparable to what would be expected in patients with severe psoriasis on systemic therapies [29]. Additionally, not only RA but also psoriasis patients (65 years of age or older) are believed to carry a two- to threefold increased risk of lymphoma [16]. Therefore, any analysis of the effect of medication on these populations must consider the risk of lymphoma specific to the disease entity. At this time the consensus is that patients receiving anti-TNF therapy for RA are not believed to have an increased risk of de novo lymphoma development that exceeds the underlying risk for the entire RA population (regardless of previous or ongoing therapy) [45, 51]. Nevertheless, not enough data are available to state definitively that anti-TNF agents such as etanercept are safe to use in patients with a history of a solid tumor or lymphoreticular malignancy. Practitioners should consider other modalities prior to initiating anti-TNF therapy with patients who have a history of malignancy (excluding nonmelanoma skin cancer).

Anti-TNF Therapies and Demyelinating Neurologic Disease

Early investigators hypothesized that blocking TNF might be an effective means of treating multiple sclerosis (MS). The TNF inhibitor lenercept (not marketed in the United States), a soluble p55 TNF-receptor fusion molecule, was evaluated in a double-blind, placebo-controlled phase II study involving 168 patients with active MS. There were no significant differences between the lenercept- and placebo-treated groups evaluated using magnetic resonance imaging (MRI), but the number of lenercept-treated patients experiencing MS exacerbations was significantly increased compared with patients receiving placebo. Furthermore, the lenercept-treated patients had MS exacerbations that occurred earlier. Finally, neurologic deficits were more severe in the lenercept treatment groups [5].

In addition, cases of new onset of MS or demyelinating neurologic syndromes (such as optic neuritis, transverse myelitis, or seizure disorder) or exacerbations of previously existent conditions have been reported in patients receiving anti-TNF therapy, including etanercept, infliximab, and adalimumab. In most cases, symptoms resolved partially or fully after discontinuation of therapy, and in a few of these patients, rechallenge with the TNF-α inhibitor resulted in reappearance of symptoms [1, 11, 20, 32].

As a result of the association between TNF-α inhibition and demyelination suggested by these reports, anti-TNF-α agents should not be initiated in patients with a history of demyelinating neurologic disease. Demyelinating neurologic syndromes associated with TNF-α inhibition are very rare, but clinicians should be vigilant for the new onset of neurologic symptoms that appear while patients are using anti-TNF-α therapies. At baseline, the practitioner should question the patient for any current neurologic symptoms or history of neurologic disease. This will assist in determining if a symptom or sign while on therapy is either pre-existing or truly new-onset.

Cardiac Safety

Both infliximab and etanercept were evaluated for their possible beneficial effects in patients with congestive heart failure (CHF). In multiple clinical trials, neither agent showed benefit when given to patients with CHF. One study suggested higher mortality in patients with CHF who received etanercept, yet another study did not corroborate this phenomenon [4]. In one study of infliximab, patients receiving a higher dose of infliximab (three doses at 10 mg/kg) had worse outcomes (hospitalization or death) [8]. Furthermore, case reports have identified a small group of people with new-onset CHF while receiving either etanercept or infliximab. Some of these patients had neither precipitating factors nor pre-existing heart disease, and some were under the age of 50 [23]. Currently, there are no published data regarding the risk of using adalimumab in the setting of CHF. But the data regarding etanercept and infliximab support caution when considering an anti-TNF therapy for patients with concomitant congestive heart failure, and that patients should be followed for new-onset cardiac signs and symptoms while on anti-TNF therapy.

Lupus-Like Syndromes

All three anti-TNF therapies are associated with the development of autoantibodies. Specifically, anti-nuclear antibodies develop in some patients receiving these therapies. The majority of the time this laboratory abnormality has no clinical significance. But case reports and postmarketing surveillance have revealed isolated cases of lupus-like syndromes (systemic and cutaneous lupus erythematosus) arising during anti-TNF therapy. Nearly all cases of reported lupus-like syndromes arising during anti-TNF therapy resolve after discontinuation of the therapy [15, 22, 40–42, 44]. Similarly to the monitoring of any systemic medication, patients should receive a thorough review of systems during follow up visits in order to detect new-onset signs and symptoms.

Other Safety Considerations

The clinical trials of etanercept, infliximab, and adalimumab have not demonstrated any new onset, clinically significant laboratory abnormalities arising while on these therapies. Indeed, the packaging information for these medications does not specifically recommend laboratory monitoring. There are rare postmarketing reports of pancytopenia arising in patients receiving etanercept. The relationship of these events to drug is unclear, yet patients with a prior history of hematologic abnormalities should be considered for another therapeutic modality. Additionally, patients receiving etanercept who develop signs or symptoms of bleeding abnormalities or infections should be thoroughly evaluated and discontinuation of etanercept should be considered.

Clinical common sense supports the practitioner obtaining a baseline blood panel that includes a complete blood count, liver function tests, and a comprehensive metabolic panel. Some clinicians advocate a baseline anti-nuclear antibody (ANA) titer and hepatitis B and C serologies. The primary justification for these tests is twofold: (1) anti-TNF agents often may be used in conjunction with other conventional agents (such as methotrexate) that need monitoring and should not be used with abnormalities of certain organ systems (i.e., methotrexate and hepatitis C), and (2) the baseline laboratory values can be compared to laboratory examinations performed during therapy and therefore either exonerate or implicate the treating drug as the etiology of a possible new-onset clinical sign or symptom. Regardless, in a patient tolerating anti-TNF therapy laboratory, monitoring for these agents need not be frequent. The author's preference for follow-up monitoring of anti-TNF therapy is repeated blood work at 2 months into therapy, and every 6 months thereafter.

All three of the anti-TNF therapies should not be given concomitantly with the drug anakinra, another approved therapy for RA. Further, concomitant methotrexate reduces the clearance of adalimumab. At this time, while specific studies have not been conducted, it does not appear necessary to adjust the dosages of the anti-TNF therapies for patients with hepatic or renal insufficiency.

Patients on anti-TNF therapy who require immunization may receive any vaccine except a live virus vaccine (i.e., vaccinia for smallpox). If such live virus vaccination is necessary consider interrupting anti-TNF therapy. For example, etanercept therapy can be discontinued 10 days prior to and restarted approximately 10 days after the vaccination. Reassure patients that discontinuation of therapy is not associated with rebound psoriasis, and that psoriasis worsening is usually very slow while off of therapy.

All three anti-TNF therapies are pregnancy class B. It is not known whether these drugs are excreted in human milk or absorbed systemically after ingestion. Until more experience is reported in pregnant and lactating women, and unless therapy with the drug is deemed medically necessary, it is prudent to have women discontinue these therapies during pregnancy and restart the drug after babies have been weaned from breastfeeding.

Conclusion

To optimize the safe use of anti-TNF therapy, dermatologists may wish to consider utilizing a checklist that helps determine if any given patient with psoriasis with or without psoriatic arthritis warrants treatment with an anti-TNF therapy: (1) avoid patients who have active and chronic bacterial infections, (2) multiple sclerosis or demyelinating neurological disease, (3) solid tumors (except for nonmelanoma skin cancers) or lymphoproliferative malignancies, and (4) congestive heart failure. Following these guidelines and providing regular follow-up, the dermatologist can confidently offer anti-TNF therapy to patients with psoriasis and/or psoriatic arthritis. Keep in mind that the overwhelming majority of patients do not possess contraindications to and do not develop adverse events while on anti-TNF therapies, and therefore the benefit to risk ratio of using these medications is quite high.

References

1. Adalimumab (2004) Package insert
2. Ameglio F, et al. (1994) Interleukin-6 and tumour necrosis factor levels decrease in the suction blister fluids of psoriatic patients during effective therapy. Dermatology 189:359–363
3. Amgen, Data on File
4. Anker S, Coats A (2002) How to RECOVER from RENAISSANCE? The significance of the results of RECOVER, RENAISSANCE, RENEWAL and ATTACH. Int J Cardiol 86:123–130
5. Anonymous (1999) TNF neutralization in MS: results of a randomized, placebo-controlled multicenter study. The Lenercept Multiple Sclerosis Study Group and The University of British Columbia MS/MRI Analysis Group. Neurology 53:457–465
6. Bonifati C, et al. (1994) Correlated increases of tumour necrosis factor-α, interleukin-6 and granulocyte monocyte-colony stimulating factor levels in suction blister fluids and sera of psoriatic patients – relationships with disease severity. Clin Exp Dermatol 19:383–387
7. Chaudhari U. et al. (2001) Efficacy and safety of infliximab monotherapy for plaque-type psoriasis: a randomized trial. Lancet 357:1842–1847
8. Chung E, et al. (2003) Randomized, double-blind, placebo-controlled, pilot trial of infliximab, a chimeric monoclonal antibody to tumor necrosis factor-alpha, in patients with moderate-to-severe heart failure: results of the anti-TNF Therapy Against Congestive Heart Failure (ATTACH) trial. Circulation 107:3133–3140
9. Cohen R, Tsang J, Hanauer S (2000) Infliximab in Crohn's disease: First anniversary clinical experience. Am J Gastroenterol 95:3469–3477
10. Elewski B, et al. (2004) Efficacy and safety of etanercept in patients with psoriasis: Results of a global phase III study. J Am Acad Dermatol 50:P159
11. Etanercept (2004) Package insert
12. Ettehadi P, et al. (1994) Elevated tumour necrosis factor-alpha (TNF-α) biological activity in psoriatic skin lesions. Clin Exp Immunol 96:146–151
13. FDA (2003) Briefing document. Arthritis advisory meeting
14. Furst D, et al. (2003) Adalimumab, a fully human anti tumor necrosis factor-alpha monoclonal antibody, and concomitant standard antirheumatic therapy for the treatment of rheumatoid arthritis: results of STAR (Safety Trial of Adalimumab in Rheumatoid Arthritis). J Rheumatol 30:2563–2571
15. Garcia-Planella E, et al. (2003) Development of antinuclear antibodies and its clinical impact in patients with Crohn's disease treated with chimeric monoclonal anti-TNFalpha antibodies (infliximab). Eur J Gastroenterol Hepatol 15:351–354
16. Gelfand J, et al. (2003) Lymphoma rates are low but increased in patients with psoriasis: results from a population-based cohort study in the United Kingdom. Arch Dermatol 139:1425–1429
17. Gottlieb A, et al. (2004) The efficacy of infliximab across a variety of subgroups with plaque psoriasis. J Am Acad Dermatol 50:P158
18. Gottlieb A, et al. (2004) Withdrawal from etanercept after successful clinical response in psoriasis patients: Disease characteristics and the durability of treatment response. J Am Acad Dermatol 50:P146
19. Gottlieb AB, et al. (2003) A randomized trial of etanercept as monotherapy for psoriasis. Arch Dermatol 139:1627–1632
20. Infliximab (2004) Package insert
21. Keystone E, et al. (2004) Radiographic, clinical, and functional outcomes of treatment with adalimumab (a human anti-tumor necrosis factor monoclonal antibody) in patients with active rheumatoid arthritis receiving concomitant methotrexate therapy: a randomized, placebo-controlled, 52-week trial. Arthritis Rheum 50:1400–1411
22. Klapman J, et al. (2003) A lupus-like syndrome associated with infliximab therapy. Inflamm Bowel Dis 9:176–178
23. Kwon H, et al. (2003) Case reports of heart failure after therapy with a tumor necrosis factor antagonist. Ann Intern Med 138:807–811
24. Leonardi C, et al. (2004) The efficacy and safety of etanercept in the re-treatment of psoriasis after relapse. J Am Acad Dermatol 50:P146
25. Leonardi CL, et al. (2003) Etanercept as monotherapy in patients with psoriasis. N Engl J Med 349:2014–2022
26. Lipsky P, et al. (2000) Infliximab and methotrexate in the treatment of rheumatoid arthritis. Anti-Tumor Necrosis Factor Trial in Rheumatoid Arthritis with Concomitant Therapy Study Group. N Engl J Med 343:1594–1602
27. Maini R, et al. (1999) Infliximab (chimeric anti-tumour necrosis factor a monoclonal antibody) versus placebo in rheumatoid arthritis patients receiving concomitant methotrexate: a randomized phase III trial. Lancet 354:1932–1939
28. Maini RN, et al. (1998) Therapeutic efficacy of multiple intravenous infusions of anti-tumor necrosis factor a monoclonal antibody combined with low-dose weekly methotrexate in rheumatoid arthritis. Arthritis Rheum 41:1552–1563
29. Margolis D, et al. (2001) The risk of malignancy associated with psoriasis. Arch Dermatol 137:778–783
30. Mease PJ, et al. (2000) Etanercept in the treatment of psoriatic arthritis and psoriasis: a randomized trial. Lancet 356:385–390
31. Mikuls T, Weaver A (2003) Lessons learned in the use of tumor necrosis factor-alpha inhibitors in the treatment of rheumatoid arthritis. Curr Rheum Rep 5:270–277
32. Mohan N, et al. (2001) Demyelination occurring during anti-tumor necrosis factor alpha therapy for inflammatory arthritides. Arthritis Rheum 44:2862–2869
33. Moreland L, Cohen S, Klareskog L (2002) Global safety and efficacy of more than 5 years of etanercept (ENBREL) therapy in rheumatoid arthritis [abstract]. Arthritis Rheum 46(Suppl):S532

34. Moreland LW, et al. (1996) Recombinant soluble tumor necrosis factor receptor (p80) fusion protein: Toxicity and dose finding trial in refractory rheumatoid arthritis. J Rheumatol 23:1849–1855
35. Nickoloff B, et al. (1991) Cellular localization of interleukin-8 and its inducer, tumor necrosis factor-alpha, in psoriasis. Am J Pathol 138:129–140
36. Ogilvie AL, et al. (2001) Treatment of psoriatic arthritis with antitumor necrosis factor-α antibody clears skin lesions of psoriasis resistant to treatment with methotrexate. Br J Dermatol 144:587–589
37. Oh CJ, Das KM, Gottlieb AB (2000) Treatment with anti-tumor necrosis factor α (TNF-α) monoclonal antibody dramatically decreases the clinical activity of psoriasis lesions. J Am Acad Dermatol 42: 829–830
38. O'Quinn RP, Miller JL (2002) The effectiveness of tumor necrosis factor α antibody (infliximab) in treating recalcitrant psoriasis. Arch Dermatol 138: 644–648
39. Sagawa Y, et al. (1993) Is sustained production of tumor necrosis factor-a relevant to the development of pustular psoriasis? Dermatology 187:81–83
40. Sarzi-Puttini P, et al. (2003) Infliximab-induced lupus in Crohn's disease: a case report. Digest Liver Dis 35:814–817
41. Shakoor N, et al. (2002) Drug-induced systemic lupus erythematosus associated with etanercept therapy. Lancet 359:579–580
42. Stratigos A, et al. (2004) Discoid lupus erythematosus-like eruption induced by infliximab. Clin Exp Dermatol 29:150–153
43. Strober B (2003) Successful treatment of psoriasis and psoriatic arthritis with etanercept and methotrexate in a patient newly unresponsive to infliximab. Arch Dermatol 140:366
44. Swale V, et al. (2003) Etanercept-induced systemic lupus erythematosus. Clin Exp Dermatol 28: 604–607
45. Symmons D, Silman A (2004) Anti-tumor necrosis alpha therapy and the risk of lymphoma in rheumatoid arthritis: No clear answer. Arthritis Rheum 50: 1703–1706
46. Uyemura K, et al. (1993) The cytokine network in lesional and lesion-free psoriatic skin is characterized by a T-helper type 1 cell-mediated response. J Invest Dermatol 101:701–705
47. van de Putte L, et al. (2004) Efficacy and safety of adalimumab as monotherapy in patients with rheumatoid arthritis for whom previous disease modifying antirheumatic drug treatment has failed. Ann Rheum Dis 63:508–516
48. Wallace K, et al. (2004) Results of the DLQI dermatology-specific quality of life measure in moderate to severe plaque psoriasis patients receiving 24 weeks of adalimumab therapy. American Academy of Dermatology Annual Summer Meeting, 2004, New York
49. Weinblatt M, Kremer J, Bankhurst A (1999) A trial of etanercept, a recombinant tumor necrosis factor receptor: Fc fusion protein, in patients with rheumatoid arthritis receiving methotrexate. N Engl J Med 340:253–259
50. Weinblatt M, Keystone E, Furst D (2003) Adalimumab, a fully human anti-tumor necrosis factor alpha monoclonal antibody, for the treatment of rheumatoid arthritis in patients taking concomitant methotrexate: the ARMADA trial. Arthritis Rheum 48:35–45
51. Wolfe F, Michaud K (2004) Lymphoma in rheumatoid arthritis: The effect of methotrexate and anti-tumor necrosis factor therapy in 18,572 patients. Arthritis Rheum 50:1740–1751
52. Zeltser R, et al. (2001) Clinical, histological, and immunophenotypic characteristics of injection site reactions associated with etanercept: A recombinant tumor necrosis factor-α receptor: Fc fusion protein. Arch Dermatol 137:893–899

B Psoriatic Arthritis

Contents

1 TNF-α Inhibitors in Psoriatic Arthritis

Philip J. Mease

Rationale

The development of targeted immunologic therapies for the treatment of inflammatory arthritides such as rheumatoid arthritis (RA) and psoriatic arthritis (PsA), has revolutionized rheumatologic care in recent years. A leading target in this advance has been the inhibition of a key pro-inflammatory cytokine, tumor necrosis factor α (TNF-α), known to be a central element in the inflammatory cascade of a variety of diseases, including autoimmune joint and skin diseases such as PsA. The end of the 1990s saw the first documentation of the dramatic effect of TNF-α inhibition in RA with the soluble receptor protein, etanercept, [1, 2], and an anti-TNF-α monoclonal antibody, infliximab [3, 4, 5]. These observations were rapidly followed by the confirmation of the ability of TNF-α inhibition to reduce signs and symptoms of early RA as well as established RA and importantly, showing evidence of ability to inhibit disease progression toward crippling disability as evidenced by inhibition of radiographic joint changes [4, 6, 7], as well as the subsequent approval of a fully human anti-TNF-α monoclonal antibody, adalimumab (see below).

Based on our understanding of the pathophysiology of PsA and psoriasis (see Chapter III), including areas of immunologic overlap with RA, there is ample rationale to assess the effects of these agents on both the joint and skin manifestations of PsA. There has been previous documentation of TNF-α upregulation in the synovial tissue, synovial fluid, serum and skin of PsA and psoriasis patients [8–15], thus making TNF-α downregulation a potentially fruitful target of immunomodulation. In the arena of joint and peri-articular inflammation and destruction, TNF-α is central to the inflammatory process via its effects, as a molecular messenger, on a wide variety of processes. It is elaborated by a number of immunoregulatory cells including macrophages, monocytes, keratinocytes, dermal dendritic cells, mast cells, and activated T cells [16, 17] TNF-α induces the expression of endothelial, keratinocyte, and dendritic cell surface receptors involved in the migration of leucocytes to inflammatory lesions, the adhesion molecules [18]. TNF-α interacts with T cell surface receptors to induce intracellular signaling via NFκB and upregulation of T cell activation, resulting in a cascading production of a variety of pro-inflammatory cytokines [17, 19] TNF-α mediates a number of processes important in inflammatory joint destruction such as stimulation of bone resorption via activation of osteoclasts, inhibition of bone formation and synthesis of proteglycan, and induction of metalloproteinases and other effector molecules which are involved in cartilage destruction [20–24]. TNF-α activity in the skin, via T cell activation and induction of a variety of cytokines, leads to increased cellular infiltration in sites of inflammation and a variety of inflammatory mediators which lead to the erythema, induration, and scale, as well as discomfort characteristic of psoriatic lesions [25]. Thus, it would appear that inhibition of this key cytokine could yield beneficial clinical effects in the inflamed joint and skin tissue of PsA. Indeed, parallel programs of study of TNF-α inhibition in PsA were conducted with the initial two TNF-α inhibitors approved for the treatment of RA, etanercept and infliximab, beginning in 1999. Several reviews of this subject have recently appeared [26, 27, 28].

Etanercept

Etanercept is a fusion protein consisting of two TNF-α p75 receptor domains and one IgG1 Fc region. The dimeric structure of the molecule allows it to bind 50–1000 times more strongly than the natural monomeric form of the TNF receptor. It is administered subcutaneously, either twice weekly or as a double dose weekly, usually at a dose of 25 mg as established in trials in rheumatoid arthritis. Etanercept has been studied in two controlled trials in PsA. Mease, et al. [29] conducted a placebo-controlled trial of etanercept in 60 patients recruited in the Seattle region who had inadequate responses to previous systemic therapies. Patients who had partial benefit for their skin lesions from methotrexate (MTX) therapy were allowed to maintain this as a background medication. Stable NSAIDs and low dose prednisone were also allowed, similar to RA study designs. Stratification of randomization was based on MTX background. Forty-seven percent of patients maintained MTX, thus creating a four arm trial with essentially equal number of patients on etanercept, 25 mg subcutaneously twice a week, or placebo, with or without MTX background. Recognizing the potential for significant oligoarticular disease, patients with as few as three tender and swollen joints could enroll, although the majority of patients had polyarticular disease, with a mean of nearly 20 tender and 15 swollen joints, as well as elevations of acute phase reactants, and signs of disability, as measured by the Health Assessment Questionnaire (HAQ). On average, patients had an approximately 20 year history of psoriasis and a 9 year history of PsA. The study design included 3 months of placebo-controlled therapy followed by 6 months of open label observation.

The primary endpoint of the study was derived from a published, large study of sulfasalazine in PsA and dubbed the Psoriatic Arthritis Response Criteria (PsARC) [29, 30]. PsARC improvement required at least 30% improvement of tender or swollen joint count and improvement of patient and/or physician global assessment. This result was achieved by 87% of the etancercept treated patients and 23% of the placebo patients. The ACR response criteria for RA was modified for use in PsA by addition of distal interphalangeal (DIP) and carpo-metacarpal (CMC) joints, known to be commonly involved in PsA. An ACR 20 response was achieved by 73% of the etanercept patients and 13% in the placebo group. ACR 50 and 70 scores were achieved by 50% and 13%, respectively, in the etanercept group and 3% and 0% in the placebo group. There was a corresponding improvement of functional disability as measured by the Health Assessment Questionnaire (HAQ) scores, previously validated in RA [31]. Mean HAQ score improved by 83% in the etanercept treated patients, compared to 3% in the placebo patients. All p values <0.0001. Thirty-four percent of patients in the etanercept group had a HAQ score of 0, i.e. showing no signs of disability. When the data was analyzed according to concomitant use of MTX, no difference in outcome was discernable between those on or off background MTX.

Patients with more than 3% body surface area involved with psoriasis (N=38), underwent Psoriasis Area and Severity Index (PASI) [32] scoring. Those in the etanercept group showed 46% mean improvement of the PASI score whereas the mean improvement in the placebo group was 9%. A 75% improvement of the PASI score was achieved by 26% of etanercept treated patients and no placebo patients (p=0.0154). During the short course of this study, there were no significant safety or tolerability issues other than mild injection site reactions which occurred more frequently in the etanercept group, dissipated with continued use of the medication, and did not lead to any study withdrawals.

In the open label phase of this study, patients who were initially in the placebo group rapidly developed PsARC and ACR scores that were similar to the initially etanercept treated patients [33]. Interestingly, with more extended use of etanercept in all PASI-evaluable patients, the median PASI improvement was 62% after six months of open label use of etanercept, suggesting that optimal effects could be seen with more prolonged exposure to the medication. Patients were allowed to adjust background medications if they so desired. Of the patients taking concomitant MTX, 43% decreased their dosage and 25% discontinued MTX. Of patients taking prednisone, 44% were able to discontinue.

The favorable results of this study led to a multi-center study of etanercept in PsA in the US, as well as studies focusing on psoriasis, detailed in Chapter X.A. The phase III PsA trial enrolled 205 patients [34]. Study design was similar to the phase II trial, except that the ACR 20 response at three months in this six-month placebo controlled trial was chosen as the primary endpoint. This response was achieved by 59% of the patients in the etanercept group and 15% in the placebo group (Fig. B1a). The PsARC response was achieved by 72% and 31% respectively. Mean improvement of the PASI score, in 66 evaluable etanercept treated patients was 42% and –8.1% in 62 evaluable placebo patients. A PASI 75 response was observed in 23% of evaluable etanercept treated patients. Favorable outcomes were also seen in quality of life and function indices in the treated patients. From a baseline score of 1.1, the HAQ score improved 0.6 units in the etanercept group, above what is considered to be a minimal clinically important difference in PsA, 0.3 [35], and 0.1 unit in the placebo group. The Medical Outcomes Study Short Form 36 (SF 36) and the EuroQOL Feeling Thermometer also showed highly significant differences in improvement between the treated and placebo group [36].

Disease progression, as evidenced by radiographic evidence of serial damage of joints, and its correlation with hastened morbidity and mortality in RA has been well documented and underlies the focus on early, more aggressive therapy in that disease [37–40]. This correlation of radiographic progression with morbid-

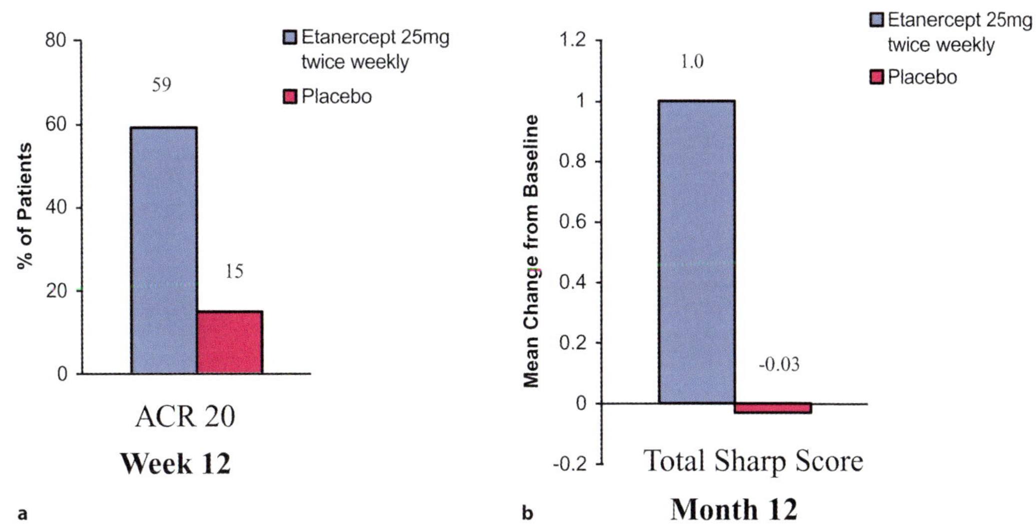

Fig. B1. a 205 PsA patients randomized to etanercept twice weekly vs. placebo. Methotrexate, nonsteroidals, and prednisone ≤10 mg allowed (p<0.0001). **b** At month 12, etanercept treated patients had no increase in Total Sharp Score, implying inhibition of progressive joint destruction (p<0.0002)

ity and mortality has not been established in PsA, nor has a fully accepted method of radiographic scoring been adopted. Retrospective assessment of radiographic progression in patients treated with MTX compared to a similar group of PsA patients not treated with MTX showed similar progression in both groups using both a Larsen and modified Steinbrocker scoring method [41].

In the etanercept phase III study, radiographs of hands and feet were obtained at baseline, six months, at entry to open label (when all patients had completed the placebo-controlled phase), and at 12 months [34, 42]. The scoring method used was the modified Sharp method [43], validated in RA, and further modified to include the DIP joints. The primary radiographic endpoint was the annualized rate of change in the Total Sharp Score (TSS). At 1 year, the group treated with etanercept had not progressed (–0.03 units) whereas the group randomized to placebo did progress (1.00 units) (Fig. B1b). Annualized changes in erosion and joint space narrowing scores also were significantly different between treatment groups. Additional radiographic assessments specific to PsA, such as periostitis, tuft osteolysis, and pencil-in-cup deformity did not change in either treatment group, perhaps because they were more "fixed" radiographic changes. The presence or absence of background MTX did not affect this analysis. Thus, for the first time in PsA, etanercept therapy has been shown to inhibit radiographic disease progression, which may be significant for long term disease outcome in this disease.

Overall safety and tolerability outcomes were similar to the experience in the phase II trial and not different from the experience with etanercept in RA [1, 2, 6, 7, 44].

Infliximab

Infliximab is a chimeric IgG1 monoclonal antibody directed against TNF; it binds to both membrane-bound and soluble TNF-α with high specificity and binding potential. It is administered IV, initially at baseline, two weeks and then 6 weeks, followed typically by infusions every 8 weeks. The usual starting dose for the treatment of RA is 3 mg/kg, although this dose may be increased and the dose frequency shortened if efficacy is inadequate at the starting dose. A series of open label observational studies with infliximab in PsA [45] and in spondyloarthropathies, in which patients with PsA were enrolled [46–47], suggested significant effect of this agent on the signs and symptoms of PsA. In the PsA specific study, 10 patients who had inadequately responded to MTX received infliximab over 54 weeks. The initial dose was 5 mg/kg at weeks 0, 2, and 6, with subsequent dosing individualized according to clinical response. Eight of 10 patients achieved an ACR 70 response by week 10, which was

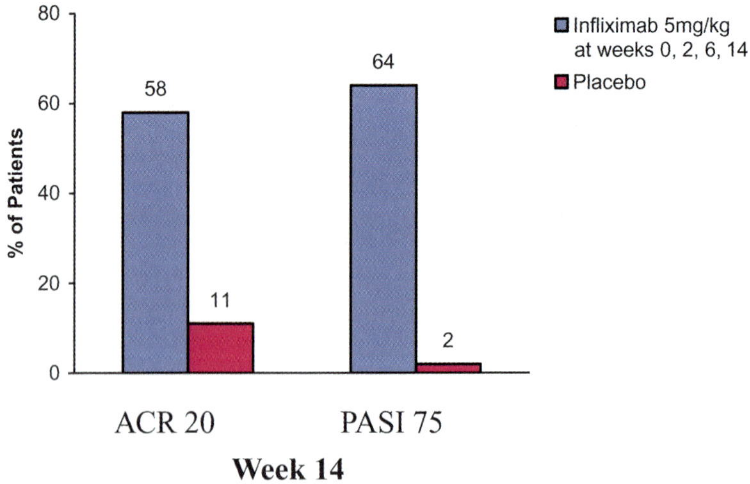

Fig. B2. Phase III trial of Infliximab in Ps/PsA. 200 psA patients randomized to infliximab 5 mg/kg at baseline and weeks 2, 6, and 14 during the placebo-controlled phase. Background DMARDs, nonsteroidals and prednisone ≤10 mg allowed (p values <0.001)

maintained by 6 patients. Joint MRI assessments showed significant reduction of inflammation. PASI scores decreased by 71% [45]. In an open spondyloarthropathy trial of 21 patients, 9 of whom had PsA, infliximab at 5 mg/kg yielded significant reduction in peripheral joint and axial symptoms [46]. Response was generally maintained over one year when infliximab was administered every 14 weeks, although symptoms began to recur prior to the next infusion, suggesting that the 14 week dosing interval was too long for optimal control of disease [47].

Based on these observations, a larger phase II, placebo-controlled trial was conducted in 104 PsA patients whose demographics and disease severity were similar to the patient group in the etanercept trials [48–49]. The dosage of infliximab was 5 mg/kg. A background DMARD was used by 64% of patients (MTX in 46%). At week 16, the primary endpoint of the study, an ACR 20 response was achieved in 69% of patients receiving infliximab, compared to 8% in the placebo group (Fig. B2). ACR 50 and 70 responses were achieved by 49% and 29% of the infliximab patients, respectively, whereas none of the placebo patients achieved these levels of response. Twenty-one patients in the infliximab group were able to have PASI evaluation, having a baseline score of ≥2.5. Mean reduction in this group was 81% and 67% achieved a PASI 75 response, whereas none did so in the placebo group ($p<0.001$). Measures of dactylitis and enthesitis showed improvement in these aspects of the disease as well. The treatment was well tolerated.

One year follow-up of this patient cohort showed sustained efficacy when infliximab 5 mg/kg was given every eight weeks [50]. ACR 20/50/70 scores were 72%/54% and 35% in those originally treated with infliximab and the originally placebo patients achieved similar results. Skin improvements were also maintained.

In this trial, radiographs of the hands and feet were obtained at baseline and 50 weeks. Since the period of placebo treatment was relatively short (14 weeks), with crossover design, the fact that no progression of joint damage was seen in either group likely reflects the similarity of benefit of 50 and 36 weeks of treatment. The calculated annual progression rate was reduced from 5.8 modified Sharp points per year of disease to 0.05 in the placebo/infliximab arm and –1.52 in the infliximab/infliximab arm [51].

A larger phase III trial (IMPACT 2) was conducted in 200 PsA patients [52]. At week 14,

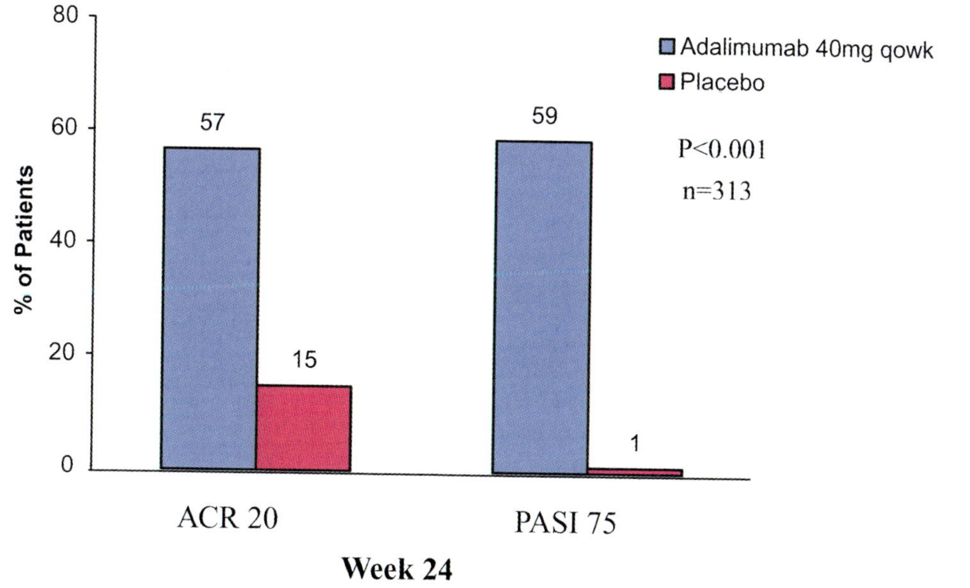

Fig. B3. Phase III trial of adalimumab in PsA. 313 PsA patients randomized to adalimumab, 40 mg qowk vs. placebo, with background MTX, nonsteroidals, and prednisone ≤10 mg allowed (p value for both <0.001)

ACR 20 response was demonstrated in 58% of the infliximab group and 11% of the placebo group (p value <0.001) The median PASI improvement in the infliximab treated, PASI evaluable, ACR 20 responders was 87% whereas it was 74% in the ACR20 non-responders, suggesting that the drug can be helpful in the skin even when the joints do not improve substantially [53]. Radiographic data from this trial is pending. Results of psoriasis studies with infliximab are detailed in Chapter X.A.1. No new side effect issues arose other than those seen in RA trials.

Adalimumab

Adalimumab is a fully human anti-TNF monoclonal antibody approved for the treatment of RA in either every other week or weekly subcutaneous dosing formats [54–57]. An open label trial of adalimumab, 40 mg every other week, in 15 PsA patients showed excellent results [58]. A large placebo-controlled trial (n=313) allowed background MTX; as in other anti-TNF trials. MTX was used by 50% of patients in both the placebo and adalimumab (40 mg every other week) arms of the study. At six months, 57% of the adalimumab treated patients achieved an ACR 20 response whereas only 15% did so in the placebo group (p<0.001) [59]. In patients evaluable for PASI scoring, PASI 50/75/90 responses were 75%/59%/42% in the adalimumab group and 12%/1%/0% in the placebo group (p<0.001). (See Fig. B3). There were no new side effects other than those seen in RA trials.

Other Anti-TNF Medications

Other anti-TNF medications are in development, such as onercept, which is a recombinant human p55 TNF-binding protein that has been tested in RA, psoriasis, and PsA. In a phase II placebo-controlled PsA trial, utilizing 50 and 100 mg three times a week, the 100 mg arm showed PsARC and ACR20 responses of 86% and 67% respectively at twelve weeks compared to 45% and 31% in the placebo arm [60].

Immunopathogenic Evidence of Benefit from TNF-α Inhibition

Several studies, recently reviewed [61], have documented the cellular and immunologic changes that result from TNF inhibition in PsA, providing a framework for understanding the clinical improvements that have been seen. Histological evaluation of synovial tissue in spondyloarthropathy, including PsA, patients treated with infliximab demonstrate reduction of synovial lining layer thickness, vascularity, endothelial expression of $a_V b_3$ and VCAM-1, and sub-lining layer expression of ICAM-1 and E-selectin. Inhibition of T cell and macrophage infiltration, but not B cell infiltration, was observed in synovial and skin biopsies [62–66]. Significant reduction in Ang2, VEGF, CD3, CD4, and CD31 have been observed in psoriatic lesions following anti-TNF therapy, correlating with clinical improvement [64]. A separate study documented reduction of VEGF as well as FLK-1 and neovessel area in synovial and skin tissue [65]. Ritchlin has documented the significant ability of anti-TNF therapy to reduce the numbers of osteoclast precursors and to inhibit osteoclast differentiation [24] These observations shed further light on the immunopathological mechanisms of psoriatic disease in skin and joints.

Safety and Tolerability

For most patients, anti-TNF medications are not associated with significant side effects and they are often regarded as safer than traditional disease modifying drugs. No routine laboratory monitoring is required. However, certain precautions, discussed below, are appropriate.

The most common side effect with etanercept in clinical trials has been injection site reactions (ISRs), occurring in up to a third of patients [34]. These are mild, transient, and eventually resolve. Somewhat fewer patients experience such reactions with adalimumab [67]. Infusion reactions with infliximab are less common and may include fever, chills, rash, headache, nausea, and chest pain; these symptoms generally respond to a slowing of the infusion rate. It is usually advisable to infuse over two hours. In such patients, it may be helpful to co-medicate with acetaminophen, steroids, or antihistamines. If a more severe reaction occurs, such as bronchospasm or anaphylaxis, then the infusion should be stopped and appropriate therapy instituted [68, 69].

Because TNF plays a central role in immune system function, some areas of surveillance for adverse effects include observation for infection, development of autoimmune disease other than the one being treated, and neoplasm.

The background infection rate in RA patients is higher than in the general population [70]. In controlled trials in RA, the rate of both routine and serious bacterial infection was similar between placebo and anti-TNF treated patients and not higher than the background rate of infection [1–7]. Despite this data, it is advisable to monitor patients with infection closely and hold anti-TNF therapy when serious infection, such as pneumonia, UTI, or cellulitis is present. Caution should be exercised when using a TNF inhibitor in patients with recurrent infections or comorbid conditions which may predispose to infection such as diabetes.

Opportunistic infection such as tuberculosis, histoplasmosis, or coccidiodomycosis although rare, may occur in patients treated with TNF inhibitors. Animal studies show that TNF has a protective effect against such infections [71]. TNF has been shown to have a role in granuloma formation and stabilization [72, 73]. These infections have been seen with each of the TNF inhibitors and appear to be more common with use of infliximab [74]. It is common practice to check a tuberculin skin test before treating with a TNF inhibitor (required with infliximab and adalimumab and advisable with etanercept), and to institute anti-TB treatment if the skin test is positive, prior to institution of anti-TNF therapy. Many of the TB cases associated with TNF antagonist therapy have been extra-pulmonary, an important point to remember in the evaluation of clinical syndromes such as fever of unknown origin, lymphadenopathy, or focal symptoms in a patient with a normal chest radiograph [75, 76].

RA patients are not at increased risk for malignancies of solid organs, and use of anti-TNF medications has not been shown to increase risk for such malignancies [77]. On the other hand, there is a 2–8 fold increased risk for lymphoma noted in various large registry studies of RA patients. In controlled trials with anti-TNF agents, the relative risk for lymphoma with etanercept was 3.47, with infliximab was 6.35, and with adalimumab, was 5.42 [78]. It can be seen that these risk rates are within the range of rates seen normally in an RA patient population. Although the risk is not statistically elevated over background, it is not known whether in individual cases, TNF inhibition may have played a role. The number of subjects treated in PsA trials with these agents is too small to make a meaningful assessment of altered risk in this disease.

Demyelinating conditions may rarely be associated with anti-TNF therapy. Cases of multiple sclerosis and optic neuritis have occurred with slightly more frequency than expected [79, 80]. TNF inhibitors should be avoided in patients with demyelinating disorders.

Although antinuclear antibodies may develop quite frequently with anti-TNF therapy, from 11–12% with etanercept and adalimumab to 52% with infliximab [69, 81, 82], the development of lupus or lupus-like disease is quite rare [83–87]. These cases tended to be mild and resolved with cessation of anti-TNF therapy.

Antibodies directed against the anti-TNF agent have been noted with each of the medications. Those associated with etanercept are not neutralizing, and they do not appear to impair effectiveness. As infliximab is a chimeric monoclonal antibody, human anti-chimeric antibodies (HACA) do form and may be neutralizing. It has been shown that concomitant use of methotrexate will reduce the frequency of HACAs. Increased HACA formation, is seen with intermittent administration of infliximab, as in Crohn's disease, and appears to be associated with decreased efficacy and increased frequency of infusion reaction [88]. Anti-human antibodies (HAHAs) occur with adalimumab administration and may be neutralizing.

TNF is elevated in congestive heart failure (CHF), a finding that prompted trials of anti-

TNF therapy in this condition [89]. The etanercept trials did not show improvement in survival, hospitalization, or New York Heart Association class [90]. When infliximab was tested in patients with Class III and IV CHF, there was a dose related increase of hospitalizations and death, leading to a warning not to use this agent in a patient with CHF [91]. Post marketing surveillance also has raised concern regarding CHF in relation to anti-TNF therapy [92].

Despite this list of potential adverse events and precautions, some serious and potentially fatal, an important perspective to maintain is that the frequency of these events is quite rare in the context of the overall use of these agents and especially in the context of their dramatic efficacy and beneficial impact on quality of life. The great majority of patients do not experience meaningful adverse effects, which may not be as readily said for the traditional disease modifying drugs, as discussed elsewhere in this text.

Practical Considerations in Anti-TNF Administration

Several questions often arise in the management of patients with TNF antagonist therapy. How does one manage the patient who only achieves partial response or appears to lose their response to an anti-TNF medication? Although etanercept and adalimumab may be given as monotherapy, as can infliximab if methotrexate is poorly tolerated, they can be administered in combination with medications such as methotrexate, leflunomide, and sulfasalazine, as well as corticosteroids and NSAIDs for potentially additive effect. The experience in RA suggests that increasing etanercept dose above 25 mg two times a week or 50 mg once a week does not yield more benefit for arthritis [93]. However there may be exceptions to this rule and the experience in psoriasis, as described by Leonardi in this text, suggests that 50 mg twice a week is more efficacious in the skin. The "standard" dose for infliximab in RA is 3 mg/kg every eight weeks, but greater benefit can be seen with higher doses, up to 10 mg/kg monthly [69]. Similarly, the "standard" dose for adalimumab is 40 mg every other week, at which dose most patients achieve adequate benefit, but greater benefit in the joints and skin may be seen with weekly dosing [82].

If a patient loses response to one anti-TNF medication, does it make sense to switch to another anti-TNF medication, or should one switch to a different class of medication? Recent studies in RA have shown that approximately 60% of patients who have not had efficacy, or have lost efficacy from a course of either etanercept or infliximab may have a good response with the other medication [94, 95]. Similar data has recently been shown when patients switch from etanercept or infliximab to adalimumab [96]. Thus, it would appear that switching amongst agents in this class is quite reasonable.

It appears safe to administer an anti-TNF medication with a traditional disease modifying drug; however, is it safe to administer it with another biologic agent? A study of the combination of etanercept and anakinra, an anti-IL1 agent, showed a higher rate of infection in the combination group, suggesting that it is not advisable to use this combination [97]. Combination with alefacept or efalizumab has not been studied. A practical consideration here is that such combinations may be prohibitively costly.

Conclusion

The development of medications that specifically target key elements of the inflammatory cascade, such as the anti-TNF agents, represents a major advance in our ability to improve the symptoms and signs and potentially inhibit or halt disease progression in psoriatic arthritis. Dramatic reductions in tenderness and swelling of joints as well as tendon insertions has allowed patients to resume their normal lives with less fatigue and dysfunction. It is not uncommon to hear patients state that their "life has been given back to them". The promise of these agents in inhibiting radiographic progression and possibly altering the natural history of the disease is now an attainable goal. Although these medications are parenterally administered, patients adapt quickly and easily to either subcutaneous or intravenous formulations and appreciate the choice. Surveillance for side effects, especially infection, must be maintained, but the lack of need for frequent laboratory monitoring and overall infrequency of adverse effects is reassuring and freeing for both the patient and physician. The effectiveness of these medications teaches us about the centrality of TNF in both the joint and skin pathophysiology. The ability of these drugs to impact both joints and skin promotes collaboration and teamwork between rheumatologists and dermatologists as both strive to improve the patient's well-being.

References

1. Moreland LW, Schiff MD, Baumgartner SW, et al. (1999) Etanercept therapy in rheumatoid arthritis. A randomized, controlled trial. Ann Intern Med 130(6):478–486.
2. Weinblatt ME, Kremer JM, Bankhurst AD, et al. (1999) A trial of etanercept, a recombinant tumor necrosis factor receptor: Fc fusion protein, in patients with rheumatoid arthritis receiving methotrexate. N Engl J Med 340(4):253–259.
3. Maini R, Breedveld FC, Kalden JR, et al. (1998) Therapeutic efficacy of multiple intravenous infusions of anti-tumor necrosis factor alpha monocolonal antibody combined with low-dose weekly methotrexate in rheumatoid arthritis. Arthritis Rheum 41: 1552–1563.
4. Maini R, St. Clair EW, Breedveld F, et al. (1999) Infliximab (chimeric anti-tumor necrosis factor alpha monoclonal antibody) versus placebo in rheumatoid arthritis patients receiving concomitant methotrexate: a randomized phase III trial. Lancet. 354:1932–1939.
5. Lipsky PE, van der Heijde DM, St. Clair EW, et al. (2000) Infliximab and methotrexate in the treatment of rheumatoid arthritis. N Engl J Med 343: 1594–1602.
6. Bathon JM, Martin RW, Fleischmann RM, et al. (2000) A comparison of etancercept and methotrexate in patients with early rheumatoid arthritis. N EnglJ Med 343(22):1586–1593.
7. Genovese MD, Bathon JM, Martin RW, et al. (2002) Etanercept versus methotrexate in patients with early rheumatoid arthritis; two-year radiographic and clinical outcomes. Arthritis Rheum 46(6): 1443–1450.
8. Ritchlin C, Haas-Smith SA, Hicks D, et al. (1998) Patterns of cytokine production in psoriatic synovium. J Rheumatol 25 (8):1544–1552.
9. Danning CL, Illei GG, Hitchon C, et al. (2000) Macrophage-derived cytokine and nuclear factor κB p65 expression in synovial membrane and skin of patients with psoriatic arthritis. Arthritis Rheum 43:1244–1256.
10. Mizutani H, Ohmoto Y, Mizutani T, et al. (1997) Role of increased production of monocytes TNF-α, IL-1β and Il-6 in psoriasis: relation to focal infection, disease activity and responses to treatments. J Dermatol Sci 14:145–153.
11. Partsch F, Steiner G, Leeb BF, et al. (1997) Highly increased levels of tumor necrosis factor-α and other proinflammatory cytokines in psoriatic arthritis synovial fluid. J Rheumatol 24:518–523.
12. Bonifati C, Ameglio F (1999) Cytokines in psoriasis. Int J Dermatol 101:783–794.
13. Ettehadi P, Greaves NW, Wallach D, et al. (1994) Elevated tumor necrosis factor-alpha (TNF-α) biological activity in psoriatic skin lesions. Clin Exp Immunol 96:146–151.
14. Mussi A, Bonifati C, Carucci M, et al. (1997) Serum TNF-alpha levels correlate with disease severity and are reduced by effective therapy in plaque-type psoriasis. J Biol Regul Homeost Agents 11:115–118.
15. Chodorowska G (1998) Plasma Concentrations of IFN-γ and TNF-α in psoriatic patients before and after local treatment with dithranol ointment. J Eur Acad Dermatol Venerol 10:147–151.
16. Wakefield PE, James WD, Samlaska CP (1991) Tumor necrosis factor. J Am Acad Dermatol 24: 675–685.
17. Feldmann M, Brennan FM, Maini RN (1995) Role of cytokines in rheumatoid arthritis. Annu Rev Immunol 14:397–440.
18. Terajima S, Higaki M, Igarashi Y, et al. (1998) An important role of tumor necrosis factor-α in the induction of adhesion molecules in psoriasis. Arch Dermatol Res 290:246–252.
19. Barnes PJ, Karin M (1997) Nuclear factor-kappaB A pivotal transcription factor in chronic inflammatory diseases. NEJM 336:1066–1072.
20. Saklatvala J (1986) Tumor necrosis factor alpha stimulates resoption and inhibits synthesis of proteoglycan in cartilage. Nature 322:547–549.
21. Bertolini DR, Nedwin GE, Bringman TS, et al. (1986) Stimulation of bone resorption and inhibition of bone formation in vitro by human tumor necrosis factors. Nature 319:516–518.
22. Shinmei M, Masuda K, Kikuchi T, Shimomura Y (1989) The role of cytokines in chondrocyte mediated cartilage degradation. J Rheumatol 6(suppl 18):32–34.

23. Dayer JM, Beutler B, Cerami A (1985) Cachectin/tumor necrosis factor stimulates collagenase and prostaglandin E_2 production by human synovial cells and dermal fibroblasts. J Exp Med 162:2163–2168.
24. Ritchlin C (2003) Mechanisims of TNF-alpha and RANKL mediated osteoclastogenesis and bone resoption in psoriatic arthritis. Journal of Clin Invest 111(6):821–831.
25. Nickoloff BJ (1999) The immunologic and genetic basis of psoriasis. Arch Dermatol 135:1104–1110.
26. Mease PJ. Psoriatic Arthritis/ Psoriasis. ch.32 in Smolen JS, Lipsky PE (eds.) Targeted Therapies in Rheumatology. Martin Dunitz, London, 2003.
27. Mease PJ (2003) Current treatment of psoriatic arthritis. Rheum Dis Clin N Am 29:495–511.
28. Mease PJ (2003) Recent advances in the treatment of psoriatic arthritis. Current Opinion in Rheumatology 15(3):205–212.
29. Mease PJ, Goffe BS, Metz J, Vanderstoep A, Finck B, Burge DJ (2000) Etanercept in the treatment of psoriatic arthritis and psoriasis: a randomized trial. Lancet 356:385–390.
30. Clegg DO, Reda DJ, Weisman MH, et al. (1996) Comparison of sulfasalazine and placebo in the treatment of psoriatic arthritis. A Department of Veterans Affairs Cooperative Study. Arthritis Rheum 39: 2013–2020.
31. Fries JF, Spitz PW, Young DY (1982) The dimensions of health outcomes: the health assessment questionnaire, disability and pain scale. J Rheumatol 9: 789–793.
32. Fredriksson T, Pettersson U (1978) Severe psoriasis–oral therapy with a new retinoid. Dermatologica 157:238–244.
33. Mease PJ, Goffe BS, Metz J, et al. (2001) Enbrel® (etanercept) in patients with psoriatic arthritis and psoriasis. Ann Rheum Dis 60 (Suppl 1):146.
34. Mease P, Kivitz A, Burch F, et al. (2004) Etanercept treatment of psoriatic arthritis: safety, efficacy, and effect on disease progression. Arthritis Rheum 50 : 2264–2272.
35. Mease P, Ganguly L, Wanke E, et al. (2004) How much improvement in functional status is considered important by patients with active psoriatic arthritis:applying the outcome meausres in rheumatoid arthritis clinical trials (OMERACT) group guidelines. Ann Rheum Dis 63(Suppl 1):391.
36. Kosinski M, Keller SD, Ware JE Jr, Hatoum HT, Kong SX (1999) The SF-36 Health Survey as a generic outcome measure in clinical trials of patients with osteoarthritis and rheumatoid arthritis: relative validity of scales in relation to clinical measures of arthritis severity. Med Care 37(Suppl 5):MS23–39.
37. Bukhari M, Wiles NJ, Lunt M, et al. (2003) Influence of disease-modifying therapy on radiographic outcome in inflammatory polyarthritis at five years: results from a large observational inception study. Arthritis Rheum 48:21–34.
38. Strand V, Sharp JT (2003) Radiographic data from recent randomized controlled trials in rheumatoid arthritis. Arthritis Rheum 48:21–34.
39. Emery P (2002) Evidence supporting the benefit of early intervention in rheumatoid arthritis. J Rheumatol 66:3–8.
40. Landewé R (2003) The benefits of early treatment in rheumatoid arthritis: confounding by indication, and the issue of timing. Arthritis Rheum 48:1–5.
41. Rahman P, Gladman DD, Cook RJ, Zhou Y, Young G, Salonen D (1998) Radiological assessment in psoriatic arthritis. Br J Rheumatol 37:760–765.
42. Ory P, Sharp J, Salonen, D, et al. (2002) Etanercept (Enbrel) inhibits radiographic progression in patients with psoriatic arthritis. Arthritis Rheum 46 (Suppl 9):S196.
43. Sharp JT, Young DY, Bluhm GB, et al. (1985) How many joints in the hands and wrists should be included in a score of radiologic abnormalities used to assess rheumatoid arthritis? Arthritis Rheum 28:1326–1335.
44. FDA Briefing Document for the March 4, 2003 meeting of the Arthritis Advisory Committee: Update on the TNF-Blocking Agents. Available at: http://www.fda.gov/ohrms/dockets/ac/03/briefing/3930B1_01_B-TNF.Briefing.pdf. Accessed October 31, 2003. 2003.
45. Antoni C, Dechant C, Hanns-Martin Lorez PD, et al. (2002) Open-label study of infliximab treatment for psoriatic arthritis: clinical and magnetic resonance imagine measurements of reduction of inflammation. Arthritis Rheum 47(5):506–512.
46. Van den Bosch F, Kruithof E, Baeten D, et al. (2002) Randomized double-blind comparison of chimeric monoclonal antibody to tumor necrosis factor alpha (infliximab) versus placebo in active spondyloarthropathy. Arthritis Rheum 46(3):755–765.
47. Kruithof E, Van den Bosch F, Baeten D, et al. (2002) Repeated infusions of infliximab, a chimeric anti-TNFalpha monoclonal antibody, in patients with active spondyloarthropathy: one year follow up. Ann Rheum Dis 61(3):207–212.
48. Antoni CE, Kavanaugh A, Kirkham B, et al. (2002) The infliximab multinational psoriatic arthritis controlled trial (IMPACT): substantial efficacy on synovitis and psoriatic lesions with or without concomitant DMARD therapy. Arth Rheum 46(Suppl 9):S381.
49. Antoni C, Kavanaugh A, Kirkham B, et al. (2005) The infliximab multinational psoriatic arhtritis controlled trial (IMPACT): substantial efficacy on synovitis and psoriatic lesions with or without concomitant DMARD therapy. Arthritis Rheum (in press), (IMPACT)
50. Antoni CE, Kavanaugh A, Kirkham B, et al. (2003) The one year results of the infliximab multinational psoriatic arthritis controlled trial (IMPACT): substantial efficacy on synovitis and psoriatic lesions with or without concomitant DMARD therapy. Arth Rheum 48(Suppl 9):S265.
51. Antoni C, Kavanaugh A, Gladman DD, et al. (2004) The Infliximab multinational psoriatic arthritis controlled trial (IMPACT): results of radiographic analyses after 1 year. Arthritis Rheum 50(Suppl 9): S450.

52. Kavanaugh A, Krueger G, De Vlam K, et al. (2004) Infliximab significantly improves joint and skin involvement in psoriatic arthritis to a substantial extent and irrespective of baseline joint involvement or MTX use: analysis of clinical response from the IMPACT 2 trial. Arthritis Rheum 50(Suppl 9): S617.
53. Mease P, Kavanaugh A, Krueger G, et al. (2004) Infliximab improves psoriasis regardless of arthritis response in patients with active psoriatic arthritis: results from the IMPACT 2 trial. Arthritis Rheum 50 (Suppl 9): S616.
54. Weinblatt ME, Keystone EC, Furst DE, et al. (2003) Adalimumab, a fully human anti-tumor necrosis factor alpha monoclonal antibody, for the treatment of rheumatoid arthritis in patients taking concomitant methotrexate: the ARMADA trial. Arthritis Rheum 48 (1): 35–45.
55. van de Putte LB, Atkins C, Malaise M, Sany J, et al. (2003) Monotherapy in the Treatment of Patients with Severely Active Rheumatoid Arthritis. Arthritis Rheum 46(suppl 9): S205.
56. Furst DE, Schiff MH, Fleischmann RM, et al. (2003) Adalimumab, a fully human anti tumor necrosis factor-alpha monoclonal antibody, and concomitant standard antirheumatic therapy for the treatment of rheumatoid arthritis: results of STAR (Safety Trial of Adalimumab in Rheumatoid Arthritis). J Rheumatol. 30(12): 2563–2571.
57. Keystone E, Haraoui B. (2004) Adalimumab therapy in rheumatoid arthritis. Rheum Dis Clin North Am 30 (2): 349–364.
58. Ritchlin C, Anandarajaha A, Totterman S, et al. (2004) Preliminary data from a study of adalimumab in the treatment of psoriatic arthritis. Ann Rheum Dis 63(Suppl 1): 403.
59. Mease P, Gladman DD, Ritchlin C, et al. (2004) Adalimumab therapy in patients with psoriatic arthritis: 24-week results of a phase III study. Arthritis Rheum 50: 4097.
60. Nikas SN, Drosos AA (2003) Onercept. Serono. Curr Opin Investig Drugs 4 (11): 1369–1376.
61. Mease P (2004) TNFalpha therapy in psoriatic arthritis and psoriasis. Ann Rheum Dis 63 (7): 755–758.
62. Tak P-P, Kraan MC, Goedkoop AY, et al. (2003) Early effects of infliximab therapy on inflammatory cells in lesional epidermis and synovial tissue if patients with psoriatic arthritis [abstract]. Arthritis Rheum 47 (Suppl 9): Abstract 339.
63. Tak P-P, Kraan MC, Goedkoop AY, et al. (2003) Infliximab reduces the expression of adhesion molecules in skin and synovial tissue of patients with psoriatic arthritis [abstract]. Arthritis Rheum 47 (Suppl 9): Abstract 605.
64. Veale DJ, Markham T, Fearon U, et al. (2003) Anti-TNF alpha therapy in psoriasis and psoriatic arthritis: clinical and angiogenic responses [abstract]. Arthritis Rheum 47 (Suppl 9): Abstract 341.
65. Canete JD, Sanmarti R, Marsal S, et al. (2003) Anti-angiogenic effects of infliximab in synovial tissue in psoriatic arthritis [abstract]. Arthritis Rheum 47 (Suppl 1): Abstract 345.
66. Kruithof E, Baeten D, Van den Bosch F, et al. (2003) Down-regulation of synovial inflammation by TNF alpha blockade with infliximab in spondyloarthropathy: a histopathological study in 20 patients [abstract]. Ann Rheum Dis 62 (Suppl 1): Abstract AB0370.
67. Devos SA, Van Den BN, De Vos M, Naeyaert JM (2003) Adverse skin reactions to anti-TNF-alpha monoclonal antibody therapy. Dermatology 206(4): 388–390.
68. Cheifetz A, Smedley M, Martin S, et al. (2003) The incidence and management of infusion reactions to infliximab: a large center experience. Am J Gastroenterol 98(6): 1315–1324.
69. Remicade® (infliximab) prescribing information. Malvern, Pa: Centocor, Inc, 2003.
70. Doran MF, Crowson CS, Pond GR, O'Fallon WM, Gabriel SE (2002) Frequency of infection in patients with rheumatoid arthritis compared with controls: a population-based study. Arthritis Rheum 46(9): 2287–2293.
71. Garcia I, Miyazaki Y, Araki K, et al. (1995) Transgenic mice expressing high levels of soluble TNF-R1 fusion protein are protected from lethal septic shock and cerebral malaria, and are highly sensitive to Listeria monocytogenes and Leishmania major infections. Eur J Immunol 25(8): 2401–2407.
72. Flynn JL, Chan J (2001) Immunology of tuberculosis. Annu Rev Immunol 19: 93–129.
73. Mohan VP, Scanga CA, Yu K, et al. (2001) Effects of tumor necrosis factor alpha on host immune response in chronic persistent tuberculosis: possible role for limiting pathology. Infect Immun 69(3): 1847–1855.
74. Ruderman EM, Markenson JA.(2003) Granulomatous infections and tumor necrosis factor antagonist therapies: update through June 2002. Arth Rheum 48 (Suppl 9): S241.
75. Keane J, Gershon S, Wise RP, et al. (2001) Tuberculosis associated with infliximab, a tumor necrosis factor alpha-neutralizing agent. N Engl J Med 345(15): 1098–1104.
76. Furst DE, Breedveld FC, Kalden JR, et al. (2004).Updated consensus statement on biological agents, specifically tumour necrosis factor alpha (TNFalpha) blocking agents and interleukin-1 receptor antagonist (IL-1ra), for the treatment of rheumatic diseases, 2004. Ann Rheum Dis 63 Suppl 2: ii2–ii12.
77. Beauparlant P, Papp K, Haraoui B (1999). The incidence of cancer associated with the treatment of rheumatoid arthritis. Semin Arthritis Rheum 29(3): 148–158.
78. Cush JJ, Kavanaugh AF. FDA Meeting March 2003: Update on the safety of new drugs for rheumatoid arthritis. Part I: The risk of lymphoma with rheumatoid arthritis (RA) and TNF inhibitors. Available at: http://www.rheumatology.org/research/hotline/0303TNFL.htm. Accessed on October 24, 2003–2003.
79. Mohan N, Edwards ET, Cupps TR, et al. (2001) Demyelination occurring during anti-tumor necrosis factor therapy for inflammatory arthritides. Arthritis Rheum 44(12): 2862–2869.

80. Robinson WH, Genovese MC, Moreland LW (2001) Demyelinating and neurologic events reported in association with tumor necrosis factor alpha antagonism: by what mechanisms could tumor necrosis factor alpha antagonists improve rheumatoid arthritis but exacerbate multiple sclerosis? Arthritis Rheum 44(9):1977–1983.
81. Enbrel® (Etanercept) prescribing information. Thousand Oaks, Calif: Immunex Corporation, 2003.
82. HumiraTM (adalimumab) prescribing information. North Chicago, IL: Abbott Laboratories, 2003.
83. Kavanaugh A, Keenan G, DeWoody K, et al. (2001) Long-term follow-up of patients treated with remicade (infliximab) in clinical trials. Arthritis Rheum 44:S81.
84. Shakoor N, Michalska M, Harris CA, Block JA (2002) Drug-induced systemic lupus erythematosus associated with etanercept therapy. Lancet 359(9306):579–580.
85. Klapman JB, Ene-Stroescu D, Becker MA, Hanauer SB (2003) A lupus-like syndrome associated with infliximab therapy. Inflamm Bowel Dis 9(3):176–178.
86. Ali Y, Shah S (2002) Infliximab-induced systemic lupus erythematosus. Ann Intern Med 137(7):625–626.
87. Debandt M, Vittecoq O, Descamps V, Le L, X, Meyer O (2003) Anti-TNF-alpha-induced systemic lupus syndrome. Clin Rheumatol 22(1):56–61.
88. Baert F, Noman M, Vermeire S, et al. (2003) Influence of immunogenicity on the long-term efficacy of infliximab in Crohn's disease. N Engl J Med 348:601–608.
89. Mann DL, McMurray JJ, Packer M, et al. (2004) Targeted anticytokine therapy in patients with chronic heart failure: results of the Randomized Etanercept Worldwide Evaluation (RENEWAL). Circulation 109:1594–602.
90. Anker SD, Coats AJ (2002) How to RECOVER from RENAISSANCE? The significance of the results of RECOVER, RENAISSANCE, RENEWAL and ATTACH. Int J Cardiol 86(2-3):123–130.
91. Chung ES, Packer M, Lo KH, Fasanmade AA, Willerson JT (2003) Randomized, double-blind, placebo-controlled, pilot trial of infliximab, a chimeric monoclonal antibody to tumor necrosis factor-alpha, in patients with moderate-to-severe heart failure: results of the anti-TNF Therapy Against Congestive Heart Failure (ATTACH) trial. Circulation 107(25):3133–3140.
92. Kwon HJ, Cote TR, Cuffe MS, Kramer JM, Braun MM (2003) Case reports of heart failure after therapy with a tumor necrosis factor antagonist. Ann Intern Med 138(10):807–811.
93. Schiff M, Mease PJ, Weinblatt M, et al. (2000) Randomized controlled trial of 25 Mg vs. 50 Mg Enbrel (Etanercept) twice weekly in rheumatoid arthritis (RA). Arth Rheum 43(Suppl 9):S391.
94. Hansen KE, Cush JJ, Patel S, Genovese MC, Schiff M (2002) The efficacy of switching from etanercept to infliximab in patients with rheumatoid arthritis. Arthritis Rheum 46:9 (Suppl):S538-A1439.
95. Haraoui PB, Keystone EC, Thorne JC, et al. (2003) The Canadian biologic observational switchover survey (BOSS): Switching from infliximab to etanercept leads to successful treatment of rheumatoid arthritis. Ann Rheum Dis. 62 (Suppl 1):Abstract 226.
96. Bombardieri S, Tzioufas AG, McKenna F, et al. (2004) Efficacy evaluation of adalimumab (Humira) in patients with single and multiple prior biologics in the ReAct trial. Arthritis Rheum 50(Suppl 9):S187.
97. Genovese MC, Cohen S, Moreland L, et al. (2003) A randomized double-blind controlled study evaluating the safety and efficacy of etanercept vs etanercept plus ankinra in patients with rheumatoid arthritis. Ann Rheum Dis 62(Suppl 1):66.

2 Other Biologic Therapy

Ja Huen Jung, Zuhre Tutuncu,
Arthur F. Kavanaugh

Introduction

Psoriatic arthritis (PsA) runs a variable course, from mild synovitis to severe progressive erosive arthropathy. Patients with polyarticular peripheral joint involvement have been reported to have a more aggressive disease course and a worse prognosis [1]. Regarding treatment, patients with severe and progressive articular disease that is not responsive to non-steroidal anti-inflammatory drugs (NSAIDs) are candidates for treatment with disease-modifying anti-rheumatic drugs (DMARDs) [2]. However, none of the traditional DMARDs available to date has been shown to be effective in the treatment of the spinal manifestations of psoriatic arthritis [3]. In addition, many patients with severe peripheral arthritis fail to respond to standard DMARDs therapy. Driven by this clinical unmet need, in conjunction with progress in biotechnology and advances in our understanding of the immunopathogenesis of PsA, there has been great interest in the development of biologic agents for the treatment of PsA and psoriasis.

Recently, data from clinical trials of the tumor necrosis factor (TNF) inhibitors etanercept, infliximab, and adalimumab in PsA have generated considerable excitement [4–7]. In rheumatoid arthritis (RA), TNF inhibitors have

X

been shown not only to control signs and symptoms of disease, but also to have disease-modifying properties by preventing progression of joint damage and preserving quality of life and functional status. The introduction of the clinic of TNF inhibitors has opened significant new avenues for the treatment of PsA. Despite the tremendous success achieved in PsA patients treated with TNF inhibitors, approximately one-third of patients with moderate to severe PsA have inadequate responses to such treatment. This has provided the impetus for the development of additional biologic agents. Several promising biologic agents, directed at targets other than TNF, are now being studied in the treatment of PsA (Table B1). These therapies are reviewed in this chapter.

In recent years, a great deal has been learned about the immunopathogenesis of psoriasis and PsA. For example, there is significant evidence that T lymphocytes, particularly CD8+ cells, play an important pathogenic role in the skin and joint manifestations of PsA. Activated T cells have been noted in the affected tissue, both skin and joint, in patients with PsA [8, 9]. In PsA synovial fluid, the demonstration of a predominance of CD8+T lymphocytes, with clonal expansion, has led to the proposal that these cells may be driving the immune responses [10]. The proposal for a primary CD8+T cell-driven immune response in PsA gains further support from the evidence that CD8+T cells also dominate the infiltrate at marrow sites adjacent to entheseal inflammation [11]. Analysis of T cell receptor beta chain variable (TCRβV) gene repertoires reveals common expansions in both skin and synovium, suggesting an important role for cognate T cell responses in the immunopathogenesis of PsA. This suggests that the inciting antigen may be related in both afflicted skin and synovium [12].

There is also substantial evidence that dysregulation of the cytokine cascade may be relevant to the immunopathogenesis of PsA. The

Table B1. Biologic agents studied or under consideration for the treatment of psoriatic arthritis. *TNF*, tumor necrosis factor; *mAb*, monoclonal antibody; *rIL*, recombinant interleukin; *IL-2R*, interleukin-2 receptor; *LFA*, leukocyte function associated antigen; *TCR*, T-cell receptor; *CTLA4Ig*, cytotoxic T-lymphocyte-associated antigen 4/immunoglobulin

Target	Agent	Comment
Suppression of inflammatory mediators		
TNF-α	Etanercept	Soluble TNF receptor fusion protein
	Infliximab	Chimeric anti-TNF mAb
	Adalimumab	Human anti-TNF mAb
IL-1	Anakinra	IL-1 receptor antagonist
IL-8	ABXIL-8	Human anti-IL-8 mAb
Modulation of the function of anti-inflammatory mediators		
IL-10	rIL-10	Recombinant human Th2 cytokine
IL-11	rIL-11	Recombinant human Th2 cytokine
Alteration of T cell interaction		
CD25 (IL-2 receptor)	Daclizumab	Humanized anti-CD25 mAb
CD2	Alefacept	Human LFA-3/IgG fusion protein
CD11a (LFA-1)	Efalizumab	Humanized anti-CD11a mAb
TCR/CD3	huOKT3γ1(ala-ala)	Humanized anti-CD3 mAb
CD80/CD86	IDEC-114	Humanized anti-CD80 mAb
	CTLA4Ig	Fusion protein of CTLA-4/Ig
CD40/CD40L	IDEC-131	Humanized anti-CD154 mAb

cytokine network in the psoriatic skin and synovium is dominated by monocyte-derived cytokines, including IL-1β, IL-10, and TNF-α, along with T cell derived cytokines such as IL-2 and INF-γ [13]. In the synovium of PsA, IFN-γ, IL-2 and IL-10 levels were found to be higher in comparison to psoriatic skin. Cytokines secreted by activated T cells and other mononuclear pro-inflammatory cells induce proliferation and activation of synovial and epidermal fibroblast, contributing to the joint damage and fibrosis that have been reported in patients with longstanding PsA.

The delineation of specific alterations in components of the immune response and inflammatory cascade provides potential targets for immunomodulatory therapies. Progress in pharmaceutical biotechnology has facilitated the synthesis of agents directed at these targets. Based upon successes in proof-of-concept animal models and ex-vivo studies, a number of these novel immunomodulatory agents have been assessed in clinical trials in PsA.

Although there are exceptions, the myriad individual components of the immune and inflammatory responses can be broadly grouped into several functional categories. This facilitates consideration of targeting these molecules in a specific condition such as an autoimmune systemic inflammatory disease like PsA. However, it is recognized that these are complex interactions among these pathways and that the targets themselves are often characterized by pleiotropy and redundancy in their function.

Therefore, it is no doubt overly simplistic to speak of alteration in one function of a molecule. A more complete understanding of the wider implications of therapy must come from careful clinical studies. In this chapter, we will focus on three main avenues for immunomodulatory intervention in PsA: (1) inhibition of the activity of proinflammatory mediators, (2) modulation of the activity of anti-inflammatory mediators, and (3) alteration of T cell function.

Inhibition of Pro-inflammatory Mediators

TNF-α, IL-1, IL-6, IL-8, and other proinflammatory cytokines have been shown to be present at elevated concentrations in the synovial fluid and synovial membranes of affected joints of patients with PsA [14]. The levels of these cytokines do not seem to be quite as high in PsA as they are in RA, but the overall pattern is similar, and their concentrations exceed those observed in non-inflammatory conditions. TNF-α is produced by multiple cells in the body, including activated T cells, keratinocytes, mast cells, and Langerhans cells [15]. However, at inflammatory sites, the majority of TNF is secreted by activated macrophages. It has been shown that TNF-α is a central cytokine that it is capable of increasing production of IL-1, IL-6, IL-8, and other molecules via activation of the nuclear transcription factor, NFκB [16, 17]. IL-1 can also cause further synthesis of cytokines and chemokines, thereby amplifying and propagating the inflammatory process. IL-6 is involved in keratinocyte proliferation, among other activities. The effects of IL-8 include T cell and neutrophil activation and chemotaxis, as well as keratinocyte proliferation. NFκB is a nuclear transcription factor that stimulates the transcription of cytokines, including TNF-α, IL-6, and IL-8, as well as adhesion molecules such as intercellular adhesion molecule-1 (ICAM-1, CD54), vascular cell adhesion molecule-1 (VCAM-1, CD106), and E-selectin (CD62-E) [18].

The available TNF inhibitors provide effective control of PsA in many cases, and other means of reducing TNF activity are also being evaluated. TNF-α converting enzyme (TACE) is a transmembrane protein that cleaves cell surface-bound TNF-α to release soluble cytokine [19]. Inhibition of TACE reduces lipopolysaccharide-stimulated TNF production and it may represent a new approach to treating inflammatory arthritis such RA and PsA.

Despite the success of TNF directed therapies in PsA, some of the patients with PsA failed to respond to TNF inhibitor therapy. Therefore additional immunomodulatory approaches are under consideration. IL-1 has been implicated as a key cytokine in the pathogenesis of joint inflammation on the basis of experimental studies in arthritis and clinical trials in RA [20]. Anakinra (IL-1ra), a homologue of the naturally occurring IL-1 receptor antagonist, has been approved for use in moderate to severely active RA.

Other IL-1 inhibiting agents are in development for the treatment of rheumatic diseases. This includes: (1) sIL-1 receptor, a recombinant soluble form of the type II "decoy" IL-1 receptor, (2) IL-1 Trap, a novel recombinant molecule consisting of IL-1 receptor type I (IL-1RI) and IL-1 receptor accessory protein (IL-1RAcP) fused to human IgG Fc, and (3) an inhibitor of IL-1 converting enzyme (ICE, also called caspase-1), a metalloproteinase that facilitates the secretion of proinflammatory cytokines IL-1β and IL-18 [21, 22]. To date, there have been no controlled clinical trials of anakinra or any other IL-1 inhibitor in PsA. However, it is reasonable that agents targeting IL-1 may be studied in the future to treat synovitis in PsA, due to their potential clinical efficacy and anti-erosive properties.

IL-6 is involved in proliferation of keratinocytes in psoriasis [23] and may contribute to cartilage destruction, bone absorption and angiogenesis. Clinical trials are underway evaluating the efficacy of two biologics directed against IL-6, a neutralizing monoclonal antibody against the IL-6 receptor and a soluble IL-6 receptor construct. A monoclonal antibody to the IL-6 receptor (MRA) blocks bioactivity of IL-6 and has shown favorable effects in patients with RA [24]. Based on these findings, the blocking of IL-6 binding to IL-6 receptor may have possible therapeutic benefit in patients with PsA.

IL-18 is a proinflammatory cytokine that can induce gene expression and synthesis of TNF, IL-1, Fas ligand (CD95L), several chemokines, and vascular adhesion molecules. Preclinical studies in arthritis models suggest that neutralizing monoclonal antibodies or recombinant human IL-18 binding protein inhibit the activity of IL-18 and can reduce inflammation [25].

Chemokines and chemokine receptors control the recruitment of leukocytes to sites of inflammation. In animal models of arthritis, various chemokine antagonists have effectively reduced synovial inflammation and leukocyte infiltration. Several chemokine antagonists, including CXCL-8/IL-8 antibody and CCR1 antagonist, are under development for the treatment of rheumatic diseases.

IL-8 may play a role in the vascular responses found in psoriasis [26]. ABX-IL8 is a fully human monoclonal antibody that binds free IL-8 and may deactivate it in the skin. In a phase II trial in patients with psoriasis, intravenous infusion of ABX-IL8 every 3 weeks resulted in significant improvement in their PASI and in histological responses [27]. Preliminary studies of this agent have been conducted in RA, with promising results. Therefore, this or other inhibitors of IL-8 may be tested in PsA.

Anti-inflammatory Cytokines

Given that cytokines function in cascades and circuits, anti-inflammatory cytokines serve an equally important role as the proinflammatory mediators, and modulation of their function may be an effective therapeutic strategy in PsA. For example, systemic therapy with IL-10 and IL-11 appear to downregulate the production of proinflammatory mediators in inflammatory diseases.

Interleukin-10

IL-10 is an important cytokine with varied effects on immunoregulation [28]. It promotes the development of a Th2-biased pattern of cytokine secretion by inhibiting IFN-γ production by T lymphocytes and natural killer cells. Of note, it has been shown that IL-10 is relatively deficient in psoriatic skin lesions, although it is present at high levels in synovium and serum from patients with PsA [13]. In an open-label, 7-week, phase II trial with recombinant IL-10 (rIL-10) in 14 patients with chronic plaque-type psoriasis, ten patients (71%) had a reduction in PASI scores of >50% [29]. The cytokine pattern in responding patients shifted from Th1-type to Th2-type. No significant changes were observed in the production of TNF, IL-6, or IFN-γ [30].

Human rIL-10 has also been studied in patients with PsA [31]. In a 4-week, double blind placebo controlled study in PsA patients, IL-10 given by subcutaneous injection produced modest but significant clinical improvement in the skin, but not in articular disease activity scores. Only minor adverse effects were observed. Interestingly, Th1-type cytokine production in vitro was suppressed and decreased T cell and macrophage infiltration in synovial tissues was observed in human rIL-10 group compared with placebo group. It has also been shown in vivo that IL-10 modulates immune responses via diverse effects on endothelial activation, as well as leukocyte recruitment and effector function. Although IL-10 exerts multiple immunomodulatory effects, clinical benefit may be greater for the skin than for the joints. Long term, appropriately powered studies will be required to clarify the potential efficacy of IL-10 in articular disease.

Interleukin-11

Recombinant human IL-11 (rhIL-11) has been shown to have anti-inflammatory activity in vitro and in vivo. It directly interacts with macrophages to reduce the production of pro-inflammatory cytokine such as TNF-α, IL-1β, and IL-12 [32, 33]. This effect is due to the inhibition of NF-κB nuclear translocation through enhanced expression of the inhibitor of NF-κB, IκB. IL-12 has a critical role in promoting and maintaining T-cell activation and inducing Th1-type cytokines such as IFN-γ in psoriasis [34]. In addition to effects on macrophages, rhIL-11 directly blocks IL-12 induced Th1 differentiation and IFN-γ production.

The rhIL-11 has been tested in 12 patients with extensive psoriasis. An open trial of rhIL-11 daily subcutaneous injection with 2.5 or 5.0 mg/kg for 8 weeks resulted in 20% to 80% improvement in PASI score in 11 patients. There was a reduction in pathological epidermal hyperplasia, expression of ICAM-1 on epidermal keratinocytes, and the number of infiltrating T lymphocytes in skin lesions [35]. However, there have not yet been any published reports on recombinant human IL-11 use in the treatment of PsA.

Alteration of T-Cell Function

IL-2/IL-2 Receptor Blockade

The role of IL-2 and the IL-2 receptor in T cell activation has been well-documented. Daclizumab is a humanized antibody to the α-subunit (CD25) of the IL-2 receptor that blocks normal IL-2 binding to this receptor. Because IL-2 is a major stimulus for T-cell growth, blockade of the IL-2 receptor could be useful in treating T cell mediated diseases such as PsA. In two centers, 19 patients with psoriasis received daclizumab at an initial dosage of 2 mg/kg, then 1 mg/kg at weeks 2, 4, 8 and 12 [36]. The results showed a consistent blockade of CD25 in peripheral blood and psoriatic skin during the first 4 weeks of therapy. Variable desaturation of receptors began after 4 weeks, which correlated with a reversal in disease improvement. Patients with a pretreatment PASI score of <36 showed a mean reduction in severity by 30% at 8 weeks. This is a treatment strategy that could be tested in PsA.

Blockade of T-Cell-Associated Molecules

In recent years, there has been intense interest in any research on blocking T cell interactions with other cell types for T cell-mediated diseases. There is evidence that costimulatory ligand-receptor pairs play an important role in the pathogenesis of psoriasis and PsA (Fig. B4).

Alefacept. CD2 is a surface antigen expressed on all classes of T cells. It interacts with lymphocyte function associated antigen-3 (LFA-3, CD58) on antigen-presenting cells, stimulating the proliferation of T lymphocytes.

Alefacept is a human LFA-3/IgG1 fusion protein that has been approved for psoriasis, and is under clinical investigation for the treatment of PsA and RA. The LFA-3 portion of alefacept binds to CD2 receptors on T cells to block the natural interaction between LFA-3 on antigen-presenting cells and CD2 on T cells. Blockade of the LFA-3/CD2 interaction, a key co-stimulato-

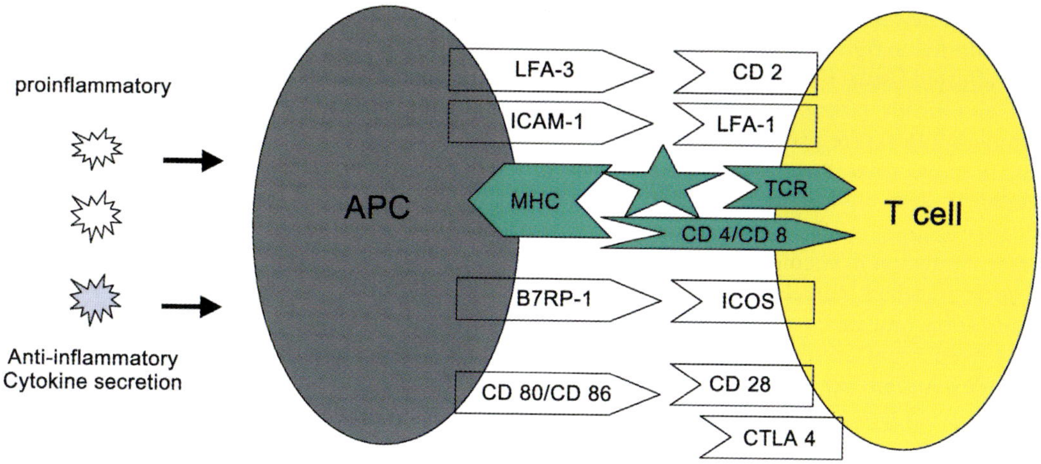

Fig. B4. Cell surface molecules mediating interactions of T cells with antigen-presenting cells. *APC,* antigen-presenting cell; *ICAM-1,* intracellular adhesion molecule-1; *LFA-1,* lymphocyte function-associated antigen 1; *MHC,* major histocompatibility complex; *TCR,* T-cell receptor; *B7RP-1,* B7-related protein-1; *ICOS,* inducible costimulator; *CTLA4,* cytotoxic T-lymphocyte-associated antigen 4. The *star* represents the putative etiologic antigen(s)

ry pathway, can inhibit T-cell activation. The IgG1 portion of alefacept can bind to FcγRIII (CD16) IgG receptors on accessory cells (e.g., natural killer cells) and may induce granzyme-mediated apoptosis. As the density of CD2 is much greater on activated memory T cells than on naive T cells, alefacept more avidly targets the memory T-cell subset [6, 37, 38].

Alefacept was evaluated as a treatment for psoriasis in multicenter, randomized, placebo-controlled, double blind study. Two hundred twenty-nine patients with chronic psoriasis received intravenous injection of alefacept at different dosages and the mean reduction in the score on the PASI 12 weeks after treatment was greater in the alefacept groups than placebo group [39]. See Chap. X.A.1 for more details of this study.

A small study suggests that alefacept may be able to improve both joint and skin symptoms in PsA. In a single center open-label study, 11 patients with PsA received intravenous 7.5 mg alefacept once weekly for 12 weeks. Synovial tissue biopsies of an index joint were obtained by arthroscopy at baseline and at week 4 and 12 [40]. Clinically, some degree of improvement in arthritis was observed in six patients (55%) at the completion of the treatment, and a similar proportion of patients achieved 50% amelioration of skin disease. CD4+, CD8+ T cells and also macrophages (CD68+) were found significantly decreased in the synovium at 12 weeks. This suggests that T cells can orchestrate macrophage activation. Alefacept has been reported to have a favorable safety profile. The changes in synovial tissue with the improvement in clinical joint scores after treatment of alefacept support the notion that T cell activation plays an important role in chronic inflammatory diseases and effective blockade of the LFA-3/CD2 interaction may be useful for treating PsA.

Efalizumab. Leukocyte function associated antigen-1 (LFA-1, CD11a/CD18) plays an important role in T cell activation and leukocyte migration [37, 41]. LFA-1 binds several ligands, including ICAM-1 and ICAM-2. This interaction is key in facilitating processes relevant to the pathogenesis of psoriasis, including the migration of T lymphocytes from the circulation into dermal and epidermal tissues, and the subsequent activation of T cells.

Efalizumab is a humanized monoclonal IgG1 antibody that binds to the α subunit of LFA-1 (CD11a), inhibiting the interaction between LFA-1 and ICAM-1. It may inhibit the inflammatory response by blocking T cells' ability to bind to endothelial cells and also to bind to APCs in the affected tissue. Efalizumab has demonstrated significant efficacy in patients who had moderate to severe psoriasis [42]. In an open-label, multicenter, dose escalation study in 39 patients with moderate to severe psoriasis, higher dosages of efalizumab produced significant clinical and histological improvement in psoriasis, which correlated with T-cell CD11a saturation and down-modulation. Efalizumab has been reported to have a favorable safety profiles. Already approved for the treatment of chronic moderate to severe plaque psoriasis, trials to determine the therapeutic potential of efalizumab for PsA are underway. Of note, recent clinical trials of efalizumab in patients with RA have been discontinued, reportedly due to unimpressive clinical responses.

huOKT3γ1 (ala-ala). A non-FcR-binding monoclonal antibody to CD3 (a component of the T-cell receptor complex), huOKT3γ1 (ala-ala), has demonstrated some therapeutic value in the treatment of PsA [9]. This compound is a modification of murine OKT3 with decreased ability to bind FcR, resulting in modulation in the function of T-lymphocytes without decreasing their number. Therefore, it may have less toxicity than conventional OKT3. In a phase I/II, open-label, dose-escalating trial involving seven patients with PsA who received huOKT3γ1 (ala-ala) for 12–14 days, six patients had an ACR70 or greater response at day 30. There was a transient, dose-dependent T cell depletion noted in seven patients and one patient developed mild cytokine release symptoms associated with elevation of IL-10. Anti-idiotypic antibodies developed in two patients. Assessment of the true efficacy and tolerability of this agent awaits controlled studies with larger number of patients.

Blockade of VLA-4. Very late activation antigen 4 (VLA-4, CD49D) is a member of the β1 integrin family of cell-adhesion molecules. Like LFA-1, interactions between VLA-4 and its ligands such as VCAM-1 have an important role in recruiting lymphocytes to sites of inflammation, stabilizing the interaction between T cell and APC and providing costimulatory signals to T cells. On the base of its action, an inhibitor of VLA-4 could be hypothesized to have immune suppressant and anti-inflammatory activity. A monoclonal antibody to VLA-4, natalizumab, has been studied in multiple sclerosis and Crohn's disease, and could be assessed in PsA.

Blockade of Costimulatory Pathways

Many drugs that target the interaction between CD28 and its two ligands are now in clinical development for the treatment of psoriasis. These include antibodies directed against CD80 and CD86, and soluble immunoglobulin fusion proteins of the extracellular domain of CD152, cytotoxic T-lymphocyte-associated antigen 4 (CTLA-4).

CD28 is a heterodimeric cell-surface protein expressed by mature T cells and binds to two ligands, CD80 (B7–1) and CD86 (B7–2) on antigen-presenting cells (APCs). Blocking of this interaction between B7 molecules and CD28/CD152 results in incomplete T cell activation and eventually T cell anergy. CTLA-4 is not expressed on resting T cells but is induced by T cell activation and serves an inhibitory role in T cell interactions. As CTLA-4 binds the same CD80/86 molecules with higher avidity, soluble forms of the molecule can compete with CD28 to block costimulatory signals. These observations led to the development of CTLA-4 immunoglobulin (CTLA4Ig), a soluble receptor construct composed of the extracellular domain of CTLA-4 and an IgG Fc fragment. CTLA4Ig has been investigated in a phase I open label study in patients with psoriasis [43]. Clinical improvement was associated with reduced cellular activation of lesional T cells, keratinocytes, dendritic cells, and vascular endothelium. This study highlights the critical and proximal role of T cell activation through the B7-CD28 costimulatory pathway in maintaining the pathology of psoriasis. Studies of CTLA-4Ig in rheumatoid arthritis have shown promising results, and studies in PsA may be anticipated in the near future.

A number of anti-CD80/86 monoclonal antibodies are in development. The anti-CD80 molecule IDEC-114 blocks costimulatory signal by binding directly to CD80. Clinical data for this drug are just beginning to emerge. In a phase I trial of IDEC-114 in 35 patients with psoriasis, there was clinical activity with 40% of patients achieving at least 50% reduction in PASI after receiving four biweekly doses [27]. However anti-CD80 agents have not been shown promising effect in phase II trials in psoriasis and lately, they are being tested in indications other than psoriasis.

Inducible costimulator (ICOS), another member of the CD28/CTLA-4 family, is an important costimulatory receptor expressed on activated T cells. ICOS may be of particular relevance to the activation of memory T cells. ICOS participates in a variety of immunoregulatory functions. In collagen-induced arthritis, ICOS regulates in vivo and in vitro expression of IL-17, a proinflammatory cytokine implicated in RA [44]. These data suggest that anti-ICOS monoclonal antibody may also provide specific T cell based therapy for inflammatory arthritides such as PsA.

Other Approaches

A placebo-controlled double-blind trial of recombinant interferon gamma in 24 patients over a period of 4 weeks reported a modest improvement in arthritis activity; however, the effect appeared transient as improvement present at 1 month was not sustained over 6 months despite continued treatment [45]. The putative efficacy of interferon gamma in PsA is clouded by the experience in cutaneous psoriasis where joint disease developed during interferon treatment and subsided following termination of therapy [46].

Future Directions

Recent biotechnologic advances have led to a creation of new strategies for treating systemic inflammatory disease with agents designed to target specific components of the immune system. With better understanding of these immune responses of the disease, the future for the potential novel biologics for PsA is very promising.

Anti-cytokine biologics (e.g., IL-1, IL-2R, IL-6/IL-6R, IL-15, IL-18, and TNF converting enzyme inhibitor), inhibitions of regulatory molecules (e.g., NFκB, p38 MAP kinase) and chemokines (e.g., CCR1, CXCR-5), co-stimulatory molecule (e.g., ICOS, VLA-4), adhesion molecules (e.g., ICAM-1, VCAM-1) are among potential future therapeutic candidates for psoriatic arthritis and other immunological disorders (Table B2). Based upon increased understanding of the angiogenic process and the demonstration of elevated level of vascular endothelial growth factor (VEGF) and plasminogen activator inhibitor-1 (PAI-1) in psoriasis, anti-angiogenic therapy such as VEGF inhibitor may also be added to the armamentarium of the highly specific immune system modulating agents. Inhibition of B-cells and complement are other structures that have scientific rational in PsA, and may be utilized in future studies.

Conclusion

To date, systemic treatment of PsA has been limited by the incomplete efficacy and suboptimal tolerability of available agents. While inhibitors of TNF have achieved impressive clinical results in PsA, there remains an unmet need. Greater understandings of immunopathogenesis of this chronic, progressive, systemic inflammatory disease, along with continued developments in biotechnology, have fueled development of novel immunomodulatory therapies for PsA. The promise of these new target agents is more specific immunomodulation that could result in enhanced efficacy with greater safety. There is also the potential for long term control of disease, which is of great relevance given the chronic nature of the disease. Proper testing of these strategies and introduction to the clinic of promising agents should improve the quality of life for patients with psoriatic arthritis.

Table B2. Future potential novel immunomodulatory therapies in psoriatic arthritis. *TACE-I,* TNF-α converting enzyme inhibitor; *NF-κB,* nuclear transcription factor κB; *MAP,* mitogen-activated protein; *BAFF-R,* B-cell activating factor receptor; *BlyS,* B-lymphocyte stimulator; *VEGF,* vascular endothelial growth factor; *ICOS/B7RP-1,* inducible costimulator/B7-related protein-1; *VLA-4,* very late antigen 4; *ICAM,* intracellular adhesion molecule 1; *VCAM-1,* vascular cell adhesion molecule 1

Mechanism	Target
Modulation of cytokines	TNF-α (including TACE-I)
	IL-1
	IL-6
	IL-18
Inhibition of regulatory molecules	NF-κB
	p38 MAP kinases
B-cell directed inhibition	CD20
	BAFF-R/BlyS
Inhibition of angiogenesis	VEGF
Inhibition of costimulatory molecules	ICOS/B7RP-1, VLA-4
Inhibition of adhesion molecules	ICAM-1, VCAM-1
Inhibition of complement	Anti-C5a

References

1. Bulbul R, Williams WV, Schumacher HR Jr (1995) Psoriatic arthritis. Diverse and sometimes highly destructive. Postgrad Med 97:97–96, 103–106, 108
2. Mease P (2003) Psoriatic arthritis/psoriasis. In: Smolen J, Lipsky P (eds) Targeted therapies in rheumatology. Martin Dunitz, London, pp 525–548
3. Pipitone N, Kingsley GH, Manzo A, et al. (2003) Current concept and new developments in the treatment of psoriatic arthritis. Rheumatology 42:1138–1148
4. Antoni C, Kavanaugh A, Kirkham B, et al. (2003) The one-year results of the infliximab multinational psoriatic arthritis controlled trial. Arthritis Rheum 48:S604
5. Braun J, Sieper J (2000) Anti-TNF alpha: a new dimension in the pharmacotherapy of the spondyloarthropathies? Ann Rheum Dis 59:404–407
6. Braun J, Sieper J (2003) Role of novel biological therapies in psoriatic arthritis. Biodrugs 17:187–199
7. Mease PJ, Goffe BS, Metz J, et al. (2000) Etanercept in the treatment of psoriatic arthritis and psoriasis: a randomized trial. Lancet 356:385–390
8. Panayi G (1994) Immunology of psoriasis and psoriatic arthritis. Baillieres Clin Rheumatol 8:419–427
9. Utset TO, Auger JA, Peace D, et al. (2002) Modified anti-CD3 therapy in psoriatic arthritis: a phase I/II clinical trial. J Rheumatol 29:1907–1913
10. Costello PJ, Winchester RJ, Curran SA, et al. (2001) Psoriatic arthritis joint fluids are characterized by CD8 and CD4 T cell clonal expansions that appear antigen driven. J Immunol 166:2878–2886
11. Laloux L, Voisin MC, Allain J, et al. (2001) Immnohistological study of enthesis in spondyloarthropathies: comparison in rheumatoid arthritis and osteoarthritis. Ann Rheum Dis 60:316–321
12. Tassiulas I, Duncan SR, Centola M, et al. (1999) Clonal characteristics of T cell infiltrates in skin and synovium of patients with psoriatic arthritis. Hum Immunol 60:479–491
13. Ritchlin C, Haas-Smith SA, Hicks D, et al. (1998) Patterns of cytokine production in psoriatic synovium. J Rheumatol 25:1544–1552
14. Partsch G, Steiner G, Leeb BF, et al. (1997) Highly increased levels of tumor necrosis factor-alpha and other proinflammatory cytokines in psoriatic arthritis synovial fluid. J Rheumatol 24:518–523
15. Giustizieri ML, Mascia F, Frezzolini A, et al. (2001) Keratinocytes from patients with atopic dermatitis and psoriasis show a distinct chemokine production profile in response to T cell-driven cytokines. J Allergy Clin Immunol 107:871–877
16. Choy EH, Panayi GS (2001) Cytokine pathways and joint inflammation in rheumatoid arthritis. N Engl J Med 344:907–916
17. Duan H, Koga T, Kohda F, et al. (2001) Interleukin-8-positive neutrophils in psoriasis. J Dermatol Sci 26:119–124

18. Gottlieb AB (2001) Psoriasis: immunopathology and immuno-modulation. Dermatol Clin 19: 649–657
19. Black RA (2002) Tumor necrosis factor-alpha converting enzyme. Int J Biochem Cell Biol 34:1–5
20. Bresnihan B, Cunnane G (1998) Interleukin-1 receptor antagonist. Rheum Dis Clin North Am 24: 615–628
21. Dinarello CA (1998) Interleukin-1 beta, interleukin-18, and the interleukin-1 beta converting enzyme. Ann N Y Acad Sci 856:1–11
22. Gabay C (2003) IL-1 trap. Regeneron/Novartis. Curr Opin Investig Drugs 4:593–597
23. Krueger J, Ray A, Tamm I, et al. (1991) Expression and function of interleukin-6 in epithelial cells. J Cell Biochem 45:327–334
24. Nurieva RI, Treuting P, Duong J, et al. (2003) Inducible costimulator is essential for collagen-induced arthritis. J Clin Invest 111:701–706
25. Plater-Zyberk C, Joosten LA, Helsen MM, et al. (2001) Therapeutic effect of neutralizing endogenous IL-18 activity in the collagen-induced model of arthritis. J Clin Invest 108:1825–1832
26. Barker JN, Jones ML, Mitra RS, et al. (1991) Modulation of keratinocyte-derived interleukin-8 which is chemotactic for neutrophils and T lymphocytes. Am J Pathol 139:869–876
27. Singri P, West DP, Gordon KB (2002) Biologic therapy for psoriasis: the new therapeutic frontier. Arch Dermatol 138:657–663
28. Asadullah K, Sterry W, Stephanek K, et al. (1998) IL-10 is a key cytokine in psoriasis. J Clin Invest 101 :783–794
29. Reich K, Garbe C, Blaschke V, et al. (2001) Response of psoriasis to interleukin-10 is associated with suppression of cutaneous type 1 inflammation, downregulation of the epidermal interleukin-8/CXCR2 pathway and normalization of keratinocyte maturation. J Invest Dermatol 116:319–329
30. Asadullah K, Friedrich M, Hanneken S, et al. (2001) Effects of systemic interleukin-10 therapy on psoriatic skin lesions: histologic, immunohistologic, and molecular biology findings. J Invest Dermatol 116: 721–727
31. McInnes IB, Illei GG, Danning CL, et al. (2001) IL-10 improves skin disease and modulates endothelial activation and leukocyte effector function in patients with psoriatic arthritis. J Immunol 167: 4075–4082
32. Leng SX, Elias JA (1997) Interleukin-11 inhibits macrophage interleukin-12 production. J Immunol 159: 2161–2168
33. Trepicchio WL, Bozza M, Pedneault G, et al. (1996) Recombinant human IL-11 attenuates the inflammatory response through down-regulation of proinflammatory cytokine release and nitric oxide production. J Immunol 157:3627–3634
34. Yawalkar N, Karlen S, Hunger R, et al. (1998) Expression of interleukin-12 is increased in psoriatic skin. J Invest Dermatol 111:1053–1057
35. Trepicchio WL, Ozawa M, Walters IB, et al. (1999) Interleukin-11 therapy selectively downregulates type I cytokine proinflammatory pathways in psoriasis lesions. J Clin Invest 104:1527–1537
36. Krueger JG, Walters IB, Miyazawa M, et al. (2000) Successful in vivo blockade of CD25 (high-affinity interleukin 2 receptor) on T cells by administration of humanized anti-Tac antibody to patients with psoriasis. J Am Acad Dermatol 43:448–458
37. Weinberg JM (2003) An overview of infliximab, etanercept, efalizumab, and alefacept as biologic therapy for psoriasis. Clin Ther 25:2487–2505
38. Weinberg JM, Tutrone WD (2003) Biologic therapy for psoriasis: the T cell-targeted therapies – Efalizumab and Alefacept. Cutis 71:41–45
39. Ellis CN, Krueger GG (2001) Treatment of chronic plaque psoriasis by selective targeting of memory effector T lymphocytes. N Engl J Med 345:248–255
40. Kraan MC, van Kuijk AWR, Dinant HJ, et al. (2002) Alefacept treatment in psoriatic arthritis. Reduction of the effector T cell population in peripheral blood and synovial tissue is associated with improvement of clinical signs of arthritis. Arthritis Rheum 46:2776–2784
41. Lebwohl M, Tyring SK, Hamilton TK, et al. (2003) A novel targeted T-cell modulator, efalizumab, for plaque psoriasis. N Engl J Med 349:2004–2013
42. Gottlieb AB, Krueger JG, Wittkowski K, et al. (2002) Psoriasis as a model for T cell mediated disease: immunobiologic and clinical effects of treatment of treatment with multiple doses of efalizumab, an anti-CD11a antibody. Arch Dermatol 138:591–600
43. Abrams JR, Kelley SL, Hayes E, et al. (2000) Blockade of T lymphocyte costimulation with cytotoxic T lymphocyte-associated antigen 4-immunoglobulin (CTLA4Ig) reverses the cellular pathology of psoriatic plaques, including the activation of keratinocytes, dendritic cells, and endothelial cells. J Exp Med 192:681–693
44. Nakahara H, Song J, Sugimoto M, et al. (2003) Anti-interleukin-6 receptor antibody therapy reduces vascular endothelial growth factor production in rheumatoid arthritis. Arthritis Rheum 48:1521–1529
45. Fierlbeck G, Rassner G (1990) Treatment of psoriasis and psoriatic arthritis with interferon gamma. J Invest Dermatol 95(Suppl 6)138S–141S
46. O'Connell PG, et al. (1992) Arthritis in patients with psoriasis treated with gamma-interferon. J Rheumatol 19:80–82

Synthesis and Conclusion XI

Kenneth B. Gordon, Eric M. Ruderman

Contents

In the introduction to this text, we noted that our experience working together in a cooperative clinic treating psoriasis and psoriatic arthritis allowed us to give our patients what we considered to be better care. We believed that the information we had derived from our own experience, working within our respective specialties, would help each of us, our trainees, and our patients to better understand the range of issues that need to be considered when making therapeutic decisions. By integrating the chapters of this book along these same lines our goal was to make the current information regarding psoriatic disease of both skin and joints readily available and relatively easy to grasp for practitioners caring for their patients. In this brief conclusion to this text, we hope to provide a synthesis of some of the most salient points raised in these chapters and apply them to the fundamental question facing each of us: how best to care for patients who suffer both from psoriasis and psoriatic arthritis.

1 The Impact of Psoriasis and Psoriatic Arthritis

At the outset, it is important to remember that each patient is different. They have unique perspectives on what is a cosmetically tolerable, as well as differing thresholds for pain. They have individual perspectives on the risks and benefits of systemic therapies, and some may have lifestyles that preclude the use of certain modalities. All of these issues should be explored before making individual treatment decisions. However, there are a few central aspects of disease that will have the most significant impact on these decisions. The most obvious is, of course, the severity of each disease, in both the acute setting and in the future. Physicians too often consider improvement of the red, scaly plaques of psoriasis or the stiff, swollen joints of psoriatic arthritis as the primary goal of treatment. However, severity of the disease from the patients' perspective is best considered in two areas: the impact of disease on their quality of life, and the natural history of disease and its potential future impact.

The impact of psoriasis and psoriatic arthritis on the patient's quality of life is covered in Chap. VII. Improving this fundamental outcome is perhaps the most important goal of the treatment of psoriasis and psoriatic arthritis. The manifestations of disease that influence quality of life for patients are distinct for these two diseases. The symptoms of psoriasis, with pain, pruritus, and bleeding, may all have a physical impact on patients' lives. However, in many patients the emotional trauma from the presence of diffuse areas of visibly abnormal skin, or even limited disease, predominates over the physical. Interpersonal relationships and body image have clearly been shown to be significantly altered. Moreover, patients with psoriasis often feel restricted in their ability to participate in many normal social functions; altered appearance can significantly influence employment and leisure activities. Improving quality of life in patients with psoriasis means reducing not only the physical symptoms of the disease, but reducing the impact of the physical lesions on emotional and societal function.

Quality of life considerations in psoriatic arthritis, while necessarily including the impact of the associated skin disease, focus on the distinct issues created by the joint disease. The key drivers for therapy, particularly during the early stages of disease, are the patient's joint symptoms. Functional limitations and joint damage must also be recognized as significant contributors to reduced quality of life. Ultimately, pain, stiffness, functional impairment, and deformity are the central components in both the physical and emotional impact of the disease. While there is clearly a significant emotional component, it is based primarily on symptoms and not on appearance, as in psoriasis. From a quality of life perspective, therefore, the predominant goals of therapy of psoriatic arthritis are the reduction of symptoms of disease and preservation of function.

The second important factor underlying a treatment plan for any disease is an understanding of the natural history and the potential for alteration of life in the future. For example, a malignancy may have few symptoms and little impact on a patient's current quality of life, but early treatment may prevent later morbidity and mortality. In general, this consideration is more critical for psoriatic arthritis than to psoriasis. In cutaneous psoriasis, there is no data to date to suggest that early treatment has a significant impact on the disease. Moreover, effective therapy for even the most severe forms of psoriasis can still result in normal appearing skin. Delays in the initiation of therapy, or a history of ineffective treatment, does not seem to alter this fact, as skin has the ability to repair itself despite significant damage.

While the natural history of disease may lack central importance in the therapy of psoriasis, it is critical in the treatment of psoriatic arthritis. Patients with progressive psoriatic arthritis clearly develop irreversible joint damage. Loss of function, not only from progressive pain and stiffness, but from permanent damage to the joints, can have a devastating impact on the patient's life. Although only a minority of patients with psoriatic arthritis may go on to significant permanent disability, aggressive treatment of disease may prevent even these. Thus, more so than psoriasis, future considerations may drive more aggressive therapy than may seem warranted by the current disease state.

2 Pathophysiology and Therapy

One of the central principles governing therapeutic choices in psoriasis and psoriatic arthritis is that both are principally inflammatory diseases. However, this principle oversimplifies the pathophysiology of these diseases and can misleadingly suggest that therapies will generally work for both conditions. Understanding the varying pathophysiological mechanisms of these diseases, as covered in Chap. III, is a critical step towards deciphering which treatments should have an impact on both conditions.

Psoriasis is a T cell mediated disease requiring the persistent presence of T cells to maintain activity. As noted in Chap. II, much of the genetic susceptibility to psoriasis is thought to be localized to the MHC locus and other areas in the genome that govern immune response. The activation of other inflammatory cells, including dendritic cells and macrophages also plays a significant role in the psoriatic inflammatory cascade and cytokine web that are central to disease development and persistence. In response to this continued T cell and innate immune activity, keratinocytes proliferate too quickly and fail to mature normally. Additionally, the vasculature dilates and proliferates. It is these keratinocyte and vascular changes that result in the clinical appearance of psoriasis. These changes in non-inflammatory cells can be reversed with appropriate therapy.

Psoriatic arthritis is also initiated by a T cell mediated, adaptive immune response, that also is likely a central factor in the genetics of the disease (Chap. II.B). This response triggers angiogenesis and inflammation in the joints, with resultant expansion of inflammatory cytokines such as TNF-α and IL-1. These and other changes, such as an elevation of the ratio of RANK ligand to osteoprotegerin, in the synovial milieu trigger recruitment and activation of osteoclast precursor cells. Osteoclast activity and cytokine-induced metalloproteinase expression by synovial lining cells are then responsible for the cartilage and bone degradation that lead to irreversible joint disease.

While the immunopathogenesis of psoriasis and psoriatic arthritis are similar, they are not identical. These seemingly subtle differences may have profound influence on the choice of treatment. Obviously, treatment directed against local T cell or keratinocyte responses, including topical treatments, phototherapy, and retinoids will have little impact on the course of psoriatic arthritis. Similarly, non-steroidal anti-inflammatory agents that do not affect T cell activity will have less of an impact on psoriasis than on inflammatory arthritis. Even agents that target T cells directly, such as cyclosporine, may be presumed to have more impact on psoriasis than psoriatic arthritis, as the persistent influence of T cells is required for psoriasis, but may be of lesser importance for arthritis. As we develop a greater understanding of the true mechanisms of biologic therapies, the areas in which they will have the greatest effect will undoubtedly become more clear. Ultimately, defining the pathophysiology of these diseases themselves will lead to greater understanding of the potential efficacy of new agents being developed.

3 The Choice of Therapy: The four Quadrant Model

All of the factors above will impact the choice of appropriate therapy for a patient. Ultimately, this choice will be determined by the clinicians' interpretation of the mechanisms of disease, as well as the evidence for the efficacy, safety, tolerability, and convenience of the medications discussed in this text. Most importantly, therapeutic decisions that incorporate the presence or absence of each disease, as well as their relative severity, will be advantageous for the patient. Aside from those patients with psoriasis or psoriatic arthritis alone, we recognized in our practice four distinct subsets of patients, identified according to the model in Fig. 1. These four groups of patients represent the most likely scenarios faced by a clinician caring for psoriasis and psoriatic arthritis: (1) limited psoriasis with mild and non-destructive psoriatic arthritis, (2) extensive psoriasis with mild and non-destructive psoriatic arthritis, (3) limited psoriasis with more severe or destructive psoriatic arthritis, and (4) more severe forms of both diseases. In addition, there may be special circumstances, such as the patient who develops progressive psoriatic arthritis while already under good control for his or her psoriasis. Obviously, these circumstances may change over time, so the clinician, whether a dermatologist or a rheumatologist, should be sure to do careful follow-up examinations. Moreover, patient responses to therapy may vary, which may influence future therapeutic interventions. However, given the information covered in the therapeutic chapters of this text, we can offer some suggested treatment approaches based on this model. These suggestions are not intended to be algorithms for care, but general observaions that can assist in making therapeutic decisions.

3.1 Quadrant 1: Limited Psoriasis, Mild, Non-progressive Arthritis

These sets of disease characteristics are probably the most common faced by a clinician. As mentioned in Chap. V.A, about two-thirds of patients with psoriasis have limited disease while a number of patients with psoriatic arthritis have no evidence of joint destruction and symptoms that can be controlled relatively easily. In these circumstances, it is probably judicious to use the most benign therapies available, even if these treatments may not alter the course of both diseases. If the psoriasis can be treated sufficiently with topical therapy or UVB and the arthritis is adequately controlled with

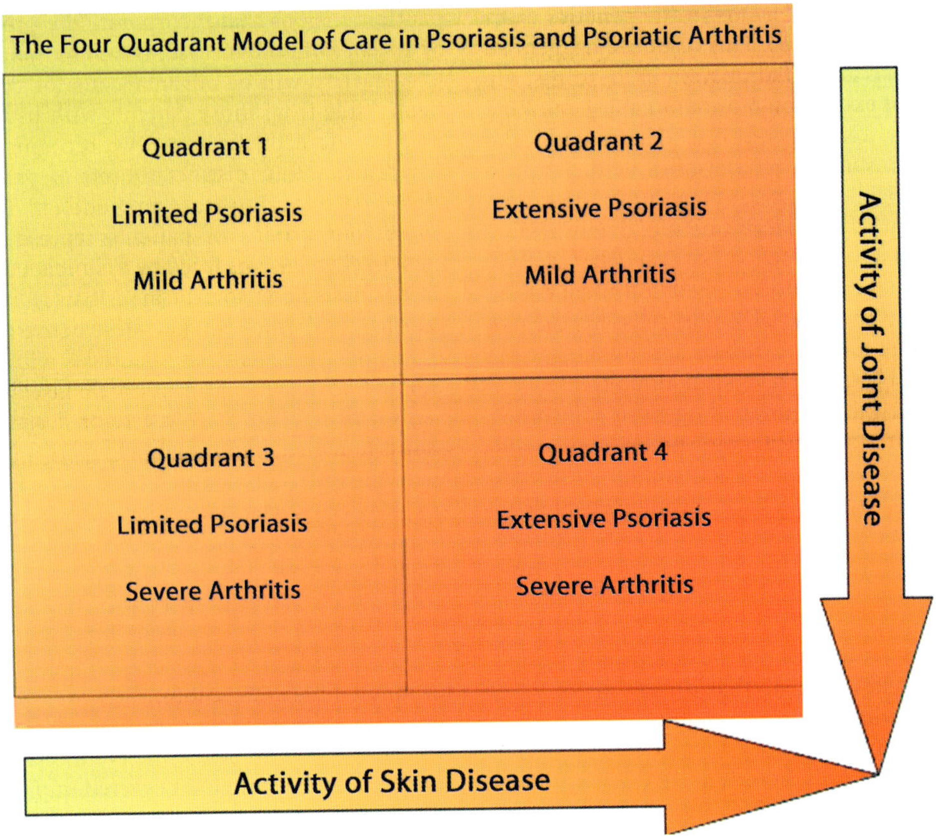

Fig. 1. The four quadrant model of care in psoriasis and psoriatic arthritis

NSAIDs, it is probably not necessary to expose the patient to the potential side effects of more invasive systemic treatments. While this approach may seem dated, and lacks the elegance of a unified treatment paradigm, this type of safe and traditional care is likely to be the best technique for patients with disease that has a limited impact on their quality of life.

3.2 Quadrant 2: Diffuse Psoriasis and Mild and Non-destructive Arthritis

In these circumstances, it is best to focus treatment on the most pressing issues, while taking agents that may be of benefit for both conditions into special consideration. In deliberating upon the choice of treatment, for example, the need for speed in the therapeutic response may be of great importance. For example, if, like most patients with psoriasis, the patient has chronic plaques, it is likely that there is no significant health need for rapid and necessarily predictable therapy for psoriasis. In these cases, it is very reasonable to select a treatment that may take time to work and may not be effective in every case. Medications that can clearly be of benefit for both psoriasis and psoriatic arthritis, methotrexate or an anti-TNF-α agent like etanercept, would be appropriate. If a patient has erythroderma, rapidly progressive plaque psoriasis, or pustular psoriasis, however, while maintaining mild psoriatic arthritis, consideration should first be given to treating the psoriasis primarily. In these circumstances, retinoids or cyclosporine may be most appropriate. Once the skin disease is under control, it then may be reasonable to slowly transition the patient to treatment that is more effective for the arthritis.

One special set of conditions should be given consideration. Since the great majority of patients with both forms of psoriatic disease will develop psoriasis first, what of the patient who develops psoriatic arthritis while on effective therapy for the skin? Our suggestion depends upon the ease with which the arthritis can be controlled. If a patient is being treated safely and effectively with phototherapy or acitretin, common sense would dictate not altering the therapy to something that may not have similar efficacy in a given patient because of the presence of arthritis that can be easily controlled. Only when the arthritis becomes difficult to control or progressive would we suggest changing therapy to accommodate the arthritis in a patient with severe psoriasis who has been stably controlled.

3.3 Quadrant 3: Limited Psoriasis and More Severe Psoriatic Arthritis

This set of circumstances requires prompt and effective therapy for arthritis to prevent progression of joint destruction. In the circumstance where there is only limited psoriasis, therapy should be directed to the arthritic component. However, since the two treatments that are likely to be most effective for joint disease also have efficacy in psoriasis, the use of either methotrexate or an anti-TNF biologic is warranted.

One potential controversy in this situation stems from fact that it often requires larger doses of medication to control the skin when compared to the joints. While the primary issue with anti-TNFs at higher dose is the cost of the medication, increasing the dose of methotrexate can lead to greater exposure and the potential for greater toxicity. An unresolved issue has been the risk of hepatotoxicity with methotrexate use in psoriatic arthritis. While all of these patients necessarily carry the additional diagnosis of psoriasis, and all the monitoring recommendations, including liver biopsy, that this entails (see Chap. IX.A.4), rheumatologists, perhaps swayed by the evidence for limited hepatotoxicity with this drug in rheumatoid arthritis, are loathe to recommend regular biopsies.

In this situation, the decision needs to be made as to whether improvement in the cutaneous component merits exposure to higher doses of medication, either synthetic or biologic. It is our opinion that, given the added risk of high doses of methotrexate, both from the standpoint of safety and tolerability, as well as the added cost of additional exposure to a biologic agent, it would make more sense to add topical therapy before increasing the dose of anti-arthritic medication.

3.4 Quadrant 4: Severe Psoriasis and Arthritis

In this circumstance, aggressive therapy should be implemented at once. Agents that impact both diseases should be considered as the primary agents of choice in patients who are under these conditions. However, acute, severe cutaneous disease may require the most rapid and effective agents to date, cyclosporine or infliximab, to get them under control. These can be started at the same time as methotrexate, or tapered to etanercept or another anti-TNF agent quickly, once the cutaneous disease is under better control. Therapy should be continued and modified as necessary until there is no further evidence of progressive arthritis and the psoriasis is controlled to the point where the impact on the patient is acceptable.

4 Conclusion

Ultimately, therapy for patients with psoriasis and psoriatic arthritis is dependent upon a multitude of factors, most of which have been touched upon in this book. Treatment decisions must come not only from an understanding of the approach to the patient with either cutaneous or joint disease, but from an appreciation of the impact of *both* on the lives of the patient. Over the past decade, and in the years to come, information and therapeutic options have expanded, and will continue to expand, to create new horizons in our understanding of what we can provide for those who suffer from these co-morbid diseases. This book is just a beginning in what we hope is a long-term cooperative effort on the part of dermatologists, rheumatologists, and primary care providers to further our care for patients who suffer from psoriasis and psoriatic arthritis.

Subject Index

Printing: Krips bv, Meppel
Binding: Stürtz, Würzburg